# ANNUAL REVIEW
# OF NURSING RESEARCH

## Volume 25, 2007

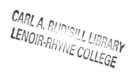

# Annual Review of Nursing Research

Volume 25, 2007

*Vulnerable Populations*

JOYCE J. FITZPATRICK, PhD, RN, FAAN
Series Editor

ADELINE NYAMATHI, ANP, PhD, FAAN
DEBORAH KONIAK-GRIFFIN, RNC, EdD, FAAN
Volume Editors

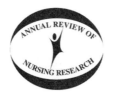

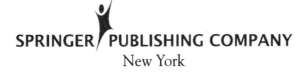
SPRINGER PUBLISHING COMPANY
New York

To purchase copies of other volumes of the *Annual Review of Nursing Reserach* at 10% off of the list price, go to www.springerpub.com/ARNR.

Springer Publishing Company, LLC.
11 West 42nd Street
New York, NY 10036

*Acquisitions Editor: Sally J. Barhydt*
*Production Editor: Carol Cain*
*Cover design by Joanne E. Honigman*
*Typeset by Apex Publishing, LLC*

07 08 09 10/ 5 4 3 2 1

ISBN-10: 0-8261-4137-4
ISBN-13: 978-0-8261-4137-8
ISSN-0739-6686

ANNUAL REVIEW OF NURSING RESEARCH is indexed in *Cumulative Index to Nursing and Allied Health Literature* and *Index Medicus*.

Printed in the United States of America by Bang Printing.

# Contents

# Contributors

Teresita L. Briones, PhD, RN
Associate Professor
University of Illinois at Chicago
Chicago, Illinois

Fang-Yu Chou, RN, PhD
Assistant Professor
San Francisco State University
School of Nursing
San Franciso, California

Esther H. Condon, RN, PhD,
FAAN
Professor
Hampton University School of
Nursing
Hampton, Virginia

Darcy Copeland, RN, MSN,
PhD(c)
University of California, Los Angeles
School of Nursing
Los Angeles, California

Dorothy Coverson, MSN, RN,
PhD(c)
Nell Hodgson Woodruff School of
Nursing
Emory University
Atlanta, Georgia

Chandice Covington, PNP, PhD
Professor and Dean of College of
Nursing
University of North Dakota
Grand Forks, North Dakota

Ruth Davidhizar, DNS, APRN, BC,
FAAN
Professor and Dean
School of Nursing
Bethel College
Mishawaka, Indiana

Bertha Davis, RN, PhD, FAAN
Professor
Hampton University School
of Nursing
Hampton, Virginia

Claudia M. Davis, RN, MN,
PhD(c)
University of California,
Los Angeles
School of Nursing
Los Angeles, California

Colleen DiIorio, PhD, RN,
FAAN
Professor
Grace C. Rollins School of Public
Health
Emory University
Atlanta, Georgia

Elizabeth L. Dixon, RN, MSN,
MPH, PhD
Assistant Professor
University of California,
Los Angeles
School of Nursing
Los Angeles, California

Jacquelyn H. Flaskerud, RN, PhD, FAAN
Professor Emerita
University of California, Los Angeles
School of Nursing
Los Angeles, California

Susan Gennaro, DSN, RN, FAAN
Florence and William Downs
  Professor in Nursing Research
New York University, College of
  Nursing
New York, New York

Joyce Newman Giger, EdD, APRN, BC, FAAN
Professor and Lulu Wolff Hassenplug
  Endowed Chair
University of California, Los Angeles
School of Nursing
Los Angeles, California

Rosa M. Gonzalez, RN, MSN, MPH
University of Miami School of
  Nursing & Health Studies
Coral Gables, Florida

Barbara Ann Greengold, RN, MSN, PhD(c)
Doctoral Student
University of California, Los Angeles
School of Nursing
Los Angeles, California

William L. Holzemer, RN, PhD, FAAN
Professor and Associate Dean for
  International Progams
University of California, San
  Francisco School of Nursing
San Francisco, California

M. Katherine Hutchinson, RN, PhD
Assistant Professor and Associate
  Director

Center for Health Disparities
  Research
University of Pennsylvania School of
  Nursing
Philadelphia, Pennsylvania

Loretta Sweet Jemmott, RN, PhD, FAAN
van Ameringen Professor in
  Psychiatric Mental Health
  Nursing
Director, Center for Health
  Disparities Research
University of Pennsylvania, School of
  Nursing
Philadelphia, Pennsylvania

Tonia Jones, RN, PhD
Nursing Research Coordinator
Kaiser Sunset
Los Angeles, California

Christine E. Kasper, RN, PhD, FAAN
Professor
Uniformed Services University of the
  Health Sciences, Graduate School
  of Nursing
Bethesda, Maryland

Janna Lesser, PhD, RN
Assistant Professor
Department of Family
  Nursing Care
University of Texas Health Science
  Center at San Antonio
San Antonio, Texas

Arlene J. Montgomery, RN, PhD
Associate Professor and Assistant
  Dean for Academic Affairs
Hampton University School of
  Nursing
Hampton, Virginia

**Malaika Mutere, PhD**
Project Director
University of California, Los Angeles
School of Nursing
Los Angeles, California

**Michelle Nelson, MSN**
Doctoral Student
Nell Hodgson Woodruff School of
Nursing
Emory University
Atlanta, Georgia

**Manuel Angel Oscós-Sánchez, MD**
Assistant Professor
Department of Family and
Community Medicine
University of Texas Health Science
Center at San Antonio
San Antonio, Texas

**Nilda P. Peragallo, PhD, FAAN**
Professor and Dean
University of Miami School of
Nursing & Health Studies
Coral Gables, Florida

**Carmen J. Portillo, RN, PhD, FAAN**
Professor
University of California, San
Francisco School of Nursing
San Francisco, California

**Linda A. Robinson, RN, CS, PhD**
Professor
University of San Diego, School of
Nursing
San Diego, California

**E. Jane Servonsky, RN, PhD, PNP**
Associate Professor

Hampton University School of
Nursing
Hampton, Virginia

**Jan Shoultz, APRN, DrPH**
Associate Professor
Department of Nursing, University of
Hawaii
Honolulu, Hawaii

**Aaron J. Strehlow, RN, PhD**
Administrator and Director of
Clinical Services
University of California,
Los Angeles
School of Nursing
Los Angeles, California

**Ora Lea Strickland, PhD, RN, FAAN**
Professor
Nell Hodgson Woodruff School of
Nursing
Emory University
Senior Editor, *Journal of Nursing
Measurement*
Atlanta, Georgia

**Lorraine Tulman, RN, DNSc, FAAN**
Associate Professor of Nursing
University of Pennsylvania, School of
Nursing
Philadelphia, Pennsylvania

**Antonia M. Villarruel PhD, FAAN**
Professor
University of Michigan School of
Nursing
Ann Arbor, Michigan

# Preface

This 25th volume in the *Annual Review of Nursing Research* (ARNR) series marks an important quarter-century anniversary. Each of the 25 volumes has been filled with chapters written by top nurse researchers. In the early volumes, it was difficult to identify content across all areas of nursing research to fill a volume. Now, and including this 25th volume, there is sufficient nursing research in one specific area to complete an entire volume.

Volume 25, 2007, is focused on nursing science in vulnerable populations. The topic is timely and important and has been identified as a priority for the nursing discipline, both for scientific development and professional practice. Further, it is a core component of the historical development of nursing. Adeline Nyamathi and Deborah Koniak-Griffin, well-known scholars in this area, serve as the volume editors. They selected the content areas for the chapters and edited these into this comprehensive volume.

The volume is composed of four parts. Part I includes two chapters, both of which set the stage for deliberations about the science of nursing in relation to specific vulnerable populations. In Chapter 1, Adeline Nyamathi, Deborah Koniak-Griffin, and Barbara Ann Greengold present an overview of the development of nursing theory and science with vulnerable populations. This chapter captures the essence of the themes that follow and challenges future nurse researchers to expand the science in the area. In Chapter 2, Ora Lea Strickland, Colleen DiIorio, Dorothy Coverson, and Michelle Nelson identify and discuss measurement issues in nursing science with vulnerable populations. Both of these chapters introduce the volume and specific content areas that are included in the chapters in Parts II through IV.

Part II is focused on diverse approaches used to build the science with research on vulnerable populations. In Chapter 3, Antonia Villarruel and Deborah Koniak-Griffin present research on lifestyle behavior interventions with Hispanic children and adults. Nilda Peragallo and Rosa Gonzalez discuss research on the prevention of infectious diseases in Chapter 4. In Chapter 5, M. Katherine Hutchinson, Bertha Davis, Loretta Sweet Jemmott, Susan Gennaro, Lorraine Tulman, Esther Condon, Arlene Montgomery, and E. Jane Servonsky delineate methods to promote research partnerships to reduce health disparities among vulnerable populations. This chapter is focused on the existing efforts to share expertise between majority institutions and historically Black universities. Chapter 6 is focused on generating science by training future scholars to address the needs of vulnerable populations. It is authored by Elizabeth Dixon, Aaron Strehlow, Claudia Davis, Darcy Copeland, Tonia Jones, Linda Robinson, Jan Shoultz, and Jacquelyn Flaskerud.

Part III is focused on integrating biologic methods in vulnerable population research. In Chapter 7, Christine Kasper delineates genomics and proteomics methodologies for vulnerable population research. In Chapter 8, Teresita Briones presents psychoneuroimmunology and related mechanisms in understanding health disparities in vulnerable populations.

The final section, Part IV, is focused on reducing health disparities among vulnerable populations. In Chapter 9, Carmen Portillo, William Holzemer, and Fang-Yu Chou discuss research on HIV symptoms. In Chapter 10, Joyce Newman Giger and Ruth Davidhizar delineate ways to promote culturally appropriate interventions with vulnerable populations. Janna Lesser and Manuel Angel Oscós-Sánchez present community-academic partnerships with vulnerable populations in Chapter 11. In the final chapter, 12, Adeline Nyamathi and Chandice Covington include discussion of research on women living with HIV/AIDs as an example of a vulnerable population in Thailand.

As with previous volumes, it is important to acknowledge the contributions of the nurse scholars who contributed the chapters for this volume. In addition, we would like to acknowledge the *ARNR* Advisory Board members who have supported this effort over the past 25 years. And, most importantly, recognition is due to the volume editors for this special volume and for the previous volumes for their efforts to advance the science of nursing through dissemination of important nursing research. Editing one of these volumes is a monumental task that involves finding colleagues willing to meet deadlines and to integrate their work into a synthesis chapter, sometimes distilling a lifetime of research and professional contributions. We thank all of you for your contributions and acknowledge your scholarship and leadership in nursing science.

*Joyce J. Fitzpatrick, PhD, RN, FAAN*
*Series Editor*

# Foreword

Vulnerability and strength are universal features of the human condition. Everyone is vulnerable to some situation, ailment, or problem. Complex and interrelated social, political, cultural, and economic factors lead to greater vulnerability for some groups. In the health care arena, the vulnerable label applied to populations refers to those groups of persons whose vulnerability increases their potential to suffer health disparities.

Usually those populations that are vulnerable for health disparities are those that experience reduced resource availability, increased risk for health problems, and thus, impaired health status leading to increased morbidity and mortality. Flaskerud and Winslow (1998) effectively described this interrelationship of resources, relative risk, and health status among vulnerable populations.

Racial and ethnic discrimination and poverty are primary factors leading to unacceptable health disparities and unequal health care services. The very young and very old, women, and groups that are typically stigmatized or marginalized also fit within the vulnerable population definition. Discrimination and inequity persist for these groups despite concerted efforts mandated at national and local levels. The Institute of Medicine (IOM) discovered disparities in the delivery of care related to the climate and procedures within service facilities and organizations as well as discrimination during patient-provider interactions. The IOM also emphasized that racial and ethnic disparities take place "in the context of broader historic and contemporary social and economic inequality" (Smedley, Stith, & Nelson, 2003, p. 19). Personal histories, experiences, cultural beliefs and practices, and world views color communication across cultural, racial, ethnic, and socio-economic divides often leading to miscommunication, misunderstanding, and intended or unintended discrimination. Improvements in the cross-cultural interaction dynamic have occurred through cultural competence training of health providers; however, to date, disparities in the health care arena have not been significantly reduced.

Beginning with Florence Nightingale, nurses have demonstrated dedication and aptitude for identifying persons, groups, and environments in need of intervention and new approaches to assessing and reducing vulnerability. This issue of *The Annual Review of Nursing Research* extends that dedication with landmark research, tests of interventions, and theoretical reviews that bring us closer to the goals of *Healthy People 2010* (U.S. Department of Health and Human Services [USDHHS], 2000) for the elimination of health disparities. Nurses are positioned within the health care delivery team to serve in leadership roles to address existing disparity and inequality for vulnerable populations. Concerted, creative, and concentrated efforts by nurses are needed, efforts that extend and expand current foci on cultural competence and community involvement. These efforts need to take into account the sometimes neglected recognition of strengths within vulnerable groups.

Although many groups who are vulnerable to health disparities experience discrimination, racism, and are often marginalized, they are not without skills and power to work effectively toward self-advocacy and improved health and well-being. The resilience and courage demonstrated by vulnerable individuals and groups provide ample evidence of the co-existence of strength in the face of vulnerability, discrimination, inequality, and disparity. Currently participatory research strategies (Flaskerud & Anderson, 1999) and community-based participatory research (Israel, Eng, Schulz, & Parker, 2005) are being employed effectively to involve vulnerable populations in health disparities research and service planning. Often however, community involvement concentrates on community-based agencies and organizations with minimal or no involvement of grass-roots community members, those persons who comprise the target vulnerable populations. Nurses can lead the way with community-based projects that involve community members in addition to community agencies and their staffs. Active partnerships between nurses and their intended intervention recipients can be used effectively to plan, implement, and evaluate research and intervention programs that truly address health care and education needs as perceived by the community. Such partnerships need to foster mutual commitment, trust, and respect. Equitable distributions of goal-setting and decision-making power evolve through shared responsibilities and mutual learning among partners. Nurses should move to the forefront in the important research needed to design and implement effective interventions with vulnerable populations capitalizing on their strengths to increase their resources, reduce their risks, and improve their health status with more equitable, quality health care.

*Adeline Nyamathi and Deborah Koniak-Griffin*

## REFERENCES

Flaskerud, J. H., & Anderson, N. (1999). Disseminating the results of participant-focused research. *Journal of Transcultural Nursing, 10*(4), 340–349.

Flaskerud, J. H., & Winslow, B. J. (1998). Conceptualizing vulnerable populations health-related research. *Nursing Research, 47*(2), 69–78.

Israel, B. A., Eng, E., Schulz, A. J., & Parker, E. A. (Eds.). (2005). *Methods on community-based participatory research for health*. San Francisco: Jossey-Bass.

Smedley, B. D., Stith, A. Y., & Nelson, A. R. (Eds.). (2003). *Unequal treatment: Confronting racial and ethnic disparities in health care*. Washington, DC: National Academies Press.

U.S. Department of Health and Human Services. (2000, November). *Healthy People 2010 (2nd ed.)*. *Understanding and improving health and objectives for improving health*. 2 vols. Washington, DC: U.S. Government Printing Office.

# PART I

## Development of Nursing Science in Vulnerable Populations Research

# Chapter 1

## Development of Nursing Theory and Science in Vulnerable Populations Research

Adeline Nyamathi, Deborah Koniak-Griffin,
and Barbara Ann Greengold

### ABSTRACT

*Inequalities with respect to the distribution of societal resources can predispose people to vulnerability, which has led to a growing concern across America. The Federal Government has taken a leadership role and has launched several initiatives to combat health inequalities experienced by vulnerable populations. The National Institute of Health and all of its institutes, including the National Institute of Nursing Research, have written strategic plans to reduce, and ultimately, eliminate such health disparities. Nursing research has been conducted in the setting of vulnerable populations; several theoretical models for studying vulnerability have been created; and interventional studies designed to reduce health disparities have been implemented. This introduction includes the following: (a) a definition of the concept of vulnerability and health disparities; (b) a discussion of the conceptual models of vulnerability and health disparity and their applications; (c) a description of the impact of federal funding on vulnerable populations research; (d) a synopsis of the contributions made by nurse researchers in the field of vulnerable populations research; and (e) an overview of the volume.*

**Keywords: vulnerability; health disparities; vulnerable populations research**

# INTRODUCTION

## Definition of Vulnerability and Health Disparities

Vulnerable populations are social groups who have increased morbidity and mortality risks, secondary to factors such as low socioeconomic status and the lack of environmental resources (Flaskerud & Winslow, 1998). Vulnerable populations also have been described as groups at risk for poor psychological, physical, or social health, such as high-risk mothers, high-risk infants, chronically ill people, and disabled persons (Aday, 1994). Women and children, ethnic people of color, gay men and lesbians, immigrants, homeless people, persons diagnosed with human immunodeficiency virus (HIV), chemically dependent people, and older people have been traditionally considered to be vulnerable populations (Flaskerud & Winslow, 1998). Erlen (2003) defines vulnerable groups as people who are less fortunate than others due to variables such as age, gender, or cultural background.

Shi and Stevens (2005) offer five reasons to focus national attention on vulnerable populations: these groups have greater health care needs; their prevalence continues to escalate; vulnerability is a societal (in contradistinction to an individual) issue; vulnerability and the nation's health and resources are interrelated; and there is a growing emphasis on equality with respect to health.

The concept of health disparity must be defined in relation to vulnerable populations in order to understand the growing national emphasis on health equality. Health disparity is defined as inequality with respect to quality of care, access to care, health status, and health outcomes (Villarruel, 2004). In a Strategic Plan on Reducing Health Disparities created by the National (National Institute of Nursing Research [NINR], 2000), health disparity is defined as differences that exist among some populations within the United States in the incidence, prevalence, mortality, and burden of disease and other adverse health events.

There is a growing effort to try to understand the relationship between vulnerable populations and health disparity, particularly among racial and ethnic minorities (Guthrie, 2005). In 1986, the publication of the Report of the Secretary's Task Force on Black and Minority Health, a landmark document, galvanized the effort to improve the health and well-being of minorities. As a result of this report, a number of descriptive studies of vulnerable groups were undertaken. Findings revealed, for example, that African American patients are less likely than Whites to receive analgesia for comparable long bone fractures (Todd, Deaton, D'Amamo, & Goe, 2000). African American women, with significantly lower income and educational levels than White women, have been shown to have a much greater prevalence of diabetes, hypertension, and angina (Appel, Harrell, & Deng, 2002). Health disparities have also been experienced by American Indians (Keltner, Kelley, & Smith, 2004).

As a result of the mounting evidence that, within the United States, vulnerable populations are experiencing health disparities, the U.S. Congress commissioned the Institute of Medicine (IOM) to study the issue of racial and ethnic disparities. The IOM reviewed over 100 studies that assessed the quality of health care provided to various racial and ethnic minority groups, holding constant variables such as access-related factors, insurance status, and personal income. As a result of their review, it was concluded that minorities are less likely than Caucasians to receive needed services, and that disparities exist in a number of disease areas, such as cancer, cardiovascular disease, HIV/AIDS, diabetes, and mental illness (IOM, 2002). Healthy People 2010, a national health promotion and disease prevention initiative, compared the incidence and prevalence of certain disease rates among vulnerable versus non-vulnerable groups. Findings revealed that the infant death rate among African Americans is more than double that of Whites; heart disease death rates are more than 40% higher for African Americans compared to Whites; Hispanics living in the United States are almost twice as likely to die from diabetes and have higher obesity and high blood pressure rates than non-Hispanic Whites; and American Indians and Alaska Natives have infant death rates which are almost double those of Whites (U.S. Department of Heath and Human Services, 2000). Further, Latino families with young children suffering from asthma often lack adequate health care resources and consequently experience high levels of disease-related morbidity (Berg et al., 2003).

The IOM also looked at the factors that contribute to health care disparities. These include cultural or linguistic barriers, fragmentation of the health care system, the types of incentives given to health care providers to contain costs, and the site of care delivery. Additional factors leading to health care disparities included prejudice against minorities on the part of the health care provider; clinical uncertainty secondary to caring for minority patients; and the presence of stereotypes held by the provider about the minority patients.

In summary, vulnerable populations often experience health care inequalities (differences in access to and provision of quality health care) that become apparent when comparing vulnerable to non-vulnerable groups. Vulnerable populations also can experience disparities with respect to health status, having greater prevalence and incidence rates for many diseases (U.S. Department of Health and Human Services, 2000). Health care disparity is inversely proportional to health status disparity among vulnerable populations; that is, the groups who receive less health care experience greater morbidity and mortality. National attention on vulnerable populations is clearly related to the growing evidence that vulnerable groups experience health disparities, which represent social injustice and bear economic costs to the United States.

## Conceptual Models of Vulnerability and Health Disparity

Although vulnerable populations have been a focus in nursing research for over 50 years (Flaskerud et al., 2002), the theoretical foundation for studies has been varied and often drawn from other fields such as psychology, medicine, sociology, and public health. Most popular among the theoretical frameworks guiding studies involving vulnerable populations are social cognitive theory, the theory of reasoned action, and the health beliefs model. While these models are very useful, they were not specifically designed to address health and illness in vulnerable populations, nor do they draw upon existing knowledge or assess perceptions of these groups. Research has shown that the lack of resources, rather than the presence of risk factors, is the best predictor of illness and premature death in vulnerable populations (Flaskerud, 1999). A report by a multidisciplinary group of expert scientists and clinicians, convened by the National Heart, Lung and Blood Institute (NHLBI) to review research on risk factors for disparities among vulnerable populations, emphasized the importance of viewing socioeconomic status and race as fundamental social causative factors that contribute to disparities through access to resources, avoidance of risks, and minimization of the consequences of disease. They noted that the specific resources and risks implicated in the relationship of these factors with health may change over time (IOM, 2002). In designing health promotion and disease management interventions, nurse researchers need to consider how the availability of resources such as income, jobs, housing, and access to health care can impact risk factors (e.g., behavioral, environmental), which, in turn, influence health status. This conceptualization of vulnerable populations requires a community health perspective as the context for nursing research.

The notion of risk underlying the concept of vulnerability was described in a multifaceted model developed by Aday (1994). She proposed that risk of vulnerability may be predicted by social status (age, sex, race, or ethnicity), social capital (family structure, marital status, voluntary organizations, social network), and human capital (schools, jobs, income, housing). One's social status confers differential availability of personal and political power and associated human and social capital for different social groups based on age, gender, race and ethnicity. Health disparities are perpetuated informally through social norms and behavioral expectations or cultural practices, or formally through legally endorsed differences in access to and quality of human resources. Social status and social capital of individuals or communities will affect the degree of investments made relative to schools, employment opportunities, housing, recreation facilities, neighborhood safety, and overall quality of life. When residents within a neighborhood unite and become involved in activities of shared interests and goals, the prospect for social and human capital formation is potentiated, and the corollary vulnerability of individual members within it is diminished (Aday, 1994). In essence, vulnerability reflects the interaction effects of many factors over which individuals may have little control. Aday proposed that the interaction among individual assets, social assets, and demographic factors contributes to a higher likelihood of poor health in the United States.

A major strength of Aday's conceptualization is that it expanded upon earlier paradigms that provided individual-level explanations of how vulnerability affects health. Individual-focused models related risk (vulnerability) to characteristics of persons such as age, race, socioeconomic level, education, beliefs systems, and knowledge. Aday included both individual and community level determinants of risk in a comprehensive interaction model.

Building upon the works of Aday (1994) and others (Link & Phelamn, 1996; Mann & Tarantola, 1996; Stanhope & Lancaster, 1996), Flaskerud & Winslow (1998) developed a population-based framework known as the vulnerable populations conceptual model (VPCM; Figure 1.1). Although similar constructs are proposed in Aday's earlier model and the VPCM, the latter is specifically designed for clinical practice, research, and policy interventions aimed at impacting links between resource limitations and effects on relative risks and subsequent health outcomes. The VPCM was developed in response to the extensive practical experience of UCLA faculty conducting research and clinical practice with socially vulnerable groups.

The VPCM proposes an interactive relationship among resource availability, relative risk, and health status of vulnerable populations. These three constructs by themselves represent neutral domains that could indicate adequate or limited strengths and resources, protection from or avoidance of risks as well as exposure or susceptibility to risk, and good health or poorer health. Vulnerable populations experience limited resources and, consequently, high relative risk for morbidity and premature mortality.

Within the VPCM, resource availability is viewed as the availability of human capital (income, jobs, education, housing), social status (prestige and power), social connection (integration into society and social networks), and environmental resources (Aday, 2001; Flaskerud & Winslow, 1998). Resource

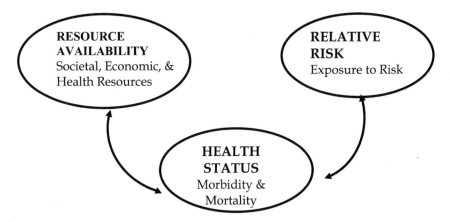

**FIGURE 1.1**    The Vulnerable Populations Conceptual Model (VPCM).

availability is determined on the community level (macro) by the quantity and quality of environmental resources, and on the individual level (micro) by social status. A critical aspect of resource availability is the ability to access the health care system. Access encompasses a wide range of issues, including financial and geographic barriers. A lack of resources increases relative risk, conceptualized as the ratio of the risk of poor health among groups who do not receive resources and are exposed to risk factors compared to those groups who do receive resources and are not exposed to these risk factors (Aday, 1994; Flaskerud & Winslow, 1998).

Relative risk reflects the differential vulnerability of different groups to poor health in that negative or stressful life events harm some people more than others. Risk factors may be behavioral (e.g., lifestyle behaviors and choices, utilization of health screening and health promotion services, exposure to or participation in stressful events such as abuse, violence, or crime) or biologic (e.g., physiologic and genetic susceptibility). Increased exposure to risk factors leads to increased morbidity and mortality in a community.

Health status of a community is indicated in disease incidence, prevalence, and morbidity and mortality rates. The continued widening gap in rates of selected infectious and chronic diseases such as HIV/AIDS and diabetes between various ethnic and racial groups (e.g., Latinos and African Americans) and Whites strongly suggests that factors other than lifestyle and behaviors, such as the availability of economic and health resources, alone or in combination with genetic predispositions, may be influencing the difference.

Investigators have used the VPCM as a basis for examining several issues, including pregnancy intentions of Latina adolescents (Escoto-Lloyd, 2005), health-related problems of preterm infants (Purdy, 2004), social environments and health disparities (Dixon, 2004), and methods to decrease distress in low-income, pregnant Hispanic women (Cohen, 2004). An extensive review of the literature provides support for the utility of the VPCM in working with rural populations (Leight, 2003).

The VPCM is applied extensively by affiliates of the UCLA School of Nursing Center for Vulnerable Populations Research (CVPR) in educational programs and research. Moreover, the VPCM provides a theoretic framework for the training of predoctoral and postdoctoral vulnerable populations fellows at the UCLA School of Nursing. All fellows in this training program are required to complete a course in vulnerable populations research, in which they are taught how vulnerable population (VP) models can be applied to a variety of research questions addressing the health problems of vulnerable populations. The application of the VP models by the fellows' individual research studies is also reviewed and discussed in group meetings of the trainees and faculty mentors. The majority of nurse scientists using the VPCM have applied it in studies examining the risks and health status of individuals rather than in investigations exploring structural and societal factors impacting health.

In the late 1980s, Nyamathi developed the Comprehensive Health Seeking and Coping Paradigm (CHSCP; Nyamathi, 1989) (Figure 1.2), which has undergone rigorous testing among vulnerable populations, such as homeless and drug-addicted persons, for more than two decades (Nyamathi, Wayment, & Dunkel-Schetter, 1993; Nyamathi, Stein, & Bayley, 2000; Nyamathi, Stein, & Swanson, 2000; Nyamathi, Stein, Dixon, Longshore & Galaif, 2003; Stein & Nyamathi, 2004). The CHSCP was originally adapted from the Lazarus and Folkman (1984) Stress and Coping Paradigm and the Schlotfeldt (1981) Health Seeking Paradigm. A broad overview of coping is provided in this complex and multidimensional framework which proposes an interactive relationship existing among several components which tap into the clients' environmental, personal, behavioral, sociodemographic, and health outcome spheres (Nyamathi, 1990). Using a nursing perspective, the health goals of the client are considered and, along with mutually designed nursing interventions, are focused on enhancing the clients' motivation to attain and maintain health and function, to prevent disease, and to attain or retain the highest possible level of health, function, or productivity (Nyamathi, 1989).

Components of the paradigm include clients' situational factors (e.g., length of time homeless) and personal factors (e.g., perceived self-esteem), resources (e.g., social support, financial and spiritual security), and sociodemographic characteristics, including acculturation. Self-esteem, for example, has been noted to be associated with positive health practices such as adherence to treatment regimens (Golin, DiMatteo, & Gelberg, 1996), as well as reduction in drug and alcohol use (Nyamathi et al., 2003). Social support, on the other hand, has been positively correlated with active coping and less likelihood of reporting

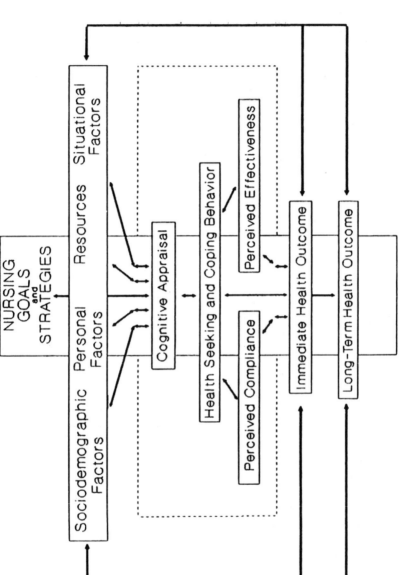

**FIGURE 1.2** Comprehensive Health Seeking and Coping Paradigm (CHSCP).

partners who use drugs (Nyamathi et al., 2003). Nursing goals and interventions are an integral part of this research- and practice-oriented paradigm that may directly influence health seeking and coping behaviors, cognitive appraisal, and health outcome. Cognitive appraisal involves consideration of threat perceived and resources available. Health seeking and coping behavior may involve problem-focused or emotion-focused coping.

The CHSCP provides a very useful framework for nurses interested in enhancing or promoting the health seeking and coping of vulnerable clients. For example, in-depth analysis of the risk and protective factors associated with ongoing drug use has revealed the interplay between support resources and psychological resources and has advanced the state of the science in the understanding of how drug use, drug problems, and drug dependence are related to social support, coping, and depression among severely impoverished adult women (Nyamathi, Leake, Keenan, & Gelberg, 2000). Using theoretical tenets of the CHSCP, Nyamathi and colleagues have discovered psychosocial and behavioral differences in homeless women and their intimate partners, an almost impossible to study subject pool considering the migratory nature of the homeless population (Nyamathi, Galaif, & Leake, 1999). Women, compared to their intimate partners, score significantly lower on mental health and self-esteem; significantly higher on depression, anxiety, and hostility measures; and similarly high on unprotected sexual activities with multiple partners and crack use. These findings provide a detailed focus for ongoing education and prevention programs.

When considering Hepatitis C infection (HCV), Stein and Nyamathi (2004) have recently revealed predictors of HCV infection among homeless adults, exposing a number of environmental predictors such as history of tattoos, being in jail or prison, and less reported variables such as use of non-injection drugs. Nyamathi's most recent testing of the model has shown that Nurse Case Managed intervention resulted in greater Mycobacterium Tuberculosis (TB) knowledge and TB chemoprophylaxis completion compared to standard intervention (Nyamathi, Christiani, Nahid, Gregerson, & Leake, 2006).

More recently, Shi and Stevens (2005) proposed a general framework to study vulnerable populations. In their model, vulnerability is influenced by individuals' predisposing, enabling, and need attributes, and also influences risk factors at an ecological or community level. These attributes reflect risk factors for poor access to health care, poor quality of care, and poor health status, as well as possible discrimination. Individual predisposing attributes include demographic factors, inherited or cultivated belief systems, and social structural variables associated with social position, status, and access to resources (i.e., race or ethnicity, gender). Examples of enabling factors include socioeconomic status associated with social position, status, access to resources, and variations in health status; individual assets (human capital) and mediating factors associated with using health care services such as health insurance, access to health care, or quality of health care. Individual need attributes include self-perceived or professional evaluated health status and quality-of-life indicators, whereas need attributes at the ecological level may include population health behaviors (e.g., smoking, exercise, diet, seat belt use), population health status trends in mortality and morbidity, and health disparities and inequalities. Predisposing, enabling, and need attributes, at both the individual and ecological levels, may each independently influence vulnerability or interact with each other to cumulatively influence vulnerability.

The concept of cumulative vulnerability is proposed within this model, referring to the belief that individuals may possess multiple vulnerability traits that heighten their risk for poor health. In essence, Shi and Stevens (2005) suggest that a gradient relationship exists between vulnerability status and health care access, quality, and health outcomes.

Gelberg, Andersen, and Leake (2000) similarly included the constructs of predisposing, enabling, and need in a Behavioral Model for Vulnerable Populations designed for studying the use of health services and health outcomes. Their model represents a major revision of the Behavioral Model (Andersen, 1968, 1995) and considers both individual and community level variables. An important and unique feature of this model is the proposed impact of satisfaction with care (e.g., general, technical quality, interpersonal aspects, financial). The predisposing vulnerable domain includes social structure characteristics such as acculturation, immigration status, and literacy; childhood characteristics (e.g., foster care, group home placement, abuse, and neglect history); residential history; living conditions (e.g., running water, heat, unsafe structures); mobility; criminal behavior and prison history; victimization; mental health; psychological resources; and substance abuse. Numerous variables are identified in the enabling vulnerable domain and the need vulnerable domain, with specific conditions of special relevance to vulnerable populations such as tuberculosis, sexually transmitted diseases, and low-birth-weight infants.

The Behavioral Model for Vulnerable Populations was tested in a prospective study designed to define and determine predictors of the course of health services utilization and physical health outcomes of homeless adults (Gelberg, Andersen, & Leake, 2000). Findings showed that better health outcomes of the homeless were predicted by a variety of variables, most notably having a community clinic or private doctor as a regular source of care. Generally, use of currently available services did not affect health outcomes. Adding predisposing and enabling domains of the vulnerable in the revised model was found to provide important supplements to traditional predisposing and enabling variables in predicting use of care.

The previously described models stress the role of the community (or ecologic system) in the development of vulnerability. The community contributes to vulnerability; thus, society is responsible for addressing the consequences of vulnerability (Shi & Stevens, 2005). In nursing practice, primary prevention strategies are most appropriately directed toward the link between social and environmental resources and risk factors (Flaskerud & Winslow, 1998). Accordingly, community-based health promotion programs may include population-focused disease prevention efforts such as broad scale immunization and cancer screenings or safety promotion for families with young children. Secondary prevention strategies may be directed toward the link between risk factors and health status; examples include HIV screening of high-risk populations of African American adolescents and young adults, and lifestyle behavior programs to prevent diabetes in overweight Latinos. Tertiary prevention strategies may be designed to prevent depletion of resources among caregivers of people with AIDS, severe mental illness, and chronic disease.

## Impact of Federal Funding on Vulnerable Populations Research

A variety of federal agencies are focusing on vulnerable populations. The National Institutes of Health (NIH, 2000) issued a draft of a strategic research plan to reduce and ultimately eliminate health disparities experienced by vulnerable groups. According to the NIH (2000), there continue to be striking disparities in the burden of illness and death experienced by Pacific Islanders, African Americans, Hispanics, American Indians, Alaska Natives, and Asians. The goal of the NIH strategic plan (2000) was to implement a national effort designed to prevent disease, promote health, and deliver appropriate care to racial and ethnic minorities, thereby reducing and eliminating health care disparities.

Within the NIH, a number of its institutes have developed strategic plans to address the issue of health disparities among vulnerable populations. The National Institute of Nursing Research (NINR) has outlined its own specific goals with respect to reducing and ultimately eliminating health care disparities among vulnerable populations. The focus of the NINR is on eliminating health disparities in terms of reducing morbidity and the burden of disease and other adverse health events among vulnerable groups. The NINR-designated vulnerable groups include African Americans, Asians, Pacific Islanders, Hispanics or Latinos, American Indians, and Native Alaskans (Phillips & Grady, 2002).

Specific to its mission, the National Institute of Allergy and Infectious Diseases (NIAID) has, as its strategic plan, the identification of several factors which cause health disparities including accessibility of health care, increased risk of disease from occupational exposure, and increased risk of disease from underlying genetic, familial, or ethnic factors (NIAID, 2000). The mission of the National Institute on Alcohol Abuse and Alcoholism (NIAAA) is to develop research and treatment interventions to help reduce and eliminate alcohol-related health disparities among vulnerable groups (Le Fauve, Lowman, Litten, & Mattson, 2003). Alternatively, the National Institute of Environmental Health Sciences (NIEHS) has looked at how poverty, environmental pollution, and health interrelate (NIEHS, 2001). According to the NIEHS, both health care access and differences in environmental and occupational exposure play a role in health disparities (i.e., a shortened lifespan and higher morbidity rates) among vulnerable populations.

The National Center on Minority Health and Health Disparities (NCMHD) is another federal agency with a mission to eliminate health disparities as they affect racial and ethnic communities. In 2003, the NCMHD awarded $65.1 million to support health services research, and to support research focusing on the elimination of health disparities among racial and ethnic minority groups and the medically underserved (U.S. Department of Health and Human Services, 2004). The NINR collaborated with the NCMHD in the development of a new initiative called Nursing Partnership Centers on Health Disparities. This initiative was designed to expand the cadre of nurse investigators involved in minority health or health disparities research, to increase the number of research projects aimed at eliminating health disparities, and to assist in developing the research careers of minority nurses by fostering the development of nursing partnerships among researchers, faculty, and students at Minority Serving Institutions (MSIs) and institutions with established health disparity research programs (NINR, 2003). Eight new Health Disparity Centers, each involving a partnership between two schools of nursing, were created through this initiative.

Across NIH, institutes fund a number of Centers of Excellence that address health disparities among vulnerable populations as well as other areas of science. In particular, NINR awards Research Center Core Grants (P30s) to interdisciplinary, collaborative nursing research programs at well-established institutional settings. At UCLA School of Nursing, the Center for Vulnerable Populations Research (CVPR) brings together a core of nurse and interdisciplinary investigators to address the needs of vulnerable populations. The mission of the center, initially funded in 1999 and now extended through 2009, is to enhance strengths of communities to eliminate health disparities faced by vulnerable populations, with a particular focus on ethnic or racial minorities and people living in poverty. Two major goals of the CVPR are to continue expanding the scientific knowledge base of health-related problems of vulnerable populations; and to expand capacity to measure, analyze, and link biologic and behavioral markers in vulnerable populations research. The infrastructure of the CVPR supports achievement of these goals through a variety of research and educational activities conducted by four cores—Administrative, BioLaboratory, Participatory Research and Community Partnership (PRCPC), and Research Support. These cores facilitate resource sharing and enhance services provided to pilot study recipients funded by the center as well as other CVPR-affiliated investigators. The team of core leaders is composed of nursing scholars and interdisciplinary scholars from the fields of medicine, public health, sociology, and statistics.

Fundamental to the philosophy of the CVPR is that in order most effectively to address health disparities among vulnerable populations, researchers must work collaboratively and in partnership with communities. For this reason, the CVPR promotes the use of participatory research methods and aims to develop science in this area by translating the knowledge, skills, and experience acquired in participatory research methods and community partnerships into practice and action. Working as partners, CVPR researchers and community representatives (vulnerable populations themselves) jointly identify problems, design and implement interventions, and evaluate and disseminate outcomes. In the end, the use of participatory methods benefits both researchers, who advance science, and vulnerable communities, whose knowledge and skills are enhanced through involvement in the research process. Furthermore, because the community has real influence on the direction of projects, community-partnered interventions are more likely to result in programs that are culturally and linguistically competent. The CVPR works to build the skills of researchers and community partners through several educational activities, including colloquia, specialized workshops, Summer Institutes, and intensive seminars on how to build community partnerships and apply participatory research methods. In addition, the CVPR utilizes multiple media to spread the word on health issues facing vulnerable populations as well as so-called best practices and innovative methods to address these issues. The CVPR Web site is located at http://www.nursing.ucla.edu/organizations/cvpr/.

Researchers affiliated with the CVPR are advancing knowledge about vulnerable populations and methods to eliminate or reduce health disparities, focusing on four areas: infectious diseases (e.g., HIV/AIDS, hepatitis, tuberculosis), chronic illness (e.g., cardiovascular disease, diabetes, asthma), substance abuse, and environmental quality (e.g., exposure to tobacco smoke, occupational hazards). The CVPR promotes and supports the integration of biologic and behavioral measures in its studies in order to produce the highest quality research. A focus on genomics and proteomics technologies for incorporation into participatory research addressing health disparities of vulnerable populations is a distinctive feature of the CVPR.

In addition to both the NIH institutes and other centers, the Federal Government has supported some key initiatives aimed at addressing health disparities among vulnerable populations. The goal of one initiative, entitled "One America in the 21st Century: The President's Initiative on Race," is to reduce health disparities among racial and ethnic minorities (U.S. Department of Health and Human Services, 2000). With the initiative Healthy People 2010, gender, race, ethnicity, education, income, disability, sexual orientation, and location of residence are variables that may determine who becomes vulnerable to health disparities. Finally, the Department of Health and Human Services (DHHS) has written an "Initiative to Eliminate Racial and Ethnic Disparities in Health," designed to improve disease prevention and to promote health care for vulnerable populations.

The IOM report *Unequal Treatment: Confronting Racial and Ethnic Disparities in Health Care* (2002) created an awareness of the fact that across America, vulnerability occurs secondary to the unequal access to and delivery of societal resources: The recent Federal Government efforts to create programs reducing and eliminating health care disparities represent an attempt to rectify this problem. The IOM report not only highlights the fact that the quality of care received by vulnerable groups across America is lower than that provided to non-vulnerable populations (Nelson, 2003), it brings forth certain ethical dilemmas. One such dilemma is that of social justice; considered to be a core ethical principle in public health nursing (Drevdahl, Kneipp, Canales, & Dorcy, 2001). Drevdahl and associates believe that nurses need to work as social activists to change the current health care disparities experienced by vulnerable groups, which are prevalent across the United States. Bekemeier and Butterfield (2005) question the usefulness of evolving policies addressing health care disparities and, instead, suggest that the time has come for nurses to take action. An intersectional perspective where change is seen as a societal, rather than an individual process, has also been proposed as another method used to achieve social justice (Guthrie, 2005).

People are entitled to equality of health care and also to cultural competency with respect to the delivery of this care (Brach & Fraser, 2000). According to Brach and Fraser, cultural competency relates to the commitment of appropriate practices and policies for vulnerable groups. They believe that vulnerable populations deserve special attention with regard to how their care is delivered. The evaluation of research strategies that adopt techniques to ensure that the care delivered to these groups is of high quality is critical. Cultural competency has the potential to reduce racial and ethnic health disparities, which can lead to social justice (Brach & Fraser, 2000).

## Vulnerable Populations Nursing Research

Vulnerable populations nursing research has been galvanized by the current social, political, and economic climate calling for reductions in health disparity (Flaskerud et al., 2002). The NIH mission—including the strategic plans of NIH institutes, the IOM report, and various other governmental initiatives—provides social and political impetus to study vulnerable populations. The escalating costs of not providing services for these groups creates an economic climate conducive to designing interventions which can mitigate morbidity-associated costs. The climate is ripe for vulnerable populations research, focused on the implementation of interventions to reduce health disparities.

Flaskerud and associates (2002) presented a review of nursing studies on vulnerable populations conducted between 1952 and 2000. In the 1950s, vulnerable populations research, for the most part, was observed to be sparse. In the 1960s, some studies were published which documented the existence of health disparities among socially vulnerable groups. One hallmark of this period was the published studies that addressed issues such as resource availability, relative risk, and health disparities. Some of these studies concluded with calls for community action to rectify inequalities, with respect to the provision of resources, for vulnerable groups. However, despite the fact that studies highlighted health disparities among vulnerable populations, the focus of the Division of Nursing was on nursing manpower, productivity, and utilization, and not on vulnerable populations research (Flaskerud et al., 2002). In the mid-1980s, progress in the field of vulnerable populations research was made, even with the major focus of funding agencies and of nursing scholars on clinical research; for example, different methods used to study vulnerable groups (i.e., focused interviews and participant observation) and new ways to characterize vulnerable populations (i.e., African Americans, Whites, social class designation, economic status) were developed.

In the mid-1980s, the National Center for Nursing Research was established, although vulnerable populations research was not a major focus of this agency. During this decade, there were some published studies that looked at socioeconomic status and ethnicity. Some of these studies were descriptive trials that examined particular vulnerable groups and their cultures, psychosocial attitudes, beliefs, and practices (Flaskerud et al., 2002).

Vulnerable populations nursing studies conducted in the 1990s were both descriptive (evaluation of the relationship between psychosocial variables and relative risk) and interventional (assessment of the effect of resource provision on health outcome). Some descriptive studies examined the relationship between health care resources and morbidity among HIV-infected women (Sowell, et al., 1997; Gentry, 1993). Intervention studies demonstrated that by the provision of resources, health outcomes could be improved.

In the past 5 years (2000–2005), there has been a proliferation of nursing vulnerable populations research, generated, in part, as a consequence of federal (i.e., the NIH, the NINR, Healthy People 2010, the IOM, the NIAAA, etc.) support. The majority of nursing research on vulnerable populations has been done by way of interventional and descriptive study design. For example, in a randomized clinical trial, Koniak-Griffin and associates (2003) provided evidence that implementation of an early intervention program by public health nurses decreases infant morbidity in families headed by minority adolescent mothers. Further, in a study assessing the impact of two randomly assigned cognitive-behavioral community-based AIDS interventions for high risk homeless African American and Latina women, participants in nurse case-managed groups revealed greater decreases in cocaine use and other illegal activities at 2-year follow-up.

The general literature reveals a number of descriptive studies that have enhanced our understanding of vulnerable populations and have broadened our understanding of the social challenges faced by these groups. For example, a program of visiting student nurses was found to be an effective way to improve health outcomes among vulnerable, community-dwelling, older adults (Masters, 2005). Increased incidence and prevalence of certain health conditions among older adults, and the impact of these conditions in terms of health-related quality of life, have also been studied (Sloss et al., 2000). Among homeless adolescents, Rew & Horner (2003) found that although these youths experience health care disparities, they possess strengths that can be identified and used to help them achieve better health. Protective strength factors, resources, and risks can be used to better understand depression among childbearing Mexican women (Heilemann, Frutos, Lee, & Kury, 2004). People with mental retardation have also been described and have been identified as vulnerable populations (Fisher, 2004). Recommendations have been made for the implementation of interventions designed to promote healthy lifestyles to improve the health status of low-income populations, suffering from hypertension and diabetes (Baumann, Chang, & Hoebeke, 2002) and immigrant Latina women at risk for these conditions (Kim, Koniak-Griffin, Flaskerud, & Guarnero, 2004).

Much of the interventional nursing research in the field of vulnerable populations is designed to address the social challenges faced by vulnerable groups (e.g., lack of resource availability in the setting of health care). In some cases, the interventions chosen by nurse scientists include educational efforts designed to prevent or reduce risky behaviors or to improve health. Koniak-Griffin and associates (2003) demonstrated that high-risk adolescent mothers who received a HIV prevention program had significantly higher levels of AIDS knowledge and were significantly more likely to use condoms, compared with their counterparts who did not receive the intervention. Lesser, Oakes, and Koniak-Griffin (2003) recommended that in order to be most effective, HIV risk reduction programs should include male partners. These programs need to address beliefs about gender and power held by both young mothers and their male partners. The benefits of providing a theory-driven, skill-based HIV/STD intervention in comparison to an information-based intervention and a health-promotion control intervention were demonstrated in a clinic-based randomized clinical trial involving sexually experienced African American and Latino adolescent girls (Jemmott, Jemmott,

Braverman, & Fong, 2005). Participants receiving the skill-based intervention reported less unprotected sexual intercourse and fewer sexual partners at the 12-month follow-up compared to those in the other two groups.

In another study an HIV self-care symptom management intervention was found to be useful in terms of health outcomes improvement among African-American mothers (Miles et al., 2003). In a large school-based study, Harrell and associates (1999) demonstrated that both classroom-based and risk-based interventions designed to reduce cardiovascular disease risk factors in children had positive effects on physical activity and knowledge, with trends toward reduced body fat and cholesterol. Further, results of a randomized clinical trial involving nurse home visitation during pregnancy and the first 2 years postpartum, showed enduring positive outcomes for black women living in an urban setting (Kitzman, et al., 2000). The enduring effects included fewer subsequent pregnancies, fewer closely spaced subsequent pregnancies, longer intervals between birth of the first and second child, and fewer months of using Aid to Families with Dependent Children and food stamps.

## Community-Based Approaches to Research With Vulnerable Populations

Community-based participatory research (CBPR) is defined as a collaborative process that equally involves all partners in a research study and treats all partners equally (Minkler, Blackwell, Thompson, & Tamir, 2003). Intervention studies can be designed to elicit community participation in vulnerable populations research (Vincent & Guinn, 2001). Without community participation, acceptance of these studies may be jeopardized (Vincent & Guinn, 2001). CBPR is often applied to vulnerable populations. For example, community-based peer-led interventions can improve the lives of Hispanics who suffer from chronic diseases (Lorig, Ritter, & Gonzalez, 2003), whereas educational interventions can result in significant improvements in self-esteem and can be used to assist people in taking responsibility for their own health (Vincent & Guinn, 2001). The IOM (2002) recommends that the community should be involved in the design and implementation of interventions to reduce health inequalities experienced by vulnerable groups. Since the IOM report was issued, there has been a dramatic increase in support of CBPR. The Centers for Disease Control and Prevention (CDC) has recently funded 25 CBPR grants that focus on health promotion and disease prevention (Minkler et al., 2003). Other federal agencies such as the NIEHS have also committed funds for the development of CBPR programs. The NIEHS has supported CBPR which looks at the effect of environmental pollutants (i.e., pesticide exposure) on health outcomes, among vulnerable groups (Arcury, Quandt, & Dearry, 2001). The NINR has addressed ways that vulnerable populations nursing research can be conducted, incorporating a community-based partnership approach (Phillips & Grady, 2002). It is no surprise that, given the federal support of community involvement in the planning, implementation, and evaluation of health interventions, CBPR studies continue to proliferate. Over the past 5 years, nursing vulnerable populations research has grown to include CBPR.

Nursing CBPR has been carried out in a variety of vulnerable population settings. However, establishing community liaisons conducive to CBPR can be challenging, due to cultural differences between investigators and vulnerable populations (Ammerman, et al. 2003). Despite the difficulties inherent in working with a vulnerable group of another race, Ammerman and colleagues observed that church leaders were able to serve as links between investigators and the community, in the implementation of CBPR within the African American community.

CBPR has been shown to be useful to gain a better understanding of vulnerable populations such as American Indians (Garwick & Auger, 2003; Holkup, Tripp-Reimer, Salois, & Weinert, 2004). The NIH mission statement (2002) identified Latinos as one group vulnerable to higher rates of diseases such as diabetes. Giachello and colleagues (2003) found that implementation of CBPR incorporating interventions such as education and social support resulted in the improvement of health outcomes among vulnerable Latino groups. *Poder es Salud* (Power for Health) is an example of CBPR designed to address health disparities in the African American and Latino communities (Farquhar, Michael, & Wiggins, 2005). *Poder es Salud* uses members of the health care community to assist in an educational effort developed to reduce language and cultural barriers, and to generate social capital. CBPR has also been successfully conducted to improve understanding of the relationship between reproductive experiences and poor birth outcomes among African American women living in Harlem (Mullings et al., 2001). Efforts are underway to promote a program of education developed to improve the health outcomes of vulnerable groups living in other areas of Harlem (Horowitz, Arniella, James, & Bickell, 2004).

In summary, there has been much progress over the past 5 decades with respect to vulnerable populations nursing research. Initially, studies were largely descriptive in nature. As it became apparent that vulnerable groups often experience inequalities in terms of health care, the research took a new turn. Interventions were designed to reduce (and ultimately eliminate) the disparities experienced by vulnerable populations. CBPR represents the most recent evolution of nursing vulnerable populations research. The goal of CBPR is to involve the community in the development and implementation of interventions designed to reduce health disparities experienced by vulnerable groups.

## REFERENCES

Aday, L. A. (1994). Health status of vulnerable populations. *Annual Review of Public Health, 15,* 487–509.

Aday, L. (2001). *At risk in America.* San Francisco, CA: Jossey-Bass.

Ammerman, A., Corbie-Smith, G., St. George, D. M., Washington, C., Weathers, B., & Jackson-Christian, B. (2003). Research expectations among African American church leaders in the PRAISE! Project: A randomized trial guided by community-based participatory research. *Research and Practice, 93(10),* 1720–1727.

Andersen, R., (1968). *Behavior models of families' use of health services.* (Research Series No. 15.) Chicago: Center for Health Administration Studies.

Andersen, R. (1995). Revisiting the behavioral model and access to care: Does it matter? *Journal of Health and Social Behavior, 36(1),* 1–10.

Appel, S. J., Harrell, J. S., & Deng, S. (2002). Racial and socioeconomic differences in risk factors for cardiovascular disease among southern rural women. *Nursing Research, 51(3),* 140–147.

Arcury, T. A., Quandt, S. A., & Dearry, A. (2001). Farm worker pesticide exposure and community-based participatory research: Rationale and practical applications. *Environmental Health Perspectives Supplements, 109(S3),* 25–35.

Baumann, L. C., Chang, M., & Hoebeke, R. (2002). Clinical outcomes for low-income adults with hypertension and diabetes. *Nursing Research, 51(3),* 191–198.

Bekemeier, B., & Butterfield, P. (2005). Unreconciled inconsistencies: A critical review of the concept of social justice in 3 national nursing documents. *Advances in Nursing Science, 28(2),* 152–162.

Berg, J., Wahlgren, D. R., Hofstetter, C. R., Meltzer, S. B., Meltzer, E. O., Matt, G. E., et al. (2003). Latino children with asthma: Rates and risks for medical care utilization. *Journal of Asthma, 40(0),* 1–11.

Brach, C., & Fraser, I. (2000). Can cultural competency reduce racial and ethnic disparities? A review and conceptual model. *Medical Care Research and Review, 57(1),* 181–217.

Cohen, J. (2004). Guiding research in health disparities of pregnant Hispanic women. *Communicating Nursing Research Conference Proceedings, 37,* 196. Western Institute of Nursing.

Dixon, E. (2004). The social ecologic model of neighborhood health. *Communicating Nursing Research Conference Proceedings, 37,* (p. 195) Western Institute of Nursing.

Drevdahl, D., Kneipp, S. M., Canales, M. K., & Dorcy, K. S. (2001). Reinvesting in social justice: A capital idea for public health nursing? *Advances in Nursing Science, 24(2),* 19–34.

Erlen, J. A. (2003). When all do not have the same. *Orthopaedic Nursing, 22(2),* 152–154.

Escoto-Lloyd, S., (2005). *Pregnancy intentions in Latina adolescents.* Unpublished doctoral dissertation, UCLA School of Nursing.

Farquhar, S. A., Michael, Y. L., & Wiggins, N. (2005). Building on leadership and social capital to create change in 2 urban communities. *American Journal of Public Health, 95(4),* 596–601.

Fisher, K. (2004). Health disparities and mental retardation. *Journal of Nursing Scholarship*, *36(1)*, 48–53.

Flaskerud, J. H., Lesser, J., Dixon, E., Anderson, N., Conde, F., & Kim, S. (2002). Health disparities among vulnerable populations. *Nursing Research*, *51(2)*, 74–85.

Flaskerud, J. H., & Winslow, B. J. (1998). Conceptualizing vulnerable populations health-related research. *Nursing Research*, *47(2)*, 69–78.

Garwick, A. W., & Auger, S. (2003). Participatory action research: The Indian Family Stories Project. *Nursing Outlook*, *51*, 261–266.

Gelberg, L., Andersen, R., & Leake, B. D. (2000). The behavioral model for vulnerable populations: Application to medical care use and outcomes for homeless people. *Health Services Research*, *34 (6)*, 1273–302.

Gentry, J. H. (1993). Women and AIDS. *Psychology and AIDS Exchange*, *11*, 1–7.

Giachello, A. L., Arrom, J. O., Davis, M., Sayad, J. V., Ramirez, D., Nandi, C., et al. (2003). Reducing diabetes health disparities through community-based participatory action research: The Chicago Southeast Diabetes Community Action Coalition. *Public Health Reports*, *118(4)*, 309–324.

Golin, C. E., DiMatteo, M. R., & Gelberg L. (1996). The role of patient participation in the doctor visit. Implications for adherence to diabetes care. *Diabetes Care*, *19(10)*, 1153–1164.

Guthrie, G. (2005). Bridging health care disparities: Addressing unmet needs of women of color. *Journal of Obstetric, Gynecologic, and Neonatal Nursing*, *5*, 385.

Harrell, J. S., McMurray, R. G., Gansky, S. A., Bangdiwala, S. I., & Bradley, C. B. (1999). A public health vs a risk-based intervention to improve cardiovascular health in elementary school children: The Cardiovascular Health in Children Study. *American Journal of Public Health*, *89(10)*, 1529–1535.

Heilemann, M. V., Frutos, L., Lee, K. A., & Kury, F. S. (2004). Protective strength factors, resources, and risks in relation to depressive symptoms among childbearing women of Mexican descent. *Health Care for Women International*, *25*, 88–106.

Holkup, P. A., Tripp-Reimer, T., Salois, E. M., & Weinert C. (2004). Community-based participatory research. An approach to intervention research with a Native American community. *Advances in Nursing Science*, *27(3)*, 162–175.

Horowitz, C. R., Arniella, A., James, S., & Bickell, N. A. (2004). Using community-based participatory research to reduce health disparities in East and Central Harlem. *The Mount Sinai Journal of Medicine*, *71(6)*, 368–374.

Institute of Medicine (IOM). (2002). *Unequal treatment: Confronting racial and ethnic disparities in health care*. Washington, DC: National Academics Press.

Jemmott, J. B., Jemmott, L. S., Braverman, P. K., & Fong, G. T. (2005). HIV/STD risk reduction interventions for African American and Latino adolescent girls at an adolescent medicine clinic: A randomized controlled trial. *Archives of Pediatric & Adolescent Medicine*, *159(5)*, 440–449.

Keltner, B., Kelley, F. J., & Smith, D. (2004). Leadership to reduce health disparities: A model for nursing leadership in American Indian communities. *Nursing Administration Quarterly*, *28(3)*, 181–191.

Kim, S., Koniak-Griffin, D., Flaskerud, J. H., & Guarnero, P. A. (2004). The impact of lay health advisors on cardiovascular health promotion: Using a community-based participatory approach. *Journal of Cardiovascular Nursing*, *19(3)*, 192–199.

Kitzman, H., Olds, D. L., Sidora, K., Henderson, C. R. Jr., Hanks, C., Cole, R. et al. (2000). Enduring effects of nurse home visitation on maternal life course: A 3-year follow-up of a randomized trial. *Journal of the American Medical Association, 282(15)*, 1983–1989.

Koniak-Griffin, D., Verzemnieks, I. L., Anderson, N. L. R., Brecht-M. L., Lesser, J., Kim, S., et al. (2003). Nurse visitation for adolescent mothers: Two-year infant health and maternal outcomes. *Nursing Research, 52*, 127–136.

Lazarus, R., & Folkman, S. (1984). *Stress, appraisal and coping.* New York: Springer Publishing.

Le Fauve, C. E., Lowman, C., Litten, R. Z. 3rd, & Mattson, M. E. (2003). Introduction: National Institute on Alcohol Abuse and Alcoholism workshop on treatment research priorities and health disparities. *Alcoholism: Clinical & Experimental Research, 27(8)*, 1318–1320.

Leight, S. B. (2003). The application of a vulnerable populations conceptual model to rural health. *Public Health Nursing, 20(6)*, 440–448.

Lesser, J., Oakes, R., & Koniak-Griffin, D. (2003). Vulnerable adolescent mothers' perceptions of maternal role and HIV risk. *Health Care for Women International, 24*, 513–528.

Link, B. G., & Phelamn, J. C. (1996). Understanding sociodemographic differences in health. The role of fundamental social causes. *American Journal of Public Health, 86 (4)*, 471–473.

Lorig, K. R., Ritter, P. L., & Gonzalez, V. M. (2003). Hispanic chronic disease self-management. *Nursing Research, 52(6)*, 361–368.

Mann, J. A., & Tarantola, D. (1996) Societal vulnerability contextual analysis. In J. A. Mann & D. Tarantola (Eds.), *AIDS in the World II: Global dimensions, social roots, and responses* (pp. 444–462). New York: Oxford University.

Masters, K. R. (2005). A student home visiting program for vulnerable, community-dwelling older adults. *Journal of Nursing Education, 44(4)*, 185–186.

Minkler, M., Blackwell, A. G., Thompson, M., & Tamir, H. (2003). Community-based participatory research: Implications for public health funding. *American Journal of Public Health, (93)8*, 1210–1213.

Miles, M. S., Holditch-Davis, D., Eron, J., Black, B. P., Pedersen, C., & Harris, D. A. (2003). An HIV self-care symptom management intervention for African American mothers. *Nursing Research, 52(6)*, 350–360.

Mullings, L., Wali, A., McLean, D., Mitchell, J., Prince, S., Thomas, D., et al. (2001). Qualitative methodologies and community participation in examining reproductive experiences: The Harlem Birth Right Project. *Maternal and Child Health Journal, 5(2)*, 85–93.

National Institute of Allergy and Infectious Diseases. (2000). *Strategic plan for addressing health disparities.* Retrieved June 8, 2005, from http://www.niaid.nih.gov/

National Institute of Environmental Health Sciences. (2001). *Health disparities research.* Retrieved June 8, 2005, from http://www.niehs.nih.gov/

National Institute of Health. (2000). *Strategic research plan to reduce and ultimately eliminate health disparities.* Retrieved June 1, 2005, from http://www.nih.gov/

National Institute of Nursing Research. (2000). *Mission statement.* Retrieved December 24, 2004, from http://www.nih.gov/ninr/research/diversity

National Institute of Nursing Research Nursing. (2003, September 9). *Nursing partnership centers on health disparities.* Retrieved December 24, 2004, from http://ninr.nih.gov/ninr/research/dea/P20s.doc

Nelson, A. R. (2003). Unequal treatment: Report of the Institute of Medicine on racial and ethnic disparities in healthcare. *Annals of Thoracic Surgery, 76*, S1377-S1381.

Nyamathi, A. (1989). Comprehensive health seeking and coping paradigm. *Journal of Advanced Nursing, 14(4)*, 281–290.

Nyamathi, A. M. (1990). Assessing the coping status of spouses of critically ill cardiac patients: A theoretically based approach. *Journal of Cardiovascular Nursing, 5(1)*, 1–12.

Nyamathi, A., Christiani, A., Nahid, P., Gregerson, P., & Leake, B. (2006). Randomized controlled trial of two treatment programs for homeless adults with latent tuberculosis infection. *International Journal of Tuberculosis & Lung Disease, 10(7)*, 775–782.

Nyamathi, A., Galaif, E., & Leake, B. (1999). A comparison of homeless women and their intimate partners. *Journal of Community Psychology, 27*, 489–502.

Nyamathi, A., Leake, B., Keenan, C., & Gelberg, L. (2000). Type of social support among homeless women: Its impact on psychosocial resources, health and health behaviors, and use of health services. *Nursing Research, 49(6)*, 318–326.

Nyamathi, A., Stein, J., & Bayley, L. (2000). Predictors of mental distress and poor physical health among homeless women. *Psychology & Health, 15*, 483–500.

Nyamathi, A. M., Stein, J. A., Dixon, E., Longshore, D., & Galaif, E. (2003). Predicting positive attitudes about quitting drug and alcohol use among homeless women. *Psychology of Addictive Behaviors, 17(1)*, 32–141.

Nyamathi, A. M., Stein, J. A., & Swanson, J. M. (2000). Personal, cognitive, behavioral, and demographic predictors of HIV testing and STDs in homeless women. *Journal of Behavioral Medicine, 23(2)*, 123–147.

Nyamathi, A., Wayment, H., & Dunkel-Schetter, C. (1993). Psychosocial correlates of emotional distress and risk behavior in African-American women at risk for HIV infection. *Anxiety, Stress, & Coping, 6*, 133–148.

Phillips, J., & Grady, P. A. (2002). Reducing health disparities in the twenty-first century: Opportunities for nursing research. *Nursing Outlook, 50*, 117–120.

Purdy, I. B. (2004). Essence of vulnerable: Generating and using knowledge for neonatal practice. *Communicating Nursing Research Conference Proceedings, 37*, 193 Western Institute of Nursing.

Rew, L., & Horner, S. D. (2003). Personal strengths of homeless adolescents living in a high-risk environment. *Advances in Nursing Science, 26(12)*, 90–102.

Shi, L., & Stevens, G. D. (2005). *Vulnerable populations in the United States*. San Francisco: Jossey-Bass.

Sowell, R. L., Seals, B. F., Moneyham, L., Demi, A., Cohen, L., & Brake, S. (1997). Quality of life in HIV-infected women in the south-eastern United States. *AIDS Care, 9(5)*, 501–512.

Schlotfeldt, R. (1981). Nursing in the future. *Nursing Outlook, 29*, 295–301.

Sloss, E. M., Solomon, D. H., Shekelle, P. G., Young, R. T., Saliba, D., MacLean, C. H., et al. (2000). Selecting target conditions for quality of care improvement in vulnerable older adults. *Journal of the American Geriatric Society, 48(4)*, 363–369.

Stanhope, M., & Lancaster, J. (Eds.). (1996). *Community health nursing: Promoting health of aggregates, families, and individuals* (4th ed.). St. Louis, MO: Mosby.

Stein, J. A., & Nyamathi, A. (2004). Correlates of hepatitis C virus infection in homeless men: A latent variable approach. *Drug & Alcohol Dependency, 75(1)*, 89–95.

Todd, K. H., Deaton, D., D'Amamo, A. P., & Goe, L. (2000). Ethnicity and analgesic practice. *Annals of Emergency Medicine, 35*, 11–16.

U.S. Department of Health and Human Services. (2000, November). *Healthy People 2010 (2nd ed.). Understanding and improving health and objectives for improving health.* 2 vols. Washington, DC: U.S. Government Printing Office.

U.S. Department of Health and Human Services. (2004). *HHS fact sheet.* Washington, DC: U.S. Government Printing Office.

Villarruel, A.M. (2004). Introduction: Eliminating health disparities among racial and ethnic minorities in the United States. In J. Fitzpatrick, A. Villarruel & C. P. Porter (eds.), *Annual review of nursing research* (pp. 1–5). New York: Springer Publishing Company.

Vincent, V., & Guinn, R. (2001). Effectiveness of a Colonial Educational Intervention. *Hispanic Journal of Behavioral Sciences, 23(2)*, 229–238.

# Chapter 2

## Advancing Nursing Science in Vulnerable Populations: Measurement Issues

Ora Lea Strickland, Colleen DiIorio, Dorothy Coverson, and Michelle Nelson

### ABSTRACT

*This study examined measurement practices of researchers in relation to vulnerable population research published in four general nursing research journals in 2004. The purpose was to identify issues and imperatives in the measurement of research variables with vulnerable populations that warrant attention. A total of 133 articles were eligible for inclusion in the study, and 428 measurement instruments were used in the studies. A content analysis of the 133 eligible articles indicated that most samples included to a greater extent more Whites than predominantly minority populations, and more adults than children. Most of the articles did not specify socioeconomic status of samples. Of the 133 eligible articles, 83 (62.4%) included samples that were comprised of a majority of racial and ethnic minorities; however, percentages of studies that focused predominately on a specific minority group were below 10% in more than 80% of studies.*

*Major findings related to measurement practices indicated inadequate specification of the measurement framework employed; lack of adequate specification of the conceptual base of measurement tools; and, a heavy reliance on the use of*

*self-report data, attitudinal and perceptual measures, and the use of questionnaires and rating scales. There was also inadequate attention to the metric qualities of laboratory physiological measures, and to reliability and validity in general. It was concluded that inadequate attention is given to measurement practices by researchers when studying vulnerable populations.*

**Keywords: measurement issues; measures; nursing measurement; reliability; validity; vulnerable populations**

# INTRODUCTION

As the nation has become aware of the problem of health disparities globally, greater concern is being raised about the availability of measurement instruments that are reliable and valid for use in research with vulnerable populations. Within nursing science, measurement practices and issues relating to vulnerable populations need to be examined in terms of the degree to which such populations have been studied, and the appropriateness of measurement practices applied to samples with members of vulnerable populations. Although assessments of measurement practices in nursing research literature was conducted in 1981 (Waltz & Strickland, 1982) and in 1985 (Strickland & Waltz, 1986; Waltz & Strickland, 1989), little attention was given to measurement practices specific to vulnerable populations.

The purpose of this chapter is to: (a) examine the measurement practices of nurse researchers in relation to vulnerable populations in articles published in four leading general nursing research journals during 2004, and (b) identify issues and imperatives in the measurement of variables with vulnerable populations that warrant attention by nurse researchers if the validity of findings from such studies are to be assured.

Within the context of this review, vulnerable populations will refer primarily to populations that are considered vulnerable due to racial and ethnic differences. However, some attention will be given to vulnerable populations issues in measurement related to age, gender, and socioeconomic status. This focus is consistent with the approach taken for Healthy People 2010 (U.S. Department of Health and Human Services [USDHHS], 2000), which has as its major goal the elimination of health disparities. It also is compatible with the Institute of Medicine (IOM) study, which found evidence of health disparities across a broad range of health problems and services based on race and ethnic background (IOM, 2003). Noting that racial and ethnic health disparities are unacceptable, the IOM urged general public awareness of the problem and recommended specific actions in the legal, policy-making, and regulatory arenas to eliminate health disparities based on different treatment of racial and ethnic minorities. If this mandate is to be adequately addressed, research focused on health disparities must be conducted with vulnerable populations, and with measurement instruments that are socioculturally and psychometrically sound when used with vulnerable populations studied.

## OVERVIEW OF MEASUREMENT WITH VULNERABLE POPULATIONS

### The Concept of Vulnerability

When the term "vulnerability" is used to refer to the health of populations, it connotes those groups with a greater than average risk for developing health problems by virtue of their marginalized sociocultural status; personal characteristics such as age, race or gender; or those who have limited access to health resources (Aday, 2001; de Chesney, 2005; Flaskerud & Winslow, 1998). From the public health perspective, a vulnerable population is more susceptible to poor mental, physical, or social health simply because of status in society. Ethnic and racial minority groups and women are considered vulnerable populations because they have typically been marginalized in society regardless of economic status and educational level achieved (Hall, Stevens, & Meleis, 1994; Koci, 2004). Immigrants and the poor are vulnerable because they often have limited access to health care due to lack of insurance or insufficient insurance coverage. Children and the elderly also are considered vulnerable because these groups are prone to specific health problems due to development or aging (de Chesney, 2005).

### State of the Science in Nursing Measurement

Assessments of the state of the science in nursing measurement conducted in 1981 (Waltz & Strickland, 1982) and in 1985 (Strickland & Waltz, 1986; Waltz & Strickland, 1989), indicated that nurse researchers were not following sufficiently recommended measurement principles and practices when studying nursing outcomes. Limitations were noted in regard to appropriate documentation of conceptual frameworks of measurement instruments, heavy reliance on self-report and attitudinal or perceptual measures, inadequate attention to reliability data within the context of the current study, and heavy dependence on old reliability or validity data, without adequate attention to whether such data were appropriate for the population studied.

The state of the science in regard to measurement with vulnerable populations has not been systematically studied. However, it is well accepted that the majority of psychosocial measurement tools have been designed and tested on non-minorities and generally well-educated populations. In addition, many instruments have been developed and tested on young adults, quite often college students. Thus, there are a limited number of reliable and valid measurement instruments that can be effectively and efficiently used with children of various ages (Strickland, 2005). For many measurement instruments, it is not clear whether they perform adequately in ethnic and racial minority groups, in persons who are not well-educated, or in the elderly. Another major limitation is that many instruments, as currently developed, are quite long and burdensome for use with clinical populations, and are not practical for use in clinical settings or for research in which participants are quite ill or frail (Strickland, 1997; 1998; 1999). Hence, the reliability and validity of instruments can be greatly compromised when they are not compatible with the population or setting in which they are used. When measurement instruments are not reliable and valid, this can lead to problems with statistical conclusion validity (Campbell & Stanley, 1963; Cook & Campbell, 1979). Therefore, the results or findings generated in studies with instruments with poor metric qualities can result in inappropriate conclusions or Type I or Type II errors.

## METHODS

Within the context of this empirical review, vulnerable populations will refer primarily to populations that are considered vulnerable due to racial and ethnic differences. However, some attention will be given to vulnerable populations issues in measurement related to age, gender, and socioeconomic status. This focus is consistent with the approach taken for Healthy People 2010 (USDHHS, 2000), which has as its major goal the elimination of health disparities. It also is compatible with the IOM study, which found evidence of health disparities across a broad range of health problems and services based on race and ethnic background (IOM, 2003). Noting that racial and ethnic health disparities are unacceptable, the IOM urged general public awareness of the problem and recommended specific actions in the legal, policy-making, and regulatory arenas to eliminate health disparities based on differential treatment of racial and ethnic minorities. If this mandate is to be adequately addressed, research focused on health disparities must be conducted with vulnerable populations, and with measurement instruments that are socioculturally and psychometrically sound when used with vulnerable populations studied.

This empirical review was conducted as part of a larger project designed to assess the measurement of research variables in nursing. A content analysis procedure was used to assess the metric qualities of measurement instruments reported in studies appearing in *International Journal of Nursing Studies, Nursing Research, Research in Nursing and Health,* and *Western Journal of Nursing Research* in 2004. These journals were selected because they are top-tiered journals, that is, referenced in index Medicus and on Medline, and are among the most frequently cited general nursing research journals. Only general nursing research journals were selected because they were more likely to reflect the state of the science in measurement across the discipline of nursing, rather than in a particular specialty area.

Studies that did not include the use of a quantitatively based measurement instruments were excluded. Only those articles that provided original quantitative findings that provided descriptions of research procedures and instrumentation within the text of the article were included in the database. Therefore, completely qualitative studies, theoretical articles, and reviews of the literature were excluded from the analysis.

A content analysis form was designed to: (a) specify characteristics of the published studies; (b) delineate the reported utilization of measurement principles and practices; (c) identify the research variables studied; and (d) identify the characteristics and metric properties of measurement tools based on the information provided in the articles. Items on the content analysis form and criteria for assessment of articles were developed based on measurement content, and principles and practices propagated by measurement textbooks (Nunnually & Bernstein, 1994; Pedhazur & Schmelkin, 1991; Waltz, Strickland, & Lenz, 2005). The content analysis form had a content validity index of 1.00 based on the item ratings of two measurement experts who held doctorates and preparation and experience in measurement and nursing research. Two raters who had been trained to use the content analysis form conducted the content analysis. An interrater reliability of 94.5 was determined based on percent agreement between the raters on five randomly selected articles. The content analysis form generated descriptive data, therefore, findings will be presented in frequencies and percentages.

## RESULTS

A total of 133 articles met the eligibility requirements for inclusion in the study, and 428 instruments were used to measure study variables. The most frequent focus of the eligible articles was nursing care or clinical practice research. However, other areas such as fundamental or basic research, nursing systems and health care delivery research, and research methods and instrument development research were well represented in the sample of articles. Of the 133 eligible articles for the study, 83 (62.4%) included samples of whom at least half were ethnic and racial minorities. A total of 248 (57.9%) of the 428 eligible instruments used in these studies were completed predominantly by ethnic and racial minorities. Table 2.1

**TABLE 2.1** Eligible Articles and Measurement Instruments from Selected Journals in 2004 by Racial/Ethnic Background

| Journals | Number of Eligible Articles | | Articles with Majority of Minorities in Sample | | All Instruments Reported | | Instruments with Majority of Minorities in Sample | |
|---|---|---|---|---|---|---|---|---|
| | Frequency | (%) | Frequency | (%) | Frequency | (%) | Frequency | (%) |
| International Journal of Nursing Studies | 47 | (35.3) | 37 | (44.6) | 115 | (26.9) | 92 | (37.1) |
| Nursing Research | 29 | (21.8) | 17 | (20.5) | 107 | (25.0) | 54 | (21.8) |
| Research in Nursing and Health | 30 | (22.6) | 17 | (20.5) | 124 | (29.0) | 64 | (25.8) |
| Western Journal of Nursing Research | 27 | (20.3) | 12 | (14.5) | 82 | (19.2) | 38 | (15.3) |
| TOTAL | 133 | (100) | 83 | (100) | 428 | (100) | 248 | (100) |

presents the number of eligible articles and measurement instruments that were included in the study from each of the selected journals and for samples of whom the majority were ethnic and racial minorities. Table 2.2 provides the distribution of articles by focus areas for all of the eligible articles and instruments for 2004 and for those articles and instruments for which the majority of the sample represented ethnic and racial minorities.

## Characteristics of Samples in the Studies

The demographic characteristics of the samples in the selected articles can serve as a barometer of the populations that nurse researchers selected to focus their research efforts and measurement endeavors. As far as demographic characteristics are concerned, most of the samples (62.4%) included racial and ethnic minorities. In addition, the majority included both genders (61.1%), and adults (69.2%) (see Table 2.3). It is noted that the number of studies with infants and children in the samples was substantially lower than those which included adults and older adults. It is also notable that the large majority of studies (78.9%) did not specify the socioeconomic status of samples. When the percentage of specific minorities included in each sample was considered, Native Americans (7.5%) were least likely to be represented and Asians or Orientals (35.3%) were most likely to be included. The larger percentages of Asians in some studies are reflective of the fact that more studies focusing on Asians were published in the *International Journal of Nursing Studies*.

The majority of articles and instruments published in the four designated journals included a sizeable number of minorities from two or more subgroups. When specific minority groups are considered separately, their representation was low. Tables 2.4 and 2.5 provide a more complete representation of the involvement of minorities in the samples and the completion of measurement instruments in the studies based on the percentage of minorities in each sample. Blacks or African Americans, Hispanics, and Native Americans comprised less than 10% of samples in more than 80% of the studies; and, comprised more than 75% of samples in less than 4% of studies. When looking at the number of measurement instruments completed by samples in these studies, Blacks or African Americans, Hispanics, Native Americans, and Asians comprised less than 10% of the samples completing tools in most studies.

## Measurement Practices and Principles Used With Instruments in Samples With a Majority of Racial and Ethnic Minorities

In order to obtain a perspective regarding the use of acceptable measurement practices in ethnic and racial minority populations in nursing journals, a careful

**TABLE 2.2**  Primary Focus of Articles and Number of Instruments Used for All Articles and Those With Majority of Minorities in Sample

| Category | All Articles | | Articles with Majority of Minorities in Sample | | All Instruments Reported | | Instruments with Majority of Minorities in Sample | |
|---|---|---|---|---|---|---|---|---|
| | Frequency | (%) | Frequency | (%) | Frequency | (%) | Frequency | (%) |
| Nursing care or clinical practice | 51 | (38.3) | 29 | (34.9) | 181 | (42.3) | 98 | (39.5) |
| Fundamental or basic research | 19 | (14.3) | 7 | (8.4) | 72 | (16.8) | 20 | (8.1) |
| Nursing education | 7 | (5.3) | 6 | (7.2) | 16 | (3.7) | 15 | (6.0) |
| Nursing systems/health care delivery | 13 | (9.8) | 11 | (13.3) | 28 | (6.5) | 22 | (8.9) |
| Research on nursing profession | 15 | (11.3) | 10 | (12.0) | 52 | (12.1) | 29 | (11.7) |
| Research methods/instrument development | 20 | (15.0) | 14 | (16.9) | 40 | (9.3) | 33 | (13.3) |
| Other | 8 | (6.0) | 6 | (7.2) | 39 | (9.1) | 31 | (12.5) |
| TOTAL | 133 | (100) | 83 | (100) | 428 | (100) | 248 | (100) |

**TABLE 2.3** Number of Articles (N = 133) Citing Specific Demographic Characteristics in Sample and Number of Instruments (N = 428) Used

| Demographic Characteristic | Articles Frequency | (%) | Instruments Frequency | (%) |
|---|---|---|---|---|
| Racial/Ethnic Background:* | | | | |
| White | 63 | (47.4) | 225 | (51.3) |
| Black or African American | 35 | (26.3) | 127 | (29.7) |
| Hispanic | 31 | (23.3) | 95 | (22.2) |
| Native American | 10 | (7.5) | 25 | (6.1) |
| Asian/Oriental | 47 | (35.3) | 122 | (28.5) |
| Other | 12 | (9.0) | 54 | (12.6) |
| Race/ethnicity not specified | 49 | (36.8) | 151 | (35.2) |
| Gender: | | | | |
| Males only | 3 | (2.3) | 6 | (1.4) |
| Females only | 28 | (21.1) | 101 | (23.6) |
| Both genders | 82 | (61.1) | 264 | (61.7) |
| Gender not specified | 20 | (15.1) | 57 | (13.3) |
| Socioeconomic Status: | | | | |
| Low SES | 4 | (3.0) | 27 | (6.3) |
| Middle class or above | 6 | (4.5) | 28 | (6.5) |
| Both low and middle class | 13 | (9.8) | 49 | (11.4) |
| Not applicable | 5 | (3.8) | 9 | (2.1) |
| Not specified | 105 | (78.9) | 315 | (73.6) |
| Age Group:* | | | | |
| Neonates | 5 | (3.8) | 7 | (1.7) |
| Infants | 3 | (2.3) | 13 | (3.0) |
| Preschool | 4 | (3.0) | 17 | (4.1) |
| School age | 7 | (5.3) | 17 | (4.1) |
| Adolescents | 15 | (11.3) | 53 | (12.7) |
| Adults | 92 | (69.2) | 299 | (69.9) |
| Older adults | 44 | (33.1) | 139 | (33.3) |
| Unable to determine | 15 | (11.3) | 34 | (8.2) |

*Percentages total more than 100% because multiple groups were represented in some studies.

**TABLE 2.4** Number of Articles (N=133) by Percent of Sample With Various Racial/Ethnic Backgrounds

| Percentage | White | | Black | | Hispanic | | Native American | | Asian/Oriental | |
|---|---|---|---|---|---|---|---|---|---|---|
| | Frequency | (%) | Frequency | (%) | Frequency | (%) | Frequency | (%) | Frequency | (%) |
| < 10% | 75 | (56.4) | 107 | (80.5) | 116 | (87.2) | 130 | (97.7) | 100 | (75.2) |
| 10 to 25% | 2 | (1.5) | 8 | (6.0) | 9 | (6.8) | 3 | (2.3) | 0 | (0.0) |
| 26 to 50% | 6 | (4.5) | 6 | (4.5) | 3 | (2.3) | 0 | (0.0) | 1 | (.07) |
| 51 to 75% | 10 | (7.5) | 7 | (5.3) | 2 | (1.5) | 0 | (0.0) | 0 | (0.0) |
| 76 to 100% | 40 | (30.0) | 5 | (3.6) | 3 | (2.3) | 0 | (0.0) | 32 | (24.1) |

Note: Percentages are in parentheses.

**TABLE 2.5** Number of Instruments (N = 428) by Percent of Sample With Various Racial/Ethnic Backgrounds

| Percentage | White Frequency | (%) | Black Frequency | (%) | Hispanic Frequency | (%) | Native American Frequency | (%) | Asian/Oriental Frequency | (%) |
|---|---|---|---|---|---|---|---|---|---|---|
| < 10% | 221 | (51.6) | 325 | (75.9) | 377 | (88.1) | 417 | (97.4) | 349 | (81.6) |
| 10 to 25% | 4 | (0.9) | 25 | (5.9) | 26 | (6.1) | 11 | (2.6) | 0 | (0.0) |
| 26 to 50% | 27 | (6.3) | 19 | (4.5) | 11 | (2.6) | 0 | (0.0) | 1 | (0.2) |
| 51 to 75% | 24 | (5.6) | 34 | (7.9) | 9 | (2.1) | 0 | (0.0) | 0 | (0.0) |
| 76 to 100% | 153 | (35.7) | 25 | (5.8) | 5 | (1.2) | 0 | (0.0) | 78 | (18.2) |

Note: Percentages are in parentheses.

analysis was done of the 248 measurement instruments that were used in samples composed of predominantly ethnic and racial minorities. Table 2.6 shows the approaches to data collection employed with these 248 instruments. From instrument descriptions in many studies, it is unclear whether a criterion- or norm-referenced approach to scoring was employed. The conceptual basis of the measurement instrument was only specified in 29.6% of cases. Moreover, there was a heavy reliance on the use of data collection via self-report (71.4%), and most data were collected with questionnaires and rating scales (79.8%). There was also more of a focus on collecting data on attitudinal or perceptual variables (44.4%) than on biochemical laboratory data (32.7%).

## Reliability Evidence

Previous attention has been directed toward the importance of describing reliability and validity data for specific instruments in order to support the credibility of research findings. Therefore, consideration was given in this review to the reporting of reliability data for each measurement instrument that was used in studies, including psychometric data collected prior to the implementation of the research study and within the context of the study itself. As displayed in Table 2.7, no reliability data were provided for 63 (25.4%) of the measurement instruments. Most of the described reliability data were based on the instrument's performance in prior studies (53.6%). When the source of reliability data is considered, only 21% of the instruments had reliability data reported from both a prior and the current study, which is the most helpful to readers. Less than half of the instruments had reliability data available regarding the instrument's performance within the current study, and only 53.6% reported reliability from a previous study. The most frequent type of reliability reported was internal consistency for both prior studies as well as the current study, followed by test-retest reliability (Table 2.8). Given that more than 35% of data collected were either biochemical or microbiological/microscopic data, it is interesting to note that laboratory precision or sensitivity data were provided for only 3.2% and 0.4% of prior and current study data, respectively.

## Validity Evidence

When validity is considered, only 21.8% of instruments had validity data available based on the current study. The major source of validity data was a prior study, with 41.5% of validity data reported from this source. Only 5.6% of validity data reflected the instrument's performance in both a prior and the current study. Validity data were not provided for 46.4% of the instruments (see Table 2.9).

In many situations, when validity data were reported, it was only mentioned without a clear specification of the nature of the validity evidence available. Table 2.9 presents the types of validity provided. Even with this liberal interpretation

**TABLE 2.6** Approaches to Data Collection and Types of Concepts Measured by Instruments Used in Samples With a Majority of Racial/Ethnic Minorities (N = 248 Instruments)

| Type of Data Collected | Frequency of Use | (%) |
|---|---|---|
| Measurement framework used: | | |
| Criterion-referenced | 27 | (10.9) |
| Norm-referenced | 3 | (1.2) |
| Both | 1 | (0.4) |
| Not specified | 217 | (87.5) |
| Approach to data collection: | | |
| Direct observation | 28 | (11.4) |
| Indirect observation | 8 | (3.3) |
| Self-report | 177 | (71.4) |
| Objective instrumentation | 19 | (7.7) |
| More than one approach | 4 | (1.6) |
| Unable to determine | 9 | (3.6) |
| Other | 3 | (1.2) |
| Type of measure:* | | |
| Achievement/cognitive | 29 | (11.9) |
| Attitudinal/perceptual | 110 | (44.4) |
| Behavioral/performance | 17 | (6.9) |
| Biomechanical | 23 | (9.3) |
| Biochemical | 81 | (32.7) |
| Microbiological/microscopic | 9 | (3.6) |
| Format of the measure:* | | |
| Anecdotal record | 2 | (0.8) |
| Interview | 10 | (4.0) |
| Questionnaire/rating scale | 198 | (79.8) |
| Review of documents | 8 | (3.8) |
| Biological | 14 | (5.6) |
| Other | 14 | (5.6) |
| More than one | 6 | (2.4) |
| Unable to determine | 16 | (6.5) |

*Some instruments had more than one approach.

**TABLE 2.7**   Reliability Data Sources for Instruments Used for Samples With a Majority of Racial/Ethnic Minorities (N = 248)

| Reliability data sources | Frequency | (%) |
|---|---|---|
| Current study | 106 | (41.7) |
| Previous studies | 133 | (53.6) |
| Both | 52 | (21.0) |
| Reliability data not provided | 63 | (25.4) |

**TABLE 2.8**   Reliability Data Provided for Instruments Used for Samples With a Majority of Racial/Ethnic Minorities (N = 248)

| | From prior studies | | From current study | |
|---|---|---|---|---|
| Type of reliability provided | Frequency | (%) | Frequency | (%) |
| None | 115 | (46.4) | 142 | (57.1) |
| Test-retest | 41 | (16.5) | 10 | (4.0) |
| Internal consistency | 75 | (30.2) | 90 | (36.3) |
| Parallel forms | 6 | (2.4) | 3 | (1.2) |
| Split half | 2 | (0.8) | 0 | (0.0) |
| Intrarater | 2 | (0.8) | 0 | (0.0) |
| Interrater | 12 | (4.8) | 7 | (2.8) |
| Instrument calibration | 1 | (0.4) | 0 | (0.0) |
| Use of laboratory precision/ sensitivity | 8 | (3.2) | 1 | (0.4) |

Note: More than one type of procedure was reported for some tools.

for reporting validity, the majority of the instruments had no data on validity obtained from prior studies (58.5%), nor for the current study (78.2%). Various types of validity testing procedures were used to determine validity of measures in prior studies; however, the most frequently cited types of validity reported were criterion-related concurrent validity (11.3%), construct validity using hypothesis testing (10.1%), factor analysis (6.8%), criterion-related predictive validity (6.4%), and posteriori content validity (6.0%). The most frequently reported type of validity for the current study was posteriori content validity (7.2%), followed by factor analysis (4.0%) (see Table 2.10).

**TABLE 2.9**    Validity Data Sources for Instruments Used for Samples With a Majority of Racial/Ethnic Minorities (N = 248)

| Validity data sources | Frequency | (%) |
|---|---|---|
| Current study | 54 | (21.8) |
| Previous studies | 103 | (41.5) |
| Both | 14 | (5.6) |
| Unable to determine source | 1 | (0.4) |
| Validity data not provided | 115 | (46.4) |

## Limitations in Measurement Practices Related to Research With Vulnerable Populations

This content analysis of research articles is the first to consider measurement practices related to the measurement of research variables with vulnerable populations. Although most articles focused on nursing care or clinical practice research, there was generally balance in the publication of research from a variety of areas of focus. The representation of vulnerable populations in samples of the studies raises concern in some areas, and hope in others.

## Measurement Implications of Characteristics of Study Samples

A major limitation related to the reporting of sample characteristics is the lack of attention to specifying the socioeconomic status of samples. Findings indicate an inattention to the specification of socioeconomic status variables beyond that of education in almost 80% of studies. The selection of measurement instruments for use in research needs to take into consideration the degree to which the measure has performed successfully in prior samples with similar characteristics. Socioeconomic background is of particular relevance for the selection of instruments in health care research and reporting of research results because this variable has consistently been associated with health outcomes (Burchard et al., 2003; Dixon, 2004; Flaskerud & Winslow, 1998; Foster & Sharp, 2002). The urgent need to test interventions designed to eliminate health disparities in persons from lower socioeconomic groups, further supports this need. Lack of specification of socioeconomic backgrounds of samples in studies does not encourage the exchange of important information that will be helpful to other researchers during their selection of measurement tools for lower-socioeconomic target populations.

**TABLE 2.10**    Validity Data Provided for Instruments Used for Samples With a Majority of Racial/Ethnic Minorities (N = 248)

| Type of validity provided/ mentioned | From prior studies | | From current study | |
|---|---|---|---|---|
| | Frequency | (%) | Frequency | (%) |
| None | 145 | (58.5) | 194 | (78.2) |
| Face validity | 8 | (3.2) | 1 | (0.4) |
| A priori content validity | 3 | (1.2) | 5 | (2.0) |
| Posteriori content validity | 15 | (6.0) | 18 | (7.2) |
| Content validity (unspecified) | 2 | (0.8) | 1 | (0.4) |
| Construct validity: Contrasted groups | 9 | (3.6) | 2 | (0.8) |
| Construct validity: Hypothesis testing | 25 | (10.1) | 4 | (1.6) |
| Construct validity: Factor analysis | 17 | (6.8) | 10 | (4.0) |
| Construct validity: Multitrait/ method | 2 | (0.8) | 1 | (0.4) |
| Validity (type unspecified) | 11 | (4.4) | 3 | (1.2) |
| Criterion-related validity: Concurrent | 28 | (11.3) | 6 | (2.4) |
| Criterion-related validity: Predictive | 16 | (6.4) | 1 | (0.4) |
| Convergent validity | 3 | (1.2) | 2 | (0.8) |
| Discriminant validity | 7 | (2.8) | 2 | (0.8) |
| IRT | 1 | (0.4) | 1 | (0.4) |
| G Theory | 1 | (0.4) | 1 | (0.4) |
| Accuracy/Specificity | 5 | (2.0) | 3 | (1.2) |

Note: More than one type of procedure was reported for some tools.

The fact that few studies included children is reason to take pause. Research is needed to study the health problems of children and sound measurement instruments are required to conduct this research validly. The fact that only about 25% of the studies in the sample focused on children of all ages is of concern and this fact has research and measurement implications. Reliable and valid measures for use with children will only evolve as more research is conducted with various age groups of children. It is possible that researchers who conduct research with children are not as likely to publish their research in general research journals. However, a similar argument can be made about older adults, a population that was adequately represented in the database, with 33% of studies focusing on older adults.

It is encouraging that the studies in the database reflected a balance in the inclusion of females and males in study samples. This allows for gender-based research results and gender-based measurement data that can be useful for advancing measurement and research.

The fact that over 60% of samples in studies included minorities also is encouraging. However, excitement about this finding is thwarted by the fact that low percentages of Blacks or African Americans, Hispanics or Native Americans (i.e., less than 10%) were included in most of these studies. Percentages of African Americans, Hispanics, and Native Americans were particularly low when these groups were considered separately. Therefore, these vulnerable groups were represented only on a limited basis. The small numbers of these minority subgroups in studies do not lend themselves to the consideration of the metric properties of measurement instruments specific to these racial groups for which such information often is lacking.

## Measurement Issues in Studies With Samples With a Majority of Ethnic and Racial Minorities

Measurement practices in samples where a majority of ethnic and racial minorities were included were limited by a lack of clarity about the concept measured or the conceptual basis of the measure; the inadequate reporting of the measurement framework employed; high reliance on self-report measures; and, a focus on studying attitudinal or perceptual variables. It is interesting that studies published in the early and mid-1980s (Waltz & Strickland, 1982; Strickland & Waltz, 1986; Waltz & Strickland, 1989) found similar results for all ethnic and racial groups. Therefore, little progress has been made in these areas in regard to measurement in studies with samples comprised of a majority of ethnic and racial minorities. When there is lack of reported clarity about the conceptual base of a measurement tool, it raises concerns about the appropriateness of instruments selected to measure variables in the study. In addition, it becomes difficult to assess the construct validity of a study because the conceptual base of measurement tools should be compatible with the conceptual framework of the research study (Strickland, 2002).

Lack of attention to the compatibility of the conceptual base of measurement instruments within the study's conceptual framework raises study construct validity issues. Inadequate clarity regarding the measurement framework employed is disappointing. Although the reader of research may assume whether a criterion- or norm-reference framework was employed, clarity about this issue would aid other researchers to make judgments about the appropriateness of statistical procedures employed and the potential usefulness of the instruments for use in other studies. High reliance of self-report measures in research could result in mono-method bias, particularly in studies where all variables are measured via self-report. High reliance on attitudinal or perceptual variables in nursing research may indicate inadequate attention to addressing health problems comprehensively in research. Since most health problems have psychological, social, and physiological components, focusing heavily on one area related to health problems can encourage nursing studies that are too myopic in its analysis and investigation of health problems. It is encouraging to see that about one third of instruments measured physiological variables with biochemical laboratory data. This finding is in contrast to results reported in the 1980s in which few measures focused on physiologic variables (Strickland & Waltz, 1986; Waltz & Strickland, 1982; Waltz & Strickland, 1989).

## Reliability and Validity Issues in Studies With Samples With a Majority of Ethnic and Racial Minorities

In 1986, Strickland and Waltz reported similar findings in relation to reliability and validity data reported in research studies in nursing journals. In this analytic review, more than 25% of measurement instruments had no reliability information reported at all. Even worse was the finding that more than 46% of instruments did not report any validity information; for others, inadequate validity information was provided. Reliability and validity evidence is crucial to ensure that measurement instruments used in studies measure variables well. It is important that specific evidence for reliability and validity be provided along with an adequate explication of the type of reliability and validity assessments conducted. This is needed so that fair judgments can be made regarding the adequacy of instruments for measuring variables with the target population. It may be argued that the space required for reporting adequate reliability and validity information in research reports would require too much space in journals. However, such information does not require much space and can be presented briefly.

The fact that most of the reliability and validity data reported were based on information from previous studies is not surprising, because such information may be obtained more easily. However, measurement error occurs each time an instrument is used, and there is no easy way to assess this without testing for reliability and validity. There also was inadequate attention to addressing reliability and validity within the context reported or the current study. In many instances, instruments were used within the studies on which it was appropriate. While it should have been easy to assess internal consistency reliability or to conduct test-retest reliability on a small sub-sample, this was not usually done. This issue also is of significance because whereas reliability is a necessary prerequisite for validity, it is not sufficient in of itself. If an instrument were shown to possess inadequate reliability, then the validity of study results would be brought into question.

In regards to validity, more attention should have been directed toward discussion of findings of relevance to the validity of the instruments used in the studies. This was particularly the case when results of studies were in concert with theory and assumptions in the literature. Such results support the construct validity of measures used based on hypothesis testing.

The low level of attention given to laboratory precision and sensitivity data is a reliability concern. Of equal concern was the lack of specificity data. Investigators who use laboratory data to measure research variables need to be cognizant that not all laboratories provide reliable and accurate results. Steps need to be taken by investigators to monitor the precision and accuracy of laboratory data to ensure valid study results.

## Translating Findings Into Practice and Implications for Future Research

The findings of this study have several implications for researchers, which could improve measurement and related research practices with vulnerable populations.

1. Researchers need to carefully provide sample characteristics when reporting research results, particularly information on socioeconomic background, age, ethnic and racial background, and other sample characteristics meaningful to those who study vulnerable populations. This would be helpful in the assessment of the usefulness of instruments used for studying similar populations.

2. More studies need to be included in general nursing research journals that include children of all age groups. This also includes the careful reporting of the measurement qualities of instruments used in relation to age group and other subject characteristics (Strickland, 2002).

3. Studies that include females and males in their samples should conduct gender-based reliability and validity assessments so that the gender-related measurement information will be available.

4. Given that measurement information related to the performance of instruments in specific ethnic groups is needed, researchers should make greater efforts to include higher percentages of specific ethnic and racial minority groups in studies, and when feasible, conduct reliability and validity assessments of instruments used based on ethnic and racial background.

5. Researchers need to take more care to explicate conceptual definitions of variables measured or the conceptual bases of measurement instruments in their reports of research investigations, so that readers will better understand the conceptual links between study conceptual frameworks and the measurement of research variables.

6. Investigators who report research need to clearly specify the measurement framework (i.e., criterion-referenced or norm-referenced) employed for the interpretation of scores on measurement tools used to encourage a better understanding of the nature of scores generated and appropriate statistical management of data.

7. Nurse researchers should continue to expand the selection of research variables in addition to attitudinal and perceptual variables, and ensure that study hypotheses also address other types of psychosocial and physiological variables that are of relevance to the study's conceptual framework.

8. Investigators need to use a variety of approaches to data collection and use self-report measures in moderation.

9. Researchers should take every opportunity to investigate the reliability and validity of measures within the context of studies in which the instruments are employed and report the results in research reports.

10. Investigators need to carefully monitor and report the metric properties of physiological measures and laboratory data used in studies including precision, sensitivity, and accuracy and specificity data.

11. Journal editors need to place more emphasis on ensuring that authors of research studies provide adequate information on measurement practices, reliability and validity, and particularly encourage authors to report measurement information in samples with vulnerable populations.

In conclusion, the state of the science in the measurement of variables with samples that include vulnerable populations in nursing indicates that inadequate attention has been given to measurement concerns. Researchers need to place more emphasis on employing good measurement principles and practices, particularly when vulnerable populations are the focus of study. Measurement instruments need to be designed and tested with vulnerable populations of various ages, socioeconomic backgrounds, race and ethnicities, and medical diagnoses. Although this review did not focus on vulnerable populations based on medical diagnoses, these populations also require appropriate consideration when measurement instruments are developed and tested.

## REFERENCES

Aday, L. (2001). *At risk in America*. San Francisco, CA: Jossey-Bass.

Burchard, E. G., Ziv, E., Coyle, N., Gomez, S. L., Tang, H., Karter, A. J., et al. (2003). The importance of race and ethnic background in biomedical research and clinical practice. *New England Journal of Medicine, 348*(12), 1170–1175.

Campbell, D. T., & Stanley, J. C. (1963). *Experimental and quasi-experimental designs for research*. Chicago: Rand McNally College Publishing Company.

Cook, T. D., & Campbell, D. T. (1979). *Quasi-experimentation: Design & analysis issues for field settings*. Boston: Houghton Mifflin Company.

de Chesney, M. (2005). Vulnerable populations: Vulnerable people. In M. de Chesney (Ed.), *Caring for the vulnerable: Perspective in nursing theory, practice, and research,* (chapter 1, pp. 3–12). Boston: Jones and Bartlett Publishers.

Dixon, E. L. (2004). Neighborhoods and adult health status: A multi-level analysis of social determinants of health disparities in Los Angeles County. *Dissertation Abstracts International, 65*(05), 2341 (UMI No. AAT3132998)

Flaskerud, J. H., & Winslow, B. J. (1998). Conceptualizing vulnerable populations health-related research. *Nursing Research, 47*(2), 69–78.

Foster, M. W., & Sharp, R. R. (2002). Race, ethnicity, and genomics: Social classifications as proxies of biological heterogeneity. *Genome Research, 12*(6), 844–850.

Hall, J., Stevens, P., & Meleis, A. I. (1994). Marginalization: A guiding concept for valuing diversity in nursing knowledge development. *Advances in Nursing Science, 16*(4), 23–41.

Institute of Medicine. (2003). *Unequal treatment: Confronting racial and ethnic disparities in health care*. Washington, DC: National Academies Press.

Koci, A. F. (2004). *Marginality, abuse and adverse health outcomes in women*. Atlanta: Emory University Press.

Nunnually, J. C., & Bernstein, I. H. (1994). *Psychometric theory* (3rd ed.). New York: McGraw-Hill.

Pedhazur, E. J., & Schmelkin, P. L. (1991). *Measurement, design, and analysis: An integrated approach*. Hillsdale, NJ: Lawrence Erlbaum Associates.

Strickland, O. L. (1997). Challenges in measuring nursing outcomes. *Nursing Clinics of North America, 32*(3), 495–512.

Strickland, O. L. (1998). Practical measurement [Editorial]. *Journal of Nursing Measurement, 6*(2), 107–109.

Strickland, O. L. (1999). The practical side of measurement. *The Behavioral Measurement Letter, Behavioral Measurement Database Services, 6*(1), 9–11.

Strickland, O. L. (2002). The importance of reporting sample characteristics in measurement studies [Editorial]. *Journal of Nursing Measurement, 10*(2), 79–81.

Strickland, O. L. (2005). Special considerations when conducting measurements with children. [Editorial], *Journal of Nursing Measurement, 13*(1), 3–5.

Strickland, O. L., & Waltz, C. F. (1986). Measurement of research variables in nursing. In Peggy L. Chinn (Ed.), *Nursing research methodology* (chapter 7, pp.79–90). Rockville, MD: Aspen Publishers.

U.S. Department of Health and Human Services. (2000, November). *Healthy People 2010 (2nd ed.). Understanding and improving health and objectives for improving health. 2 vols.* Washington, DC: U.S. Government Printing Office.

Waltz, C., & Strickland, O. (1982). Measurement of nursing outcomes: State of the art as we enter the eighties. In W. E. Field (Ed.), *Measuring outcomes of nursing practice, education, and administration: Proceedings of the First Annual SCCEN Research Conference, December 4–5, 1981* (pp. 47–62). Atlanta: Southern Council on Collegiate Education for Nursing, Southern Regional Education Board.

Waltz, C. F., & Strickland, O. L. (1989). Issues and imperatives in instrumentation in nursing research. In I. L. Abraham, D. M. Nadzam, and J. J. Fitzpatrick (Eds.), *Statistics and quantitative methods in nursing: Issues and strategies for research and education* (chapter 15, pp. 202–214). Philadelphia: W. B. Saunders Company.

Waltz, C. F., Strickland, O. L., & Lenz, E. (2005). *Measurement in nursing and health research.* New York: Springer Publishing Company.

# PART II

Diverse Approaches
in Building the State
of the Science in
Vulnerable Populations
Research

# Chapter 3

## Lifestyle Behavior Interventions With Hispanic Children and Adults

Antonia M. Villarruel and Deborah Koniak-Griffin

### ABSTRACT

*Chronic diseases are the leading causes of death and disability in the United States and account for 7 of every 10 deaths. While the etiology of chronic diseases is multifactorial, individual modifiable behaviors play an important role in both risk and prevention. Hispanics are disproportionately affected by chronic diseases and are a growing and significant population. The purpose of this chapter is to analyze and critique behavioral lifestyle interventions conducted with adolescent and adult Hispanics. Specific recommendations for continued research and policy are provided.*

Keywords: physical activity; Hispanics; adolescents and adults; interventions

## INTRODUCTION

Chronic diseases are the leading causes of death and disability in the United States and account for 7 of every 10 deaths. The five leading chronic diseases—cardiovascular disease (CVD), cancers, stroke, chronic obstructive pulmonary diseases, and diabetes—affect the quality of life of 90 million Americans and account for more than two-thirds of all deaths in the United States (National Center for Chronic Disease Prevention and Health Promotion, 2005). According to the Centers for Disease Control and Prevention (CDC), CVD, cancer, and stroke together account for almost 60% of all deaths in the United States (CDC, 2004a). In addition to personal and family hardship, there is an economic impact of chronic disease. In 2004, health care costs for people with chronic diseases accounted for almost 75% of the nation's health care budget (CDC, 2004a). While management of chronic diseases is one of the most common and costly health problems in the United States, these diseases are also among the most preventable.

The etiology of chronic disease is complex and multifactorial. Yet a consistent relationship has been found between individual, modifiable behaviors (e.g., smoking, lack of physical activity, poor nutrition) and risk of developing chronic disease. In their seminal report, McGinnis and Foege (1993) described the main modifiable risk factors for disease and defined them as "actual causes of death." However, an epidemiological shift from infectious disease to chronic disease, including substantial lifestyle changes during the 1990s, led to a reassessment of the modifiable factors that contributed to death in the United States for 2000 (Mokdad, Marks, Stroup, & Gerberding, 2004). According to the estimates of these authors, the actual leading causes of death were related to tobacco use (18.1%) and poor diet and physical inactivity (15.2%). Moreover, a substantial number of people demonstrate multiple chronic conditions, such as high blood pressure and high cholesterol, and modifiable risk factors such as tobacco use and poor diet and inactivity which increase their chances of developing chronic diseases and subsequent morbidity and mortality (Greenlund et al., 2004). For example, the 2003 Behavioral Risk Factor Surveillance System (BRFSS) survey found that over 37% of all adults had multiple risk factors for CVD and stroke and that considerable disparities in the types and numbers of risk factors existed for racial and ethnic groups (Hayes et al., 2005). Given the significance of chronic diseases in general, and specifically in racial and ethnic minority populations, and the importance of lifestyle behaviors in prevention of disease and complications, the purpose of this chapter is to analyze behavioral lifestyle interventions conducted with adolescent and adult Hispanics.

### Chronic Disease and Hispanics

Hispanics comprise a significant portion of the U.S. population. According to the 2000 census (U.S. Bureau of Census, 2000), Hispanics are the largest and most rapidly growing minority group in the country (Hispanics 13.7%; African Americans 12.5%). It is expected that by 2050, 25% of all American residents will be of Hispanic descent (CDC, 2004b). Furthermore, 16% of all children under the age of 18 are Hispanic, the largest racial and ethnic minority group in this age range (Flores et al., 2002).

While there has been significant growth in the Hispanic population, this group continues to be disproportionately affected by preventable chronic diseases (Sharp et al., 2003). Although the risk factors are similar, there are important disparities between Hispanic and non-Hispanic populations. Compared to non-Hispanic Whites, Hispanics in the United States are more likely to die from stroke (18%), chronic liver disease and cirrhosis (62%), diabetes (41%), HIV (152%), and homicide (128%) (CDC, 2004b).

Further, evidence suggests that Mexican Americans, the largest subgroup of Hispanics, have CVD mortality rates equal to or greater than those of non-Hispanic Whites (Pandey, Labarthe, Goff, Chan, & Nichaman, 2001); among women, definitive coronary heart disease mortality was 40% greater among Mexican Americans than non-Hispanic Whites. This finding, supported by results of the San Antonio Heart Study, is contrary to the prediction of the so-called Hispanic paradox, which suggests that Hispanics have lower all-cause and CVD mortality rates despite increased rates of diabetes and obesity and lower socioeconomic status (Hunt et al., 2003). The prevalence of CVD among Mexican Americans is about 28% (American Heart Association, 2003a).

Several modifiable risk factors contribute to CVD and other chronic diseases, including obesity, physical inactivity, and cigarette smoking. Obesity is a leading health issue among Hispanics. Between 1999 and 2002, 19% to 33% of Hispanic adults were obese. In addition, 73% of Mexican American adults were overweight, of which 33% were classified as obese (Flegal, Ogden, & Carroll, 2004). Specifically, Mexican American males were 11% more likely to report being overweight and 7% more likely to be obese than non-Hispanic White males, whereas Mexican American women were 26% more likely to be overweight and 32% more likely to be obese (CDC, 2004b).

Obesity is also a major health issue affecting Hispanic children. According to data from the 1999–2000 National Health and Nutrition Examination Survey (NHANES), among male youth, the highest overweight and obesity prevalence is found in Mexican American boys (ages 6 to 11), 43% and 27.3% respectively, and Mexican American adolescent males (ages 12 to 19), 44.2% and 27.5% respectively (Ogden, Flegal, Carroll, & Johnson, 2002). This is of particular concern given the increased prevalence of Type II diabetes among Hispanic youth (Dietz, 2001; Flores et al., 2002).

In the last decade, Type II diabetes has more than tripled to 8.2% of the total Hispanic population (CDC Youth Media Campaign, 2005). One in three children born in 2000 will develop diabetes during their lifetime, and overall, Hispanic children are 1.5 times more likely than non-Hispanic Whites to develop the disease (CDC, 2004a).

## Behavioral and Lifestyle Risk Factors Among Hispanics

Current standards for prevention and management of chronic diseases recommend that individuals not smoke or quit smoking, stay within their recommended weight range, and maintain healthy diets. However, there are many difficulties in promoting individual behavior change among racial and ethnic minority populations. For example, many modifiable behaviors such as tobacco use are less prevalent among Hispanics, whereas others, including physical inactivity and poor nutrition, are widespread. In relation to smoking, approximately 17% of the Hispanic population smoke, with higher rates among men (22.8%) than women (12%). This rate is lower when compared to the national estimate of smokers (23%) and also lower when compared with African Americans (24%) (National Center for Health Statistics, 2005).

In another example, regular physical activity is one of the principal recommendations to develop and maintain a healthy lifestyle. Regular physical activity has been shown to reduce the risk of developing heart disease, diabetes, and hypertension. However, in 2002, 25% of adults and 32% of children, aged 9 to 13 years, reported no leisure-time physical activity (CDC, 2003, 2004a). Physical inactivity was more prevalent among Hispanics (37%) and Blacks (33%) than among Whites (22%) (CDC, 2004a). According to data from the American Heart Association, 57% of Hispanic females 18 years of age and older are sedentary as compared to 36% of non-Hispanic Whites (AHA, 2003b). This partially explains the dramatic increase in the prevalence of overweight and obesity among the population.

Perceptions of physical activity and obesity are important factors in determining actual behavior. In a qualitative study, Juarbe (1998) found that, despite the existence of a covert overweight image among immigrant Mexican women, women were aware of the need for heart-healthy behaviors. The Mexican women perceived appropriate exercise and dietary knowledge as an essential condition either to being reluctant to or to committing to the decision to diet or exercise. In a subsequent study involving 143 Hispanic women aged 40 to 79 years, Juarbe and associates (2002) found that a complex process influences these older women's decision to engage in physical activity. Participants perceived little or no time for social interactions outside the home and family because of their multiple role responsibilities, despite their ability to articulate perceived benefits of physical activity, for example, health promotion and improved fitness. Other nurse researchers have observed that Mexican American women view physical activity as prescriptive, important for restoring health, and cite family responsibilities and family attitudes as factors that promote or prevent them from exercising (Berg, Cromwell, & Arnett, 2002).

Nevertheless, there is variation among Latinos in relation to behavioral lifestyle patterns, including physical activity. For example, data on 671 first-generation Latina immigrants, aged 20 to 50 years, and participating in the Women's

Cardiovascular Health Network Project, revealed that social-environmental factors, such as knowing people who exercise or seeing people exercise in the neighborhood, were more likely among women who reported any physical activity or who met national recommendations for physical activity than their counterparts (Eyler et al., 2003). Environmental factors such as vehicle traffic and street lighting were not strongly correlated with physical activity, although living in a community where places to exercise were available was a correlate. Younger age, good general health, and high self-efficacy were the most consistent personal correlates associated with physical activity. Unexpectedly, Voorhees and RohmYoung (2003) found women primarily born in Central or South America were significantly less likely to be active if they reported knowing people who exercise, if they reported that there are people in their neighborhood who exercise, if they belonged to community groups, or if they attended religious services. In this sample, women who reported their neighborhood as safe from crime were more likely to be active. No statistically significant relationships were found between activity level and personal influences. Results from this study increase awareness about the complex relationship between physical activity and personal or perceived social and physical environmental factors in urban Hispanics.

Acculturation, or the extent to which immigrant groups adopt the culture of the host country, has been a factor attributed to the variation in lifestyle behaviors among Latinos. A comprehensive literature review showed level of acculturation to be an important correlate of health behaviors; however assessment of acculturation is generally lacking in physical activity studies (Marquez, McAuley, & Overman, 2004). Further, acculturation is defined in various ways in studies reported in the literature, and many studies generalize the findings of one subgroup to all Hispanics. Results from the third National Health and Nutrition Examination Survey (NHANES III), which involved a diverse sample, revealed that Spanish-speaking Mexican Americans had higher prevalence of physical inactivity during leisure time than those who spoke mostly English, independent of place of birth. The researchers concluded that acculturation seems to be positively associated with participation in leisure-time physical activity (Crespo, Smit, Carter-Pokras, & Anderson, 2001). The influence of acculturation of health-promoting lifestyle behaviors of Spanish-speaking Hispanic adults was examined by a team of nurse researchers (Hulme et al., 2003). Their findings indicate that acculturation, along with perceived health status and demographics, explained a very small portion of the variance (12%) in overall lifestyle behaviors.

Food choices are also an important factor in the prevention of chronic diseases. A diet that includes five or more servings of fruits and vegetables and is low in saturated fats plays a key role in maintaining good health. However, more than 75% of adults in the United States report not eating the recommended amount of fruits and vegetables (CDC, 2004a). The majority of Hispanics do not eat the recommended number of servings of fruits and vegetables (Potter et al., 2000).

Food choices are influenced by culture, preferences, and availability—all of which vary by Hispanic subgroup and geographic location. In a study of Mexican American children in Texas, Suminski, Poston, and Foreyt (1999) found a high prevalence of children who consume higher than recommended amounts of fat and saturated fats, and only half of the recommended amounts of fruits and vegetables. Examination of fat intake among women participating in the Women's Health Trial Feasibility Study in Minority Populations revealed higher fat intakes from dairy foods, red meat, and vegetables or salads and less from fish and other foods among Hispanics compared to Whites and Blacks (Kristal, Shattuck, & Patterson, 1999). In both instances, there was inadequate intake of essential food groups and nutrients among the study participants.

In summary, chronic diseases are a major health issue for the U.S. population and specifically for Hispanics. Lifestyle factors, such as diet and physical activity, are important influences in the onset and progression of chronic diseases. Thus interventions aimed at supporting healthy behaviors among Hispanics are needed. The purpose of this chapter is to analyze interventions conducted with adolescent and adult Latinos in addressing lifestyle behaviors for Latinos without diagnosed diseases such as diabetes or hypertension. We will review these studies and provide direction for future research and policy.

## METHODS

Separate electronic literature searches were conducted to identify studies published between 1999 and 2005 involving samples of Hispanic children and adults. The first literature search was conducted using the data bases of Pro-Quest, Medline, CINAHL, Wilson Select Plus, and PubMed. In this search, the following key words with various logical connections were used: Hispanic/Latino adolescent health promotion, lifestyle, exercise/physical activity, diet, smoking, mental health.

For the adolescent search, approximately 300 articles were found containing the search terms. Articles pertaining to adults or to adolescent sex, pregnancy, condom use, or HIV were deleted. Of the remaining 46 articles, 24 were deleted because they were qualitative or survey design, five were reviews of literature, and 12 either had no demographics specified, included an unspecified number of Latinos, or had a sample of less than 30% Latino. A total of five articles were included in Table 3.1

A similar process was employed for the second electronic search for studies with adult samples using the data bases of PubMed and CINAHL. The following key words were used: Hispanic/Latino adult health promotion, lifestyle behaviors, exercise/physical activity, diet/nutrition, smoking, cardiovascular risk reduction/disease prevention, and intervention. Results of the *adult* search yielded approximately 500 articles containing the search terms. A majority of these articles were eliminated due to one or more of the following reasons: the samples included less than 25% Hispanic adults or persons diagnosed with a chronic disease; or the study was descriptive and did not test an intervention. Of the remaining 40 articles, 29 were excluded because qualitative or survey designs were employed or a review of the literature was presented. The remaining 11 articles met the selection criteria and are included in Table 3.1.

# RESULTS

The majority of adolescent studies included in this review dealt with physical activity and nutrition ($n = 4$). Latinos comprised 29 to 93% of the total sample. Latinos were the majority group in two studies, with only one study designed primarily for Latinos. Only one study was conducted with Spanish dominant youth (Gonzales et al., 2004). Three studies were conducted in school settings and targeted individual behaviors; only one study was a family intervention. All studies utilized a quasi-experimental design. No Latino ethnic variables (e.g., acculturation, years in United States) were included in the studies. Further, in studies that comprised a significant sample of Latinos and adolescents of other ethnicities, no subgroup analyses were conducted.

The adult studies provide an interesting contrast to those involving samples of youth. Surprisingly, 82% of the adult studies included in this review reported samples composed of 75 to 100% Hispanics. Interventions focused on lifestyle behaviors: nutrition plus physical activity/exercise ($n = 5$); physical activity/exercise alone ($n = 2$); nutrition alone ($n = 2$); smoking cessation ($n = 1$); and a combination of nutrition and another area (i.e., breast health) ($n = 1$). The research methods varied in scientific rigor from pre-test to post-test with no comparison group to experimental designs.

Randomized clinical trials were implemented in half of the studies. The interventions were largely community-based ($n = 8$), however other settings were also used, including: an adult education program ($n = 1$), a university ($n = 1$), and mixed modalities ($n = 1$). The primary program interveners were lay health advisors (LHA), often referred to as *promotoras*; however, involvement of health professionals also was reported. The intervention approaches employed included one-to-one interaction with LHAs, group education, mass media approaches, and other activities (e.g., walking).

Several of the intervention programs were specifically designed for Latinos. A large number of the interventions were culturally tailored or adapted for Hispanics and delivered in Spanish ($n = 6$), which was generally the preferred language,

**TABLE 3.1** Articles Meeting Selection Criteria for Hispanic Lifestyle

| Citation | Sample Size | Ethnicity | Intervention Design | Outcome Variables | Results |
|---|---|---|---|---|---|
| **Adult studies** | | | | | |
| *Salud para su corazon*: A community-based Latino cardiovascular disease prevention and outreach model. Alcalay, R., Alvarado, M., Balcazar, H., Newman, E., & Huerta, E. (1999). *Journal of Community Health, 24, 359–379.* | 344 at baseline, 328 at posttest; ½ male and ½ female; 50% 18-34 years; 50% 35–54 years | All Hispanic | Community-based intervention with pretest-posttest evaluation; one condition Intervention: television telenovela, public service announcements, radio programs, brochures, motivational videos to raise awareness about cardio vascular disease (CVD) & promote healthy lifestyles | Multiple item survey instrument with items measuring CVD risk factors (e.g., smoking, high BP, high blood cholesterol, overweight, physical inactivity) and cardiovascular disease (CVD) preventive health behaviors | Participants in the targeted community were more aware about risk factors for CVD and had increased their knowledge about ways to prevent heart disease (19% gain in knowledge); no differences in pre- and posttest comparisons found for health behavior; time interval between pre-post test not specified |
| Evaluation of *Salud para su corazon* (Health for your heart)—National Council of La Raza promotora outreach program. Balcazar, B., | 223 Hispanic families (320 individual family members) | All Hispanic | Pre–post test design without a control group, implemented in seven sites across United States Intervention: *Salud para su corazon* | Primary—change in heart-healthy behaviors self-reported on written questionnaires (e.g., PA, weight, cholesterol and fat, salt and sodium) | Findings support the effectiveness of the promotora model in improving heart-healthy behaviors; positive changes observed for the families' practices |

| Citation | Sample | Population | Design/Intervention | Measures | Results |
|---|---|---|---|---|---|
| Alvarado, M., Hollen, M. L., Gonzalez-Cruz, Y., & Pedregón, V. (2005, July). *Prevention of Chronic Disease, 2*, A09, 1-9. | | | to reduce risk for CVD; interveners were *promotoras* delivering 7–8 lessons in 2-hour sessions | | of heart-healthy behaviors, particularly for the items on practices related to cholesterol and fat; improvements also found for PA and weight reduction/control |
| Interpersonal and print nutrition communication for a Spanish-dominant Latino population: *Secretos de la buena vida*. Elder, J. P., Ayala, G. X., Campbell, N. R., Slymen, D., Lopez-Madurga, E. T., Engelberg, M., & Baquero, B. (2005). *Health Psychology, 24*, 49–57. | 357 Hispanic women (mean age 39.7 years); 95% of sample born in Mexico, low levels of acculturation, income and education | All Hispanic | Randomized trial with 3 conditions over the course of 12 weeks: lay health advisor providing personalized dietary counseling plus tailored print materials; tailored print materials only; or off-the-shelf print materials (control) | Primary—calories from fat and daily grams of fiber; Secondary—total energy intake, total and saturated fat intake and total carbohydrates, weight, BMI, waist-to-hip ratio | From baseline to 12-weeks postintervention women receiving promotora condition had significantly lower levels of energy intake, total fat and saturated fat, and total carbohydrates; no significant group differences for percent calories from fat or for daily intake of fiber; women in all 3 groups reduced their BMI by modest amounts |

*(Continued)*

**TABLE 3.1** Articles Meeting Selection Criteria for Hispanic Lifestyle (*Continued*)

| Citation | Sample size | Ethnicity | Intervention design | Outcome variables | Results |
|---|---|---|---|---|---|
| **Adult studies** | | | | | |
| Results of Language For Health: Cardiovascular disease nutrition education for Latino English-as-a-Second-Language students. Elder, J. P., Candelaria, J. I., Woodruff, S. I., Criqui, M. H., Talavera, G. A., & Rupp, J., W. (2000). *Health Education and Behavior*, 27, 50–63. | 817 men and women, more than 18 years of age (mean age 31 years); largely immigrant population | 90% Hispanic, 10% other ethnicities; 41% of Hispanics were males | Two-group repeated measures design Intervention: "Language for Health," a heart healthy nutrition education for Latinos integrated into five 3-hour ESL classes Control: Stress management (comparable length) | 13 physiological (BP, lipid panel, weight, waist:hip ratio) and psychosocial (nutrition knowledge, attitudes, self-reported fat avoidance behaviors) variables measured at baseline, 3-month posttest and 6-month follow-up | Intervention group showed greater decrease in total HDL cholesterol ratio at posttest only, nonsignificant (NS) change at 6-month follow-up; systolic BP decreased over time for both groups; fat avoidance increased over time for the intervention participants; NS findings for weight, waist: hip ratio; overall effects of intervention modest and short-term |
| Results of *Mujeres felices por ser saludables*: A dietary/ breast health randomized clinical trial for Latino women. | 256 women, aged 20–40 years old, very low acculturated; 89% of women were of Mexican descent | All Hispanic | Randomized intervention (n=127) and control (n=129) groups Intervention group: group | 24-hour diet recalls breast self-exam (BSE) practices and proficiency | At 8-month follow-up, intervention group reported lower dietary fat and higher fiber intake; a higher proportion |

| | | | | |
|---|---|---|---|---|
| Fitzgibbon, M. L., Gapstur, S. M., & Knight, S. J. (2004). *Annals of Behavioral Medicine, 28,* 95–104 | | format designed for low-accultur-ated Hispanics, 16 90-min. sessions focusing on diet and breast health; based on social cognitive theory and trans-theoretical model Control group: General health information via mail for same time period | | reported practic-ing BSE at recom-mended interval and showed improved BSE proficiency compared to control group |
| *La Vida Caminando:* A community-based physical activity program designed by and for rural Latino families Grassi, K., Gonzalez, M. G., Tello, P., & He, G.(1999). *Journal of Health Education, 30,* S-13, S7. | 359 recruited; complete data available on 202; adults aged 18–55 years; 88–91% females, varying by site; overall, 72% Hispanic; 36% identified Spanish as primary language | Percent Latinos in four sites varied from 33% to 90% (overall 72%) | Community-based intervention with pretest-post-test evaluation implemented in 4 small rural cities in central CA; one condition Intervention: *La Vida Cami-nando*—four meet-ings of "walking clubs" held during a 3-month period | Self-report on type (e.g., walking, gar-dening, bicycling) and frequency of PA (minutes spent per day and days per week) and barriers to PA; measure developed by California Dept. of Health Services and administered via interviewers | Comparison of baseline data with 6- and 12-month follow-up outcomes showed a decrease in mean number of hours spent walk-ing; no significant difference in 6- and 12-month findings; work schedules and family responsi-bilities represented a significant barrier |

*(Continued)*

**TABLE 3.1** Articles Meeting Selection Criteria for Hispanic Lifestyle (*Continued*)

| Citation | Sample Size | Ethnicity | Intervention Design | Outcome Variables | Results |
|---|---|---|---|---|---|
| **Adult studies** | | | | | |
| | | | for PA training and discussion about healthy nutrition and other ways to reduce the risk of disease; written materials provided in English/Spanish; family focused; participants could repeat attending clubs | | to PA; a variety of factors believed to influence findings, including measurement problems |
| Evaluation of individually tailored interventions on exercise adherence. Keele-Smith, R., & Leon, T. (2003). *Western Journal of Nursing Research, 25,* 623–640. | 114 women and 35 men, aged 18 to 59; faculty, staff and students in a New Mexico university | 42.3% Hispanic, 50.3% white, .7% African American, 2.7% Asian, 0.7% Native American | Randomized intervention and comparison group Intervention group: education and monitoring with individualized written exercise prescription Control group: monitoring only with weekly phone contacts | Self-reported frequency and duration of exercise measured weekly (duration=current average time per exercise session across all types of exercise calculated in minutes; frequency=the current total times per week for all types of current exercise); weight and body fat; scores on the Exercise Motivation Questionnaire | After 5 weeks, more participants in the intervention group were exercising at recommended levels compared to those in the comparison group; no pretest to posttest differences found on weight or percentage of body fat; consistent exercisers had significantly higher motivation scores than did inconsistent exercisers |

| Citation | Sample | Ethnicity | Design | Measures | Findings |
|---|---|---|---|---|---|
| Effects of two frequencies of walking on cardiovascular risk factor reduction in Mexican American women. Keller, C., & Treviño, R. P. (2001). *Research in Nursing and Health*, 24, 390–401. | 36 Mexican American women 18–45 years old, premenopausal, BMI>25% and sedentary | Hispanic | Quasi-experimental design with two randomly assigned treatment groups and one comparison group; treatment groups differed in frequencies of prescribed walking (3 days versus 5 days per week) over a 24-week period | Physiologic (blood lipids, body composition) and self-reported exercise maintenance | Walking for 30 min., 3 days a week resulted in increased in serum HDL-C and reductions of serum cholesterol and body fat estimated by skin-fold sum; efficacy of intervention supported with women moving from sedentary behavior to active behavior |
| The impact of lay health advisors on cardiovascular health promotion using a community-based participatory approach. Kim, S., Koniak-Griffin, D., Flaskerud, J. H., & Guarnero, P. A. (2004). *Journal of Cardiovascular Nursing, 19,* 192–199. | 250 women and 6 men, largely immigrant and poor | All Hispanic | Intervention consisted of three group sessions delivered in Spanish by lay health advisors (promotoras): PA, maintaining a smoke-free environment, and healthy nutrition Control: None | Study examined the feasibility of recruiting and training LHAs to provide a CVD risk-reduction intervention and to collect research data and evaluated the effects of the intervention on lifestyle behavior (PA, healthy nutrition, and smoke-free environment) | Findings revealed significant pretest to posttest improvements in overall lifestyle behaviors and in the subsets of nutrition behavior, PA behavior and smoke-free behavior by self-report; for PA successes were expressed as feeling a sense of well-being and weight loss, incorporating family members into exercise routines |

(*Continued*)

**TABLE 3.1** Articles Meeting Selection Criteria for Hispanic Lifestyle (*Continued*)

| Citation | Sample Size | Ethnicity | Intervention Design | Outcome Variables | Results |
|---|---|---|---|---|---|
| **Adult studies** | | | | | |
| Provider counseling, health education, and community health workers: The Arizona WISE-WOMAN Project Staten, L. K., Gregory-Mercado, K. Y., Ranger-Moore, J., Will, J. C., Giuliano, A. R., Ford, E. S., & Marshall, J. (2004). *Journal of Women's Health, 13*, 547–556. | 217 uninsured women > 50 years with data at baseline and 12 month follow-up; all participants of the National Breast & Cervical Cancer Early Detection Program | 75% Hispanic | Experimental design with random assignment to one of three intervention groups: provider counseling (PC)-active control; PC + health education (HE) classes; PC + HE + community health worker (CHW) support; all groups seen by nurse practitioner | Physiologic—height, weight, waist, and hip circumference, BP, blood glucose, cholesterol, and triglyceride levels Behavioral—24-hour dietary recall, self-reported PA | PA—All intervention groups showed an increase in self-reported weekly minutes of moderate-to-vigorous PA, with no significant differences among groups; Nutrition – Significantly more women who received PC + HE + CHW support progressed to eating 5 fruits and vegetables per day, compared to those in other groups |
| Evaluation of a culturally appropriate smoking cessation intervention for Latinos. Woodruff, S. I., Talavera, G. A., & | 313 Spanish-speaking Hispanic smokers, > 18 years of age; 51% female; 78% born in Mexico, 16% U.S.-born; low level of | All Hispanics | Randomized two-group trial Intervention: *Proyecto Sol*, a culturally appropriate 3-month program delivered by pro- | Physiologic (past abstinence by expired carbon monoxide [CO] and behavioral (self-administered smoking behavior | Postintervention, validated (CO) past week abstinence rates were more than twice as high in the intervention group (20.5%) than the |

| Citation | Sample | Design/Intervention | Measures | Results |
|---|---|---|---|---|
| Elder, J. P. (2002). *Tobacco Control, 11,* 361–367. | acculturation; 272 participants at follow-up | motores, including four home visits plus telephone contacts; Comparison: Referral to Spanish language California Smokers' Helpline | survey) measures at baseline and 1 week after the intervention | comparison (8.7%); the primary predictor of abstinence was number of cigarettes smoked per day at baseline; differential attrition higher for intervention group |

**Children/Adolescent Studies**

| Citation | Sample | Design/Intervention | Measures | Results |
|---|---|---|---|---|
| Prevention of the epidemic increase in child risk of overweight in low-income schools: The El Paso coordinated approach to child health. Coleman, K. J., Tiller, C. L., Sanchez, J., Heath, E. M., Sy, O., Milliken, G, & Dzewaltowski, D. A. (2005). *Archives of Pediatric and Adolescent Medicine,159,* 217–224. | 896 third grade children (473 control schools [224 girls and 249 boys] and 423 CATCH schools [199 girls and 224 boys]) | 93% Hispanic | Child and Adolescent Trial for Cardiovascular Health (CATCH) An untreated, matched control group design with repeated dependent pretest and posttest samples | Outcomes: Risk of overweight or overweight, BMI, waist-to-hip ratio, yards run in 9 minutes, passing rates for Fitnessgram national mile standards, moderate to vigorous PA and vigorous PA in gym class, and percentage of fat and sodium in school lunches. |

Girls in control schools had significant increases in percentage of risk of overweight or overweight from third (26%) to fifth (39%) grades, as did girls in CATCH schools (30%–32%); however, the rate of increase for girls in the CATCH schools was significantly lower (2%) compared with the rate for control girls (13%)

*(Continued)*

**TABLE 3.1** Articles Meeting Selection Criteria for Hispanic Lifestyle (*Continued*)

| Citation | Sample Size | Ethnicity | Intervention Design | Outcome Variables | Results |
|---|---|---|---|---|---|
| | | | | | A similar pattern was seen for boys, with a rate of increase in CATCH schools of 1% (40%–41%), which was significantly less than the 9% increase (40% to 49%) for control boys. |
| **Children/Adolescent Studies** | | | | | |
| Dance for health: Improving fitness in African American and Hispanic adolescents. Flores, R. (1995). *Public Health Reports*, *110 (2)*, 189. | 81 seventh-grade boys and girls | 43% Hispanic; 44% African American; 13% other | Controlled trial intervention and control groups. Intervention group: health education 2x/week, dance-oriented phys ed. 3x/week. Control group: health education 2x/week, usual PA (mostly playground activity) | Outcomes: Timed mile run; resting heart rate (HR), sex-adjusted BMI; attitudes toward PA | Dance for Health was an effective program to improve health and reduce weight in minority students. The program appears to be more effective with girls than boys. Students in the intervention had a significant lowering of BMI and resting HR compared with students in the usual activity group. |

| | | | | |
|---|---|---|---|---|
| Preventing poor mental health and school dropout of Mexican American adolescents following the transition to junior high school. Gonzales, N. A., Dumka, L. E., Deardorff, J., Jacobs C. S., & McCray, A. (2004). *Journal of Adolescent Research, 19,* 113–131. | 27 families, 13 in the Spanish group and 14 in the English group No control group | 4.5% African American (*n* = 1), 4.5% Anglo (*n* = 1), 86.5% Mexican American (*n* = 19), and 4.5% other (*n* = 1) | Intervention consisted of 9 group sessions: adolescent stress management; increased parent use of appropriate discipline, adequate monitoring, and support; family cohesion | Study tested three proximal mediators of the intervention: (a) adolescent skills to cope with stress, (b) parenting skills, and (c) family cohesion. Analysis: Qualitative process evaluations, paired t-tests for pre-post test change | Findings revealed significant pretest to posttest changes in adolescent coping and parenting, two proximal mediators targeted in the intervention for their potential to reduce later risk for dropout and mental health disorders in high school. Adolescents reported significantly fewer symptoms of depression at posttest. Maternal reports showed a significant change in the expected direction in their use of inconsistent discipline practices and supportive parenting, but not monitoring, and a significant decrease in adolescents' problem behaviors. |

*(Continued)*

**TABLE 3.1** Articles Meeting Selection Criteria for Hispanic Lifestyle (*Continued*)

| Citation | Sample Size | Ethnicity | Intervention Design | Outcome Variables | Results |
|---|---|---|---|---|---|
| **Adult Studies** | | | | | |
| A controlled evaluation of a school-based intervention to promote physical activity among sedentary adolescent females: Project FAB. Jamner, M. S., Spruijt-Metz, D., Bassin, S., & Cooper, D. M. (2004). *Journal of Adolescent Health, 34,* 279–289. | 47 adolescent females 10th or 11th grade Intervention n=25 Control group n=22 | 53% non-Hispanic White, 29% Hispanic, 8% Asian, and 3% other | Study participants enrolled in a special PE class available only to study members. This class met 5 days per week for 60 minutes | Used focus groups and modification of existing program. Outcome measures: Physical fitness and PA, body composition, self-efficacy, social support, enjoyment, barriers Analyses: one-way ANOVA, t-tests | The intervention had a significant effect on cardiovascular fitness ($p = .017$), lifestyle activity ($p = .005$), and light ($p = .023$), moderate ($p = .007$), and hard ($p = .006$) activity. All changes were in a direction that favored the intervention. There was no effect of the intervention on psychosocial factors related to exercise |

| Study | Sample | Demographics | Design/Intervention | Measures | Results |
|---|---|---|---|---|---|
| California Project LEAN's Food on the Run Program: An evaluation of a high-school-based student nutrition advocacy and physical activity program. Agron, P., Takada, E., & Purcell, A. (2002). *Supplement to the Journal of the American Dietetic Association, 102,* S103–S105. | $N=220$ student advocates from 20 high schools throughout California Mean age: 16 30% boys; 70% girls No control group | 37% White 31% Hispanic 10% African American 13% Asian American 2% Native American 5% Other | Non-experimental: peer-education format; student advocates pretest Intervention: training on basics of nutrition; physical activities; necessary steps to create environmental changes; coordinating and carrying out 5–7 activities throughout school year; posttest end of school year. Post intervention survey of FOR site coordinators | Student advocates: Nutrition: Knowledge, attitudes, and behaviors PA: Knowledge, attitudes, & behaviors Site coordinators: # of lessons taught; time spent on each lesson; # of weeks spent on training; time spent on program per week; # of hours spent on activities outside of training No theory identified | PA: Increased knowledge ($p < .01$) Increased positive attitudes ($p < .05$) No change in PA behaviors. Nutrition: Increased knowledge ($p < .05$) Increased positive attitudes ($p < .001$) Increased healthful eating behaviors ($p < .01$) FOR site coordinators—Program implementation: Ave. # lessons = 6; Ave. time per lesson = 55.25 min.; Ave. weeks on advocate training = 9; Ave. # hours on activities outside of training = 20 hrs. |

even for bilingual participants. In one study, the culturally tailored content was purposely delivered in English; whereas, in another study, language preference determined the mode of delivery. Language used for intervention delivery was not described in two of the studies. Recruitment strategies within communities involved direct contact during local events, use of social networks, and telephone contacts. Acculturation and other ethnic variables such as place of birth or years in the United States were measured in less than half of the studies; those studies describing acculturation levels had samples with low scores, indicating maintenance of non-U.S. cultural practices. Outcome variables were not analyzed in relation to acculturation scores, perhaps because of the lack of variance in scores.

In the following section, interventions addressing major lifestyle behaviors (physical activity, nutrition, and smoking) are presented.

## Studies Involving Children and Adolescents

There were mixed results among the physical activity and nutrition interventions which targeted children and adolescents. All interventions were effective with girls, and when gender comparisons were made, interventions were more effective with girls than boys. Two of the interventions had significant effects on physical activity behavior (Flores, 1995; Jamner, Spruijt-Metz, Bassin, & Cooper, 2004), whereas one had demonstrated effects on obesity risk (Coleman et al., 2005). A strength of these studies is that all but one (Agron, Takada, & Purcell, 2002) included objective measures of physical activity (e.g., peak oxygen uptake, resting heart rate).

No explicit theory was used in any of the interventions, but concepts from behavioral theories, such as attitudes, self-efficacy, and social support were included. Only two studies reported changes in these concepts pre- and postintervention. One study reported no change in exercise self-efficacy, perceived barriers, and social support postintervention, despite changes in cardiovascular fitness and lifestyle activity (Jamner et al., 2004).

Two studies directly targeted Latino children and adolescents. One of these was a small efficacy trial designed to assess the impact of a "Dance for Health Program" on increasing aerobic capacity, weight gain, and attitudes toward physical activity and physical fitness with Latino and African American low-income adolescents (Flores, 1995). Physical education classes in a middle school were randomly assigned to the intervention condition, a 12-week program consisting of three 50-minute aerobic dance sessions in addition to a cardiovascular health-education curriculum. Students in the control condition received their regular physical activity classes. Pre- and posttest measures were obtained for body mass index (BMI), physical fitness, and attitudes related to physical activity. Girls, but not boys, in the intervention condition had a significant lowering of BMI and resting heart rate as compared with the control group. Interestingly, boys in the intervention group had a less favorable attitude toward physical activity than those in the control group. While efforts were made to select culturally appropriate music and to develop a culturally specific curriculum, efforts may also be needed to include gender-specific activities.

One study conducted with school-age children (Coleman et al., 2005) is of particular significance in that it is an effectiveness trial of an existing intervention conducted primarily with Hispanic children ($n$ = 93%). The intervention tested was an NIH funded comprehensive nutrition and physical activity curriculum, the Child and Adolescent Trial for Cardiovascular Health (CATCH). Four schools were randomly selected from those that agreed to participate in this study, and control schools were matched based on district and geographic location. Schools assigned to the intervention condition were provided with CATCH curricular materials, training, and a stipend to conduct the intervention and purchase necessary equipment. Control schools were provided with a smaller monetary incentive. Individual child measures (e.g., BMI, aerobic fitness, anthropometry) and also school level measures (e.g., cafeteria meal quality and physical activity during physical education class) were included. These measures were obtained pre-intervention and at two subsequent yearly data points. While there were mixed results in some outcome measures (e.g., cafeteria food quality, aerobic fitness), children in the intervention schools had a lower increase in the risk of being overweight or obese than did children in the control schools. As this was an effectiveness trial, the emphasis on the intervention was not fidelity, but rather adaptation. More studies are needed that test both new and existing interventions with this at-risk population.

A unique physical activity and nutrition intervention conducted by Agron, Takada, and Purcell (2002) addressed behaviors from a policy and environmental advocacy perspective. In this pre-post test design, student advocates ($n$ = 220) from more than 20 schools were recruited and trained in basic nutrition and physical activity, as well as on how to advocate for environmental and policy changes at the school. Students conducted activities, including advocacy efforts, with school personnel, and educational activities with students were designed to increase healthy options and choices. Outcome measures were obtained from the student advocates pretraining (at the beginning of the school year) and at the end of the school year, approximately 9 months later. Results indicated that student advocates had increased knowledge and attitudes related to nutrition and physical activity, but only self-reported changes in nutrition behaviors. While the approach is innovative, a measure of physical activity and nutrition behaviors of the students in the schools is warranted.

## Studies Involving Adults

Interventions and outcome measures varied widely among studies focusing on physical activity or nutrition. Thus, only limited comparisons can be made across studies. For example, in some studies outcomes were measured by self-reported behaviors, whereas in others, more objective physiologic measures such as hip-to-waist ratios and BMIs were included.

One of the five studies focusing on promoting healthy nutrition and physical activity employed a bilingual community-based and theory-driven intervention model involving mass media (e.g., public service announcements on television, radio programs, and brochures) rather than direct services to individuals (Alcalay, Alvarado, Balcazar, Newman, & Huerta, 1999). This model known as *Salud para su Corazón* (Health for Your Heart) was designed and implemented by the National Heart, Lung, and Blood Institute and involved training of *promotoras*. An agency-community partnership, under the leadership of the Community Alliance for Heart Health, guided all phases of this project. An evaluation survey showed that participants in the target community had substantial increases in awareness of risk factors for CVD and of ways to prevent heart disease. There were no differences between the pre- and posttest respondents with respect to current health behaviors.

In contrast, another intervention (also known as *Salud para su Corazón*), designed to change heart-health behaviors through structured educational classes delivered by *promotoras* at seven sites, was observed to have a positive influence on several outcomes (Balcazar, Alvarado, Hollen, Gonzalez-Cruz & Pedregón, 2005). In particular, dietary improvements were reported related to intake of foods known to be high in cholesterol and fat, as well as in physical activity and weight.

Further support for the effectiveness of *promotoras* in helping immigrant Latinos to improve lifestyle behaviors was provided in a study conducted by Kim, Koniak-Griffin, Flaskerud, and Guarnero (2004), which involved a three-session outreach program that was evaluated by a pre-posttest design. In this study, significant improvements were found for self-reported nutrition, physical activity and exercise, and creating a smoke-free environment. In a clinical trial focusing on both nutrition and exercise, community-health workers (CHW, also referred to as *promotoras*) were employed, along with health professionals, as part of the WISEWOMAN project (Staten et al., 2004). Results demonstrated that participants receiving three types of interventions (provider counseling; provider counseling and health education; or provider counseling, health education and CHW support) increased in self-reported minutes of moderate-to-vigorous physical activity, with no significant differences between groups. Significantly more women who received the more comprehensive intervention involving CHW support progressed to eating five fruits and vegetables per day compared to participants in the other two groups.

Less favorable outcomes were found in another multisite study involving a pre-posttest design with participants who received *La Vida Caminando* (the

Walking Life), an intervention consisting of formal meetings of walking clubs (Grassi, Gonzalez, Tello & He, 1999). Although information about nutrition was incorporated into this intervention, no nutrition outcome measures were used. Findings showed that at 6-month follow-up, there was a significant decrease in perceived barriers to physical activity, and the intervention was successful in decreasing many of the commonly reported barriers such as exercise programs being too expensive. Despite this favorable change in perception, both personal and family barriers interfered with participants' ability to increase their physical activity. At follow-up, a decrease in mean number of hours spent walking was reported.

*Promotoras* also have been used in interventions to promote smoking cessation with Hispanic adults. "*Proyecto Sol,*" a 3-month culturally appropriate smoking intervention based on social cognitive constructs and delivered in the smoker's home by *promotoras*, was found to positively affect smoking behaviors (Woodruff, Talavera, & Elder, 2002). Unlike the previously described studies, outcomes in this randomized, two-group trial involving 313 Spanish speaking smokers were objectively measured using validated (carbon monoxide) abstinence rates. Among participants in the intervention group, the rate of abstinence was more than twice as high as in the comparison (Smokers' Helpline) group. Because outcomes were measured only at about 1 week after intervention, the long-term impact of the program could not be determined.

Two studies evaluated interventions for promoting a healthy dietary lifestyle among Hispanics. One of these was a randomized trial involving 357 Hispanic immigrant women who maintained non-U.S. cultural practices (Elder et al., 2005). Similar to several of the previously described studies, *promotoras* were employed in this project to evaluate a 12-week, tailored nutrition communication intervention. Women were randomly assigned to one of three conditions: tailored newsletters delivered and weekly home visits or telephone calls by *promotoras* for a period of 12 weeks (*promotora*); tailored print only, delivered by mail (tailored); or off-the-shelf Latino-targeted materials, also delivered via mail (control). Four repeated assessments, conducted over an 18-month period, included measurement of percent calories from dietary fat and number of grams of dietary fiber. A strength of this study was the inclusion of an acculturation measure as well as measures of height, weight, BMI, waist and hip circumference, and waist-hip ratio. Multiple comparisons revealed that the *promotora* condition achieved significantly better levels of nutritional outcomes (e.g., lower levels of energy intake, total fat and saturated fat, and total carbohydrates), compared with either the tailored or control groups. The near obese women in all three groups reduced their BMI by modest amounts, with no significant differences among the groups. The latter finding points to the need for greater effort to prevent obesity and to treat the overweight and the obese. Acculturation status of the sample was believed to partially explain the lack of intervention effects on dietary fiber.

Applying an innovative approach to nutrition education, Elder and associates (2000) integrated their intervention into an English-as-a-second-language (ESL) curriculum for recent Hispanic immigrants with low literacy levels. The participants ($n = 732$) were exposed to either nutrition education or stress management classes (attention-placebo group) delivered during up to five, 3-hour ESL classes. Data were collected at baseline, 3-month posttest, and 6-month follow-up. Physiological measures evaluated included blood pressure (BP), total and high-density lipoprotein (HDL) cholesterol, waist and hip circumference, and weight. Self-report surveys were used to assess participants' nutrition-related knowledge, attitudes, and fat avoidance behaviors. Of the physiological and behavioral dependent variables measured, the nutrition intervention was observed to be more effective than the control in changing total HDL ratio, systolic BP, self-reported fat avoidance, and nutrition knowledge. Unfortunately, some of the effects were short-term and disappeared at the 6-month follow-up. Unique to this study was the examination of Spanish-language literacy and intervention effects. Nutrition knowledge was found to be greater among those with medium and high Spanish literacy than among those with low literacy.

Dietary interventions also have been integrated with breast health promotion and tested within a randomized clinical trial involving 20- to 40-year-old, very low-acculturated Latinas (Fitzgibbon, Gapstur, & Knight, 2004). In this community-based study, the 8-month multicomponent education program, delivered most often in Spanish, was compared with health education materials that were mailed on a schedule parallel to the intervention. Behavior change theories and social cognitive theory were incorporated in the development of the intervention. Unlike several of the previous studies, this intervention involved a nutritionist and trained breast health educator, both of whom were bilingual and bicultural. Results showed that participants in the breast health and dietary group (*Mujeres Felices por ser Saludable*) reported lower dietary fat and higher fiber intake as well as improved breast health. Long-term maintenance of behavior change was not evaluated in this study.

The remaining two studies focus on physical activity and exercise with differing samples. Students, faculty, and staff of mixed ethnic and racial backgrounds were involved in a New Mexico university-based evaluation of a 5-week education-plus-monitoring or monitoring-only intervention (Keele-Smith & Leon, 2003). An experimental pre-posttest design was employed. Participants in the experimental group received an individualized exercise prescription plan that included an exercise information brochure plus suggestions for type, frequency, and duration of exercise and strategies for increasing compliance. The prescription for exercise was derived from participants' scores on the Exercise Motivation Question (EMQ), a measure of individuals' motives for exercising. Those in the comparison group received the same information brochure without an individualized exercise prescription. Weekly contacts for 5 weeks were made with all participants; however, additional individualized exercise follow-up was conducted with those in the experimental group. The study was based on reversal theory, which proposes individuals are inherently inconsistent and that they reverse back and forth between opposing states of mind that influence how certain motivational variables such as arousal are experienced. Self-report and objective measures (e.g., weight, percentage of body fat) were outcome variables. Hispanics (n = 63) composed 42% of the 149 rather young and healthy participants in the sample, with one-half of the total group being White.

Findings post intervention revealed that significantly more participants were exercising at recommended levels in the education-plus-monitoring group than the monitoring-only group (Keele-Smith & Leon, 2003). Further, the experimental group had significantly more consistent exercisers and fewer inconsistent exercisers than did those in the comparison group. Weight loss and percentage of body fat measurements did not differ among groups, possibly due to the limited length of the treatment conditions. Outcomes and EMQ scores among participants of differing ethnic and racial groups were not compared.

In the second exercise study, Keller and Treviño (2001) employed a quasi-experimental repeated measures design (two randomly assigned treatment groups and one self-selected comparison group) to compare the effects of two different walking frequencies, while holding exercise intensity and duration constant. The sample was composed of sedentary, pre-menopausal, overweight Mexican American women (n = 36) who were evaluated for selected physiologic measures (blood lipids, body composition) and exercise maintenance regimens following the 24-week intervention. Walking for 30 minutes, 3 days a week, resulted in increases in serum HDL-C and reductions of total serum cholesterol and body fat estimated by skin-fold sums. Clinically meaningful fat loss was not observed, perhaps due to the short length of the intervention. Sustained participation in the exercise protocol was achieved in the lower-frequency, but not the higher-frequency regimen, according to women's activity logs. Findings support the effectiveness of low-intensity exercise and expand knowledge about the quantification of lower limits of beneficial exercise. For Hispanic and other minority women, maintaining a lower level of exercise intensity may be more achievable, as it is less time consuming and easier to maintain as part of their lifestyle.

## SUMMARY

The limited intervention studies included in this review support the rigorous development and testing of culturally appropriate interventions addressing lifestyle behaviors such as physical activity and nutrition (Marquez, McAuley, & Overman, 2004). Despite the limited numbers of studies, there are a few promising trends. For example, efforts were made by many investigators to address specific language and cultural needs of Hispanics. *Promotoras* were the most frequently employed interveners in studies testing culturally appropriate interventions designed to improve lifestyle behaviors of Hispanic adults. Their effectiveness was generally evidenced by improvements in one or more outcome variables. Further testing of the effectiveness of *promotoras* in randomized controlled designs is needed.

Studies in this review illustrate the difficulty of achieving favorable changes in physiologic measures such as body fat and weight, particularly for short-term interventions. Further, only short-term effects for selected outcome variables were reported in some studies, pointing to the need either for boosters or lengthier interventions and attention to building supportive environments.

Findings need to be considered in light of some of the limitations of the group of studies reviewed. First, all of the studies involving children and adolescents were school-based. There is an important subgroup of Hispanics who do not attend school regularly, who may have different needs and issues. Secondly, the samples in many studies were composed solely or predominantly of women. Few of the adult studies included men. Finally, in considering the findings of adult studies, it is important to note that this review was limited by the exclusion of important studies involving samples of participants with chronic diseases. Thus is it possible that a selection bias occurred, with greater yield of studies having healthier, younger samples. Despite this limitation, participants in many of the reported studies had risk factors for CVD and diabetes, such as overweight or obesity issues and sedentary lifestyles.

## Implications for Research and Policy

This review demonstrates that during the past 5 years, publication of databased articles related to interventions to promote healthy lifestyle behaviors (nutrition and diet, exercise and physical activity, and smoking cessation and smoke-free environments) among Hispanics has been quite limited. More than double the number of studies has been conducted with Latino adults compared to Latino children. Further, the majority of research has been conducted by non-nurses, although nurses have conducted some studies or are included in the investigative team.

The scarcity of research in this area is of particular concern for several reasons. The issue of lifestyle behaviors is likely to become a more prominent public health concern, as the Hispanic population continues to increase over the next several decades. Continued nursing research in the area of lifestyle behaviors is needed. Specific areas for recommendation include:

- More randomized control trials are needed. In particular, the body of knowledge about smoking cessation and exposure to secondary smoke is scant.

- Trials should include a combination of behavioral and physiologic measures, as conflicting findings exist with regard to results of dietary surveys. Johnson, Soultanakis, and Matthews (1998) demonstrated underreporting to be strongly associated with increased body fatness in low-income women using the USDA multiple-pass 24-hour recall (with 3 steps consisting of a quick list, detailed description, and review). Interestingly, women who scored higher on a literacy test (Wide Range Achievement Test) for reading and spelling recalled their food intake more accurately. However, Conway and colleagues demonstrated effectiveness of the USDA 5-step multiple-pass recall method within 10% of mean actual intake on the previous day, reporting, in fact, that obese women recalled food intake more accurately than overweight or normal-weight women (Conway, Ingwersen, Vinyard, & Moshfegh, 2003). The latter investigators reported, however, that their sample (n = 49) as a population overestimated their energy and carbohydrate intakes by 8–10%.

- Lifestyle behavior and preventive interventions that are culturally tailored and linguistically appropriate for Hispanics offer the greatest potential for positively impacting lifestyle behaviors.

- The majority of intervention studies for children and adolescents have occurred in school settings. While this is an important context, more studies to evaluate the effectiveness of family approaches in lifestyle behaviors are needed.

- Behaviors are influenced by context. Choices can be enhanced or limited by certain environments. The effect of environmental interventions such as increasing food availability and decreasing barriers to physical activity on individual choices should be further examined.

Based on the review of existing studies, there are several recommendations for policy that can be made. First, there is a continued need to ensure that health related information is not only culturally tailored, but is available in languages other than English, and considers the literacy level of clients. Second, given the limited level of physical activity in children, and specifically in Hispanic children, organized physical activity needs to be included in the school curriculum. Third, given the efficacy of *promotoras* in supporting healthy lifestyle behaviors, ways to integrate their services into current health care delivery systems should be considered.

In summary, given the multifactorial etiology of chronic diseases, there should be multilevels of interventions directed at promoting healthy lifestyle behaviors. While individual choice is important, the building of environments to support behavior should be included as a comprehensive health promotion strategy. This approach should be considered for all populations, nonetheless, special consideration and intervention approaches need to be provided for Hispanics and adolescents, given their unique history, culture, language, and shared strengths.

## REFERENCES

Agron P., Takada E., & Purcell, A. (2002). California Project LEAN's Food on the Run Program: An evaluation of a high-school based student advocacy nutrition and physical activity program. *Journal of the American Dietetic Association, Supplement, 102*(3), S103-S105.

Alcalay, R., Alvarado, M., Balcazar, H., Newman, E., & Huerta, E. (1999). *Salud para su corazon*: A community-based Latino cardiovascular disease prevention and outreach model. *Journal of Community Health, 24,* 359–379.

American Heart Association. (2003a). Statistical fact sheet—populations: Hispanics and cardiovascular diseases. Retrieved May 15, 2003, from http://www.americanheart.org/

American Heart Association. (2003b). Statistical fact sheet—risk factors: Overweight and obesity. Retrieved May 17, 2003, from http://www.americanheart.org/

Balcazar, H., Alvarado, M., Hollen, M. L., Gonzalez-Cruz, Y., & Pedregón, V. (2005, July). Evaluation of *Salud para su corazón* (Health for Your Heart)—National Council of La Raza *Promotora* Outreach Program. *Prevention of Chronic Disease* [serial online]. Retrieved from http://www.cdc.gov/pcd/issues/2005/july/04_0130.htm

Berg, J., Cromwell, S., & Arnett, M. (2002). Physical activity: Perspectives of Mexican American and Anglo American midlife women. *Health Care for Women International, 23,* 894–904.

Centers for Disease Control and Prevention [CDC]. (2003). Physical activity levels among children aged 9–13 years—United States, 2002. *Morbidity and Mortality Weekly Report, 52,* 785–788.

Centers for Disease Control and Prevention [CDC]. (2004a). *The burden of chronic diseases and their risk factors: National and state perspectives, 2004.* Retrieved June 30, 2005, from http://www.cdc.gov/nccdphp/burdenbook2004

Centers for Disease Control and Prevention [CDC]. (2004b). Health disparities experienced by Hispanics—United States. *Morbidity and Mortality Weekly Report, 53,* 935–937.

Centers for Disease Control and Prevention [CDC]. Youth Media Campaign (2005). Active children, active families brochure—Hispanic. Retrieved June 30, 2005, from http://www.cdc.gov/youthcampaign/materials/adults/hispanic_version.htm

Coleman, K. J., Tiller, C. L., Sanchez, J., Heath, E. M., Sy, O., Milliken, G., et al. (2005). Prevention of the epidemic increase in child risk of overweight in low-income schools: The El Paso coordinated approach to child health. *Archives of Pediatric Adolescent Medicine, 159,* 217–224.

Conway, J. M., Ingwersen, L. A., Vinyard, B. T., & Moshfegh, A. J. (2003). Effectiveness of the US Department of Agriculture 5-step multiple-pass method in assessing food intake in obese and nonobese women. *American Journal of Clinical Nutrition, 77*(5), 1171–1178.

Crespo, C. J., Smit, E., Carter-Pokras, O., & Anderson, R. (2001). Acculturation and leisure-time physical inactivity in Mexican American adults: Results from NHANES III, 1988–1994. *American Journal of Public Health, 91,* 1254–1257.

Dietz, W. H. (2001). Overweight and precursors of type 2 diabetes mellitus in children and adolescents. *Journal of Pediatrics, 138*(4), 453–454.

Elder, J. P., Ayala, G. X., Campbell, N. R., Slymen, D., Lopez-Madurga, E. T., Engelberg, M., et al. (2005). Interpersonal and print nutrition communication for a Spanish-dominant Latino population: *Secretos de la buena vida. Health Psychology, 24,* 49–57.

Elder, J. P., Candelaria, J. I., Woodruff, S. I., Criqui, M. H., Talavera, G. A., & Rupp, J. W. (2000). Results of language for health: Cardiovascular disease nutrition education for Latino English-as-a-second-language students. *Health Education and Behavior, 27,* 50–63.

Eyler, A. A., Matson-Koffman, D., Young, D. R., Wilcox, S., Wilbur, J., Thompson, J. L., et al. (2003). Quantitative study of correlates of physical activity in women from diverse racial/ethnic groups: The Women's Cardiovascular Health Network Project. *American Jouran of Preventive Medicine, 25,* (3Si), 93–103.

Flegal, K. M., Ogden, C. L., & Carroll, M. D. (2004). Prevalence and trends in overweight Mexican American adults and children. *Nutrition Reviews, 62* (7, Part 2), S144-S148.

Flores, G., Fuentes-Afflick, E., Barbot, O., Carter-Pokras, O., Claudio, L., Lara, M., et al. (2002). The health of Latino children: Urgent priorities, unanswered questions, and a research agenda. *Journal of the American Medical Association, 288,* 82–90.

Flores, R. (1995). Dance for health: Improving fitness in African American and Hispanic adolescents. *Public Health Reports, 110*(2), 189–193.

Fitzgibbon, M. L., Gapstur, S. M., & Knight, S. J. (2004). Results of *Mujeres felices por ser saludables*: A dietary/breast health randomized clinical trial for Latino women. *Annals of Behavioral Medicine, 28,* 95–104.

Gonzales, N. A., Dumka, L. E., Deardorff, J., Jacobs, C. S., & McCray, A. (2004). Preventing poor mental health and school dropout of Mexican American adolescents following the transition to Junior High School. *Journal of Adolescent Research, 19,* 113–131.

Grassi, K., Gonzalez, M. G., Tello, P., & He, G. (1999). *La vida caminando*: A community-based physical activity program designed by and for rural Latino families. *Journal of Health Education, 30,* S-13, S7.

Greenlund, K. J., Zheng, Z. J., Keenan, N. L., Giles, W. H., Casper, M. L., Mensah, G. A., et al. (2004). Trends in self-reported multiple cardiovascular disease risk factors among adults in the United States, 1991–1999. *Archives of Internal Medicine, 164,* 181–188.

Hayes, D. K., Greenlund, K. J., Denny, C. H., Croft, J. B., Keenan, N. L., et al. (2005). Racial/ethnic and socioeconomic disparities in multiple risk factors for heart disease and stroke—United States, 2003. *Mortality and Morbidity Weekly Report, 54,* 113–116.

Hulme, P. A., Noble Walker, S., Effle, K. J., Jorgensen, L., McGowan, M. G., Nelson, J. D., et al. (2003). Health promoting lifestyle behaviors of Spanish-speaking Hispanic adults. *Journal of Transcultural Nursing, 14,* 244–254.

Hunt, K., Resendez, R., Williams, K., Haffner, S., Stern, M., & Hazuda, H. P. (2003). All-cause and cardiovascular mortality among Mexican-American and non-Hispanic white older participants in the San Antonio Heart Study—evidence against the "Hispanic Paradox." *American Journal of Epidemiology, 158,* 1048–1057.

Jamner, M. S., Spruijt-Metz, D., Bassin, S., & Cooper, D. M. (2004). A controlled evaluation of a school-based intervention to promote physical activity among sedentary adolescent females: Project FAB. *Journal of Adolescent Health, 34,* 279–289.

Johnson, R. K., Soultanakis, R. P., & Matthews, D. E. (1998). Literacy and body fatness are associated with underreporting of energy intake in US low-income women using the multiple-pass 24-hour recall: A doubly labeled water study. *Journal of American Diet Association, 98*(10), 1136–1140.

Juarbe, T. (1998). Cardiovascular disease-related diet and exercise experiences of immigrant Mexican women. *Western Journal of Nursing Research, 20,* 765–782.

Juarbe, T., Turok, X., & Perez-Stable, E. (2002). Perceived benefits and barriers to physical activity among older Latina women. *Western Journal of Nursing Research, 24,* 868–886.

Keele-Smith, R., & Leon, T. (2003). Evaluation of individually tailored interventions on exercise adherence. *Western Journal of Nursing Research, 25,* 623–640.

Keller, C., & Treviño, R. P. (2001). Effects of two frequencies of walking on cardiovascular risk factor reduction in Mexican American women. *Research in Nursing and Health, 24,* 390–401.

Kim, S., Koniak-Griffin, D., Flaskerud, J. H., & Guarnero, P. A. (2004). The impact of lay health advisors on cardiovascular health promotion using a community-based participatory approach. *Journal of Cardiovascular Nursing, 19,* 192–199.

Kristal, A. R., Shattuck, A. L., & Patterson, R. E. (1999). Differences in fat-related dietary patterns between black, Hispanic and white women: Results from the Women's Health Trial Feasibility Study in Minority Populations. *Public Health Nutrition, 2,* 153–262.

Marquez, D. X., McAuley, E., & Overman, N. (2004). Psychosocial correlates and outcomes of physical activity among Latinos: A review. *Hispanic Journal of Behavioral Sciences, 26,* 195–229.

McGinnis, J. M., & Foege, W. H. (1993). Actual causes of death in the United States. *Journal of the American Medical Association, 270,* 2207–2212.

Mokdad, A. H., Marks, J. S., Stroup, D. F., & Gerberding, J. L. (2004). Actual causes of death in the United States, 2000. *Journal of the American Medical Association, 291,* 1238–1245.

National Center for Chronic Disease Prevention and Health Promotion. (2005). *Centers for Disease Control and Prevention—NCCDPHP.* Retrieved from www.cdc.gov/ nccdphp

National Center for Health Statistics. (2005). *Health of Hispanic/Latino population.* Retrieved June 30, 2005, from http://www.cdc.gov/nchs/fastats/hispanic_health.htm

Ogden, C. L., Flegal, K. M., Carroll, M. D., & Johnson, C. L. (2002). Prevalence and trends in overweight among US children and adolescents, 1999–2000. *Journal of the American Medical Association, 288*(14), 1728–1732.

Pandey, D. K., Labarthe, D. R., Goff, D.C., Chan, W., & Nichaman, M. Z. (2001). Community-wide coronary heart disease mortality in Mexican Americans equals or exceeds that in non-Hispanic whites: The Corpus Christi Heart Project. *American Journal of Medicine, 110,* 81–87.

Potter, J. D., Finnegan, J. R., Jr., Guinard, J. X., Huerta, E. E., Kelder, S. H., et al. (2000, November). 5-A-Day for better health program evaluation report. Bethesda, MD: National Institutes of Health, National Cancer Institute (NIH Publication No. 01-4904).

Sharp, T. A., Grunwald, G. K., Giltman, K. E. K., King, D. L., Curtis, J., Jatkauskas, C. J., et al. (2003). Association of anthropometric measures with risk of diabetes and cardiovascular disease in Hispanic and Caucasian adolescents. *Preventive Medicine, 37*, 611–616.

Staten, L. K., Gregory-Mercado, K. Y., Ranger-Moore, J., Will, J. C., Giuliano, A. R., Ford, E. S., et al. (2004). Provider counseling, health education, and community health workers: The Arizona WISEWOMAN Project. *Journal of Women's Health, 13*, 547–556.

Suminski, R. R., Poston, W. S., & Foreyt, J. P. (1999). Early identification of Mexican American children who are at risk for becoming obese. *International Journal of Obesity, 23*, 823–829.

U.S. Bureau of Census, U.S. Department of Commerce. (2000). *Differences in population by race and Hispanic or Latino origin for the United States: 1990 to 2000.* Table 4; PHC-T-1.

Voorhees, C. C., & Rohm Young, D. (2003). Personal, social, and physical environmental correlates of physical activity levels in urban Latinas. *American Journal of Preventative Medicine, 25*(3 Suppl. 1), 61–68.

Woodruff, S. I., Talavera, G. A., & Elder, J. P. (2002). Evaluation of a culturally appropriate smoking cessation intervention for Latinos. *Tobacco Control, 11*, 361–367.

# Chapter 4

## Nursing Research and the Prevention of Infectious Diseases Among Vulnerable Populations

Nilda Peragallo and Rosa M. Gonzalez

### ABSTRACT

*Racial and ethnic minorities, women and infants, youth, and other special needs populations have been found to be disproportionately affected by infectious disease morbidity and mortality, particularly Human Immunodeficiency Syndrome/Acquired Immunodeficiency Syndrome (HIV/AIDS) and other sexually transmitted diseases (STDs). Being a vital component of the health care delivery system, nurses play an important role in improving the health of these vulnerable populations. Twenty-six studies reporting results from evaluations of prevention strategies targeting HIV/AIDS and other STDs among vulnerable populations were reviewed. The more effective interventions appeared to be those that tailored their program content to the specific risk factors of their target population and included skills training in their curriculum. Although nurses have contributed significantly in understanding the risk factors of vulnerable groups in the United States through cross-sectional research studies, more research is needed in the evaluation of intervention programs that use this knowledge to develop and implement prevention programs, particularly at a population-based level.*

Keywords: HIV/AIDS; prevention strategies; infectious disease; vulnerable populations

# INTRODUCTION

## Purpose and Background

One of the major goals of Healthy People 2010 is to eliminate health dispari-ties affecting vulnerable groups in the United States, particularly those found with infectious diseases including HIV/AIDS and other STDs (Department of Health and Human Services [DHHS], 2004). In line with this national objec-tive, the National Institute of Nursing Research (NINR) is concentrating its efforts on supporting research focusing on cost-effective measures that target health disparities and vulnerable populations (National Institute of Nursing Research [NINR], 2005). Being a vital part of the health care delivery system, nurses have the responsibility to not only provide direct care to individuals affected by these diseases, but also to address risk factors that may be pres-ent at the population level. By studying population-based characteristics and developing, implementing, and evaluating interventions that target infectious diseases among vulnerable populations, nursing has begun to address this issue. The purpose of this review is to summarize existing nursing research evaluat-ing interventions that prevent infectious diseases among vulnerable popula-tions, particularly HIV/AIDS and other STDs, and to make recommendations on how the nursing field could further contribute to addressing this problem through research and practice.

## Defining Vulnerable Populations

Studies have found that various groups in the United States are disproportion-ately affected by infectious disease morbidity and mortality. HIV/AIDS and other STDs are among the various infectious diseases for which this health disparity has been found to be most outstanding. In fact, the Centers for Disease Con-trol and Prevention (CDC) has identified racial and ethnic minorities, women, infants, adolescents and youth, men who have sex with men and people enter-ing correctional facilities to be of particular interest when addressing HIV and other STDs (Centers for Disease Control and Prevention [CDC], 2003). The vulnerable groups discussed in this chapter include racial and ethnic minori-ties (African American, Hispanics/Latinos), women and infants, youth, groups from low socioeconomic status backgrounds (homeless, inner-city residents, low-income), and groups with special health issues (mentally ill, attendees of STD clinics). Although men who have sex with men and injection drug users have been found to be at high risk for HIV/AIDS, important studies on these populations were not included in this review. The decision to exclude these vulnerable populations was made because of space limitations in this review and with recognition that a comprehensive evaluation of intervention studies targeting men who have sex with men and injection drug users merits a separate chapter.

Certain racial and ethnic minority groups have been found to be at an increased risk for infectious diseases. In 2003, the CDC reported that African Americans were diagnosed with AIDS at almost 10 times the rate than Whites. In fact, although African Americans only comprise 12.3% of the U.S. population in 2000, they account for 40% of the total estimated AIDS cases that have been reported since the beginning of the epidemic. In 2001, HIV/AIDS was the leading cause of death among African American females between 25 and 34 years of age and among the top four leading causes of death for both African American men and women between 20 and 54 years of age (CDC, 2005a). This health disparity is also found among Hispanics. The AIDS rate for Hispanics is 4 times the rate among Whites. Similarly, comprising 14% of the United States (including Puerto Rico), Hispanics, in 2003 accounted for 18% of the total diagnosed AIDS cases up to 2003 (CDC, 2005b). The same pattern is seen with other STDs. For example, in 2003, African Americans and Hispanics reported 11 and 2 times higher rates, respectively, of gonorrhea than their White counterparts. Primary and secondary syphilis also have been found to be more prevalent among these two minority populations (CDC, 2003).

Women are also increasingly becoming a large proportion of the population living with HIV/AIDS. While women constituted 14% of the adults and adolescents diagnosed with HIV/AIDS in 1992, this percentage has grown to 22% in 2003 (CDC, 2004). Minority women have been found to be especially at risk. While Hispanic women had 6 times the AIDS diagnosis rate when compared to White women in 2003, African American women had 25 times the rate of Whites (CDC, 2005a). It has also been noted that there has been an increase in the incidence of other STDs such as chlamydia between 2002 and 2003 (CDC, 2003).

Although the incidence of AIDS diagnosis in the United States is declining, there have not been comparable declines in the HIV incidence rates among youth. According to HIV/AIDS surveillance data collected in 25 states in the United States, at least half of the cases of new HIV infection are among people under 25 years of age (CDC, 2002). Within this group, a greater proportion of the cases were reported among women, 61% as compared to 39% among men. Minority youth have also been found to be at an increased risk for HIV/AIDS. In fact, African Americans account for 56% of all HIV infections ever reported among youth between 13 and 24 years of age (CDC, 2002). The same pattern is seen among adolescents and youth with other STDs. Surveillance data show that

15 to 19 year old women and 20 to 24 year old men had higher rates of chlamydia when compared with other ages groups (CDC, 2002).

Other groups that have been identified as vulnerable include the homeless, mentally ill, and substance using persons. It is difficult to determine the impact of each of these factors on sexual risk behaviors because of the comorbidity that exists among them. Research attempting to describe the specific role that each of these conditions plays on STD and HIV risks have had conflicting results. Several studies have determined that depression, especially serious depression, is strongly associated with drug use but not other STD and HIV risk behaviors (McCusker, Goldstein, Bigelow, & Zorn, 1995; Rahav, Nuttbrock, Rivera, & Link, 1998). Other studies have concluded that mental illness is associated with a higher prevalence of risky sexual practices such as "knowing one's sex partner for less than one day" or "feeling forced into sex" (Coverdale & Turbott, 2000). Prolonged homelessness, when controlled for mental illness, has also been found to be a strong predictor of risky sexual behavior among men (Rahav et al., 1998).

## Review of the Infectious Disease Nursing Literature

Few nursing articles evaluate intervention studies targeting the prevention of infectious diseases such as HIV/AIDS and other STDs among vulnerable populations (Dancy, Marcantiono, & Norr, 2000; Flaskerud, Nyamathi, & Uman, 1997; Jemmott, Jemmott, & Fong, 1998; Koniak-Griffin, Lesser, Nyamathi, et al., 2003; Lesser et al., 2005; Nyamathi, Flaskerud, Leake, Dixon & Lu 2001; Peragallo et al., 2005). The vast majority of the articles included in nursing journals explore risk factors associated with infectious diseases among specific groups (Koniak-Griffin & Brecht, 1995; Koniak-Griffin, Lesser, Uman, & Nyamathi, 2003; Nyamathi et al., 2001; Plowden, Fletcher, & Miller, 2005; Villarruel, Jemmott, Jemmott, & Ronis, 2004). Others focus on disease management and treatment (Chou, Holzemer, Portillo, & Slaughter, 2004; Williams et al., 2005); especially nursing interventions targeting tuberculosis (Crespo-Fierro, 1997; Mayo, White, Oates, & Franklin, 1996). Other nursing articles explore the impact of living with infectious diseases such as HIV/AIDS and its stigma (Duffy, 2005) or the impact of HIV/AIDS on caretakers (Guenter, Majumdar, & Willams, 2005).

## METHODS

CINAHL (Cumulative Index to Nursing and Allied Health Literature), Medline and Expanded Academic Index were searched via Ovid to identify nursing interventions focusing on the prevention of infectious diseases among vulnerable populations from January 1, 1995 to March 1, 2005. Key search terms used included *infectious diseases, communicable diseases, interventions, nursing interventions, vulnerable populations, HIV/AIDS, STDs, primary prevention,* and *infectious diseases.* Names of researchers known in the field of infectious diseases and nursing research were also searched. Two hundred forty articles were originally selected which dealt with prevention of STDs, HIV/AIDS, Hepatitis A and C, and other infectious diseases. Articles were selected based on the following inclusion criteria: (a) prevention approach, (b) evaluation through experimental or quasi-experimental design, (c) interventions taking place in the United States, (d) vulnerable group as target population, and (e) potential nursing intervention. *Potential nursing intervention* was used instead of *actual nursing intervention* because only seven interventions were described as specific nursing interventions or implemented by nurses (Dancy et al., 2000; Flaskerud et al., 1997; Jemmott et al., 1998; Koniak-Griffin, Lesser, Nyamathi, et al., 2003; Lesser et al., 2005; Nyamathi et al., 2001; Peragallo et al., 2005). Exclusion criteria included the following: (a) interventions targeting men who have sex with men and injection drug users, (b) review articles and meta-analyses, and (c) pharmacologic prevention interventions. Because the majority of the interventions targeting hepatitis and tuberculosis described immunization programs and medication therapies, these were not included in the review. A total of 26 articles meeting the selection criteria were selected for in-depth study and included in the review Table 4.1.

## RESULTS

### Interventions Targeting Youth

Seven of the prevention studies reviewed specifically targeted adolescents and youth (Coyle, Kirby, Marin, Gomez, & Gregorich, 2004; DiClemente et al., 2004; Jemmott et al., 1998; Kirby et al., 2004; Koniak-Griffin, Lesser, Uman, et al., 2003; Lesser et al., 2005; Rotheram-Borus, Gwadz, Fernandez, & Srinivasan, 1998). All of these interventions included risk-reduction strategies and skills-focused content, most of which used the Social Cognitive Theory (SCT) to help develop the curriculum. In the study conducted by Coyle et al. (2004), 19 middle schools comprised of mostly Hispanic males and females (N = 2829) were randomized to either an STD and pregnancy prevention intervention based on the SCT and Social Inoculation Theory or standard HIV/AIDS education. Over the span of three academic years, experienced health educators and HIV infected persons taught students in the experimental group about limit setting, refusal skills in both nonsexual and sexual situations, condom skills, and consequences of unplanned intercourse through individual and group sessions. Although there was a positive intervention effect on reported sexual intercourse during the last 12 months for

**TABLE 4.1** Studies Evaluating STD & HIV Prevention Interventions

| Author and Year | Sample | Design | Intervention Characteristics | Outcome Measures and Main Results |
|---|---|---|---|---|
| **Youth** | | | | |
| Coyle et al. (2004) | Middle school H, M & F N = 2829 19 schools | Random-ized Control Trial (RCT) by school | 20 session/3 yr individual and group sessions led by health educators, HIV infected persons; based on SCT & Social Inoculation Theory. Negotiation skills; limit setting and refusal in nonsexual, sexual, and dating situations; knowledge: understanding consequences of unplanned sexual intercourse; condom demonstration | Intervention effect on decreasing ever having sex during all follow up periods among boys<br><br>No intervention effects on girls or on condom use by group or time, ever having sexual intercourse, or number of partners |
| DiClemente et al. (2004) | Community clinic, 14-18 AA, F (sexually experienced) N = 522 | RCT by individual | Four 4-hr weekly small group sessions led by peer educators matched on ethnicity and gender; based on SCT and Theory of Gender and Power<br><br>HIV knowledge, communication and negotiating skills, condom use skills, healthy relationships | Intervention effect to reduce incidence of chlamydia, but not trichomonas or gonorrhea (at 12 mo), on increased proficiency in condom use, consistent condom use, frequency of protected sex, likelihood to put condom on partner, and decreased likelihood of new sex partner (at 6 and 12 mo) |
| Jemmott et al. (1998) Nursing Research | Middle school AA, M & F N = 659 | RCT by individual | Four 1-hr weekly small group sessions led by adult and peer facilitators matched on ethnicity; based on SCT, TPB, and TRA. HIV knowledge, self-efficacy, hedonistic beliefs, negotiation and condom use skills vs. abstinence only | Abstinence intervention effect to reduce frequency of sexual intercourse at 3 mo but not at any longer follow up periods. Safer-sex intervention effective in increasing frequency of condom use (at 3, 6, and 12 mo), 100% condom use (at 3 mo) |

| Kirby et al. (2004) | High school Ethnically diverse, M & F, N = 3869 20 schools | RCT by school | 20 session/2 yr individual, group, and school-wide sessions led by teachers and peers; based on SCT, Social Influence Theory, and Models of School Change  HIV/STD knowledge, condom negotiation, communication skills (with parents and partners) | Intervention effect on decreased frequency of unprotected sex, increased condom use during last act of intercourse with stronger effect on males, Hispanics, and subgroups with high-risk sexual behaviors  No intervention effect on delay of sexual debut |
|---|---|---|---|---|
| Koniak-Griffin et al. (2003) Nursing Research | High school H, F, H, AA (pregnant, low SES) N = 497 4 school districts | RCT by school; yearly alternating assignment of intervention | Four 2-hr class sessions led by nurses; based on SCT and TRA  Project CHARM: Four-session intervention led by nurses in alternative schools to promote sexual responsibility, accountability and political awareness of the impact of HIV/AIDS in their communities; maternal protectiveness as motivator to promote positive behavior change | Intervention effective in increasing intentions to use condoms, AIDS knowledge and decreasing risky sexual behaviors (at 12 mo) |
| Lesser et al. (2005) Nursing Research | Inner-city community, parenting adolescents & male partners N = 98; 49 couples | Prospective longitudinal trial | Six small-group sessions led by teams of male-female facilitators; culturally sensitive and theory-based intervention for couples  HIV awareness, understanding vulnerability to HIV infection, attitudes and beliefs about HIV and safer sex, building condom use skills, refusal skills, and conflict negotiation, contraception and disease prevention | Increased intentions to use condoms and decreased episodes of unprotected vaginal sex among male and female participants in the intervention group compared to those receiving a standard control condition (Note: findings based on case-available analysis) |

*(Continued)*

**TABLE 4.1** Studies Evaluating STD & HIV Prevention Interventions (*Continued*)

| Author and Year | Sample | Design | Intervention Characteristics | Outcome Measures and Main Results |
|---|---|---|---|---|
| **Youth and Adults** | | | | |
| Branson et al. (1998) | STD clinic, 77%, 13–34 Blacks, F & M, N = 964 | RCT by small group | Four 1-hr biweekly small group sessions; booster session at 2 months led by counselors; based on IMB skills model for AIDS risk reduction Information, motivation, and behavioral skills | No intervention effect for rate of development of new infection, intention to use condoms, frequency of intercourse, number of partners |
| Flaskerud et al. (1997) Nursing Research | WIC center 14–86, H, F family & friends N = 508 | Prospective longitudinal | Individual counseling and small group sessions led by community health workers matched on ethnicity, gender, and language (dose not specified); based on conceptualization of cultural competence, women as traditional health educators and pubic health approach HIV testing, risk-reduction, and pregnancy counseling; condom and negotiation skills, cleaning needles, free condoms; referral and advocacy | Intervention effect to decrease frequency of unprotected sex acts (at 12 mo) |
| Kamb et al. (1998) | STD clinics 14+, diverse ethnicity M & F Heterosexual, HIV negative N = 5758 | RCT by individual | PROJECT RESPECT: Four 20–60 min individual brief or enhanced counseling sessions/ 1–4 weeks led by matched and unmatched counselors; based on TRA action and SCT HIV testing, counseling, and prevention, goal setting and risk reduction long-term plan. Content tailored to individual's personal risks, self-efficacy, attitudes, and perceived norms | Brief and enhanced counseling intervention effect to reduce diagnosis of new STDs; increase 100% condom use (at 3 and 6 mo) and safe sex practices (at 6 and 12 mo.) No intervention effect on frequency of condom use or condom use during last sex act |
| Bolu et al. (2004) | Subset analysis N = 4328 | | PROJECT RESPECT | Both brief and enhanced counseling interventions effective to reduce diagnosis of new STD |

| | | | PROJECT RESPECT | |
|---|---|---|---|---|
| Pealer et al. (2004) | Subset analysis N = 2239 | | | No counselor or counselor-client effect on new STD or intervention completion |
| Lauby et al. (2000) | Urban, 15–35 AA, F (sexually active) N = 1836 (1993); N = 1889 (1996) | Controlled trial by matched communities | 2 yr community-wide, individual and small group activities led by peers & community organizations; based on Transtheoretical Model of Behavior Change, SLT and Diffusion of Innovation<br><br>Condom literature and distribution; role-model stories, safer-sex education | Intervention effect to decrease no condom use, no communication about condoms with main partner and to increase attempt to get partner to use condom<br><br>No intervention effect on condom use during last sex, 100% condom use or condom use with non-main partners |
| Nyamathi et al. (2001) Nursing Research | Shelters, 15–50, AA,H, F & their sexual partners N = 633 | RCT by shelter | Six 1-hr sessions over 6 weeks, small group sessions led by Nurse Case-Manager (NCM) or matched peer; based on Comprehensive Health Seeking and Coping Paradigm (CHSCP) vs culturally sensitive Standard program<br><br>HIV/AIDS knowledge, condom use, negotiating skills, & coping strategies | Significant improvements were observed in the three groups in risky drug and sexual behaviors, and cognitive and psychological resources<br><br>Nurse-led group revealed significant greater improvement than counterparts in self-esteem |
| Rotheram-Borus et al. (1998) | Community-based agency 13–24, H, AA M & F N = 151 | RCT by individual | Seven 1.5 hr or three 3.5 hr biweekly small group sessions led by experienced HIV leader, at least one facilitator in group was matched on gender and ethnicity; based on HBM, Peer Influence Model, and Learning Theory<br><br>HIV knowledge, social cognitive factors, negotiation and condom use skills, and goal setting | Seven session intervention effective to decrease number of sexual partners and risky sex acts<br><br>No intervention effect observed for condom skills |

(Continued)

**TABLE 4.1**  Studies Evaluating STD & HIV Prevention Interventions (*Continued*)

| Author and Year | Sample | Design | Intervention Characteristics | Outcome Measures and Main Results |
|---|---|---|---|---|
| Shain et al. (1999) Nursing Involvement | Research clinic 14–45, MA, AA, F N = 617 | RCT by individual | Three 3-4 hr weekly small group sessions led by counselors matched on ethnicity/race and gender; based on ARRM (AIDS Risk Reduction Model) Risk recognition, commitment to change risk factors, partner communication, condom negotiation, and condom use | Intervention effect to decrease acquisition of single and multiple STD infections; multiple sex partners and higher-risk sex (6 and 12 mo) |
| **Adults** | | | | |
| Boyer et al. (1997) | STD clinic 18–35, ethnic minorities, M & F N = 399 | RCT by individual | Four 60-min individual sessions/4 wks led by matched, trained counselors based on ARRM (AIDS-Risk Reduction Model); cognitive/behavioral approach HIV/STD knowledge and communication; identification and modification of risk factors | Intervention effect to increase percent of protected sex acts and to decrease the number of sexual encounters and reasons to not use a condom & increase intention (3 mo) among men only and get partner to use a condom (5 mo) No effect on number of new STDs |
| Dancy et al. (2000) Nursing Research | Community 20–44, AA, F Low-income N = 280 | RCT by community | Six 90-min weekly group sessions and booster led by peers; based on Behavioral Change model (SCT, TRA, and HBM) Components of sexuality and social norms in relationships, STD/HIV knowledge, risk reduction strategies, steps in decision making relating to condom use | Intervention effect on HIV protective behavior (at 6, not 9, months) No intervention effect on percent of women sexually active and community preventative behaviors |

| | | | | |
|---|---|---|---|---|
| Harvey et al. (2004) | Community clinic 18–25, H, F, & partner N = 146 couples | RCT by couples | Three 2.5 hr weekly small group sessions led by matched and trained facilitators; based on Fishbein's Integrated Behavior Change Model, IMB model of HIV/AIDS risk reduction<br><br>Perceived vulnerability, HIV/STD information, strategies for safer sex, condom skills training with interactive skills-based activity | No intervention effect on frequency of unprotected vaginal sex acts, consistent condom use, percent of protected sex acts, or contraceptive use |
| Kalichman et al. (1995) | Inner-city community mental health center 31–47, M & F; N = 52 | RCT by individual | Four 90-min weekly small group sessions led by matched trained counselors; based on Cognitive-Behavioral and Skills Instruction Models<br><br>HIV/AIDS education, risk-reduction skill development, communication and interpersonal assertiveness skills, repetition, and reinforcement of skills | Intervention effective to increase condom use and condom use intention, condom use after alcohol consumption, intention to insist on condom use with resistant partner (2 mo)<br><br>Intervention effect to increase likelihood to talk to partners about safer sex and AIDS |
| Kalichman et al. (1996) | Inner-city community Adults AA, F; N = 87 | RCT by individual | Four biweekly small group sessions led by trained facilitators based on Theory of Behavior Change<br><br>HIV education and sensitization, communication skills, and self-management skills instruction | Intervention effect to increase likelihood to refuse unprotected sex<br><br>No intervention effect on condom use, intention to use condoms |
| Kalichman et al. (1999) | STD clinic 18–50, AA, M, (Heterosexual) N = 117 | RCT by individual | Two 3-hour biweekly small group sessions (with video tapes) led by community based providers; based on IMB model with enhanced motivational components<br><br>Risk reduction information, motivational, sexual communication, and condom skills | Intervention effect to increase partner communication and intention to plan ahead for sex at 6 mo and to use and carry a condom at 3 mo, but not at 6 mo |

*(Continued)*

**TABLE 4.1** Studies Evaluating STD & HIV Prevention Interventions (*Continued*)

| Author and Year | Sample | Design | Intervention Characteristics | Outcome Measures and Main Results |
|---|---|---|---|---|
| NIMH (1998) | Public STD & PC clinics) Adults, AA, H, M, F N = 1564; 37 clinics | RCT by individual | Seven 90–120 min biweekly or 1, 1-hr small group session led by certified trainers; based on Behavioral Theory<br><br>Risk reduction content based on best practices; outcome expectancies, skills, and self-efficacy | Intervention effect to reduce the number of unprotected vaginal and anal intercourse acts, increase 100% condom use and percent of condom use during vaginal or anal intercourse (12 mo) and report fewer STD symptoms<br><br>No intervention effect on incidence of gonorrhea (12 mo) |
| O'Donnell et al. (1998) | STD clinic: mean age = 30 AA, H, M N = 1904 | RCT by day of clinic visit | Dose unclear; video-viewing with/without group discussion led by clinic counselor; based on formative research approach<br><br>HIV/STD and condom use information and condom use | Intervention effect to reduce incidence of new STDs but no treatment advantage for group discussion |
| Peragallo et al. (2004) Nursing research | Urban community: 18–44, H, F Sexually active N = 657 | RCT by individual | Six 2-hr weekly small group sessions led by HIV peer counselor matched on ethnicity and gender; based on SCT<br><br>Information on HIV/AIDS/ STDs, condom use skills, sexual communication and negotiation, violence prevention, risk awareness, and risk management; peer support for behavior change | Intervention effect to increase condom use and intention, partner communication skills (at 3 and 6 mo)<br><br>No intervention effect for 100% condom use |

| Study | Setting/Sample | Design | Intervention | Outcomes |
|---|---|---|---|---|
| Raj et al. (2001) | Community center & clinic, 18–35 H, F N = 162 | RCT by clinic | Twelve 90–120 min weekly small group sessions led by community health educator; based on SCT, Freirian Empowerment Adult Education Model, Self-in-Relation Theory, Diffusion of Innovation Theory; Theory of Gender and Power<br><br>HIV/STD information, substance use, partner violence, body image, and socio-structural health risk factors information | Intervention effect to increase safer sex negotiation skills<br><br>No intervention effect on frequency of condom use |
| Sikkema et al. (2000) | Inner-city housing developments Adult, AA, H, F, N = 690; 18 Housing developments | RCT by matched development | Four 90-min individual and small group workshops for popular opinion leader facilitators and community activities /12 mo based on models of HIV risk reduction<br><br>AIDS prevention messages; safe-sex materials & free condom distribution; woman-to-woman conversations | Intervention effect to increase condom availability, percent of protected sex acts<br><br>No intervention effect on AIDS or condom use conversations with partner |

Race/ethnicity: AA = African American, H = Hispanic/Latino, MA = Mexican Americans, Gender: M = male, F = female boys, this was not seen among girls. The intervention was ineffective in increasing condom use, decreasing history of sexual intercourse, and number of sexual episodes and partners.

The intervention described by Jemmott et al. (1998) also targeted middle school students. In this study, African American students (N = 654) were randomized to an HIV abstinence intervention, a safer-sex intervention or a health promotion education program. Because both interventions were developed using the SCT, Theory of Planned Behavior (TPB), and Theory of Reasoned Action (TRA), both groups focused on self-efficacy and skills development. Adult and peer African American facilitators led small groups, which discussed either abstinence or condom use and negotiation and hedonistic beliefs for two, 4-hour weekly sessions. While the abstinence intervention was most effective in reducing the frequency of sexual intercourse at the 3-month follow-up, the safer-sex intervention was most effective in increasing 100% condom use during this same follow-up period. However, these two intervention effects were not sustained at 6- and 12-month follow-up periods. Both the safer-sex intervention and the abstinence intervention were effective in increasing the frequency of condom use at 12 months.

Kirby et al. (2004) randomized 20 ethnically diverse high schools (N = 3,869) to either a school-wide HIV/STD intervention that was based on the SCT, Social Influence Theory (SIT), and Models of School Change, or a knowledge-based curriculum. Trained teachers and peers taught male and female students, by means of individual and group sessions in the experimental group, general HIV/STD knowledge, skills in sex refusal, condom use, and partner and parent communication over two years. The school-wide intervention also included school organization, curriculum and staff development, parent education, and school-community linkages. This intervention was effective in decreasing the frequency of unprotected sex and increasing condom use during the last intercourse but was ineffective in delaying sexual debut. This was the only youth study that also assessed intervention effects by gender, ethnicity and race, and high-risk behaviors. The intervention was found to be more effective for males, Hispanics, and sub-groups with high-risk behaviors.

Koniak-Griffin, Lesser, Nyamathi et al. (2003) targeted predominantly Hispanic, pregnant females, and young mothers from four low-income high school districts (N = 497) in Project CHARM (Children's Health and Responsible Mothering). Schools were randomized to the experimental intervention (HIV prevention program) or a health promotion program. Nurses led four, 2-hour classes, based on the SCT and TRA, where they discussed the impact of HIV/AIDS on pregnant women and their children, prevention of disease during pregnancy and the postpartum period, sexual responsibility and accountability, and political awareness of the impact that HIV has on their communities. The program emphasized the role of maternal protectiveness in motivating adolescents to make healthy sexual decisions and reduce risky sexual behavior. An intervention effect was found with increasing AIDS knowledge and condom use intention, and decreasing self-reported sexual risk-taking behaviors at 12 months.

In a subsequent two-phase community-academic collaboration, a culturally sensitive HIV prevention program for teen mothers and their male partners (N = 98; 49 couples) was designed and pilot tested for feasibility (Lesser et al., 2005). The couple-focused HIV prevention program, designed by collaborating partners, was well accepted by inner-city Latino adolescent fathers and mothers and was realistic for implementation in the community setting. Preliminary descriptive findings on the distribution of scores of available participants at the 3- and 6-month follow-up evaluations showed a pattern of increasing intentions to use condoms and decreasing episodes of unprotected vaginal sex among male and female participants in the experimental group compared to those receiving a standard control condition. DiClemente et al. (2004) targeted sexually experienced African American females between the ages of 14 and 18 from four community health agencies (N = 522). Participants were randomized to either an HIV intervention or a health promotions program. Although the content delivered in this study was also developed from the SCT, this is the only intervention which incorporated the Theory of Gender and Power. African American female peer educators led small groups that discussed HIV content, condom use and negotiation skills, partner communication, as well as healthy relationships over four 4-hour weekly sessions. This intervention was effective in reducing the incidence of chlamydia, the likelihood of reporting new sex partners, increasing condom use during last intercourse, the frequency and consistent use of condoms within the last 30 days, proficiency in condom use demonstration, and likelihood of putting a condom on their partner at 6- and 12-month follow-ups. There were no intervention effects on the incidence of trichomonas or gonorrhea at the 12-month follow-up evaluation.

In the study conducted by Rotheram-Borus et al. (1998), Hispanic and African American male and females between the ages of 13 and 24 (N = 151) recruited from a community agency were randomized to one of two HIV interventions. As this study was specifically testing for the impact of the number and length of sessions had on outcome measures, both experimental groups received the same curriculum. Content included HIV knowledge, social cognitive factors, negotiation skills, and condom use and goal setting and was based on the Health Belief Model (HBM) and the Peer Influence Model. Learning Theory was used to guide the manner in which the content was delivered. Experienced HIV leaders and at least one facilitator matched on gender and ethnicity led small groups for either seven 1.5 or three 3.5 biweekly sessions. Participants of the seven-session intervention were more likely to report fewer sexual partners, risk acts, and had higher condom use skills demonstration scores than the three-session intervention and control condition. There were no intervention effects on substance abuse.

## Interventions Targeting Youth and Adults

Six studies included both adolescent and adult participants. Three of these studies specifically targeted females from ethnic and racial minorities (Flaskerud et al., 1997; Lauby, Smith, Stark, Person, & Adams, 2000; Shain et al., 1999). In a study conducted by Shain et al. (1999), the AIDS Risk Reduction Model (AARM) was used to develop an STD prevention program focused on helping 14- to 45-year-old Mexican American and African American females from an STD research clinic (N = 617) recognize their risk and commit to changing risky sexual behaviors. Mexican American and African American female counselors led three, 3–4 hour weekly small group sessions that covered condom use skills and negotiation and partner communication. Participants in the experimental group were less likely to acquire single and multiple STDs, less likely to be non-compliant to the STD treatment protocol, and less likely to engage in higher risk sexual behaviors (i.e., multiple partners) than individuals receiving standard STD risk-reduction counseling at 6- and 12-month follow-up periods.

The participants (N = 508) in the study conducted by Flaskerud et al. (1997) were Hispanic females attending Women's Infant and Children (WIC) nutrition programs; their ages ranged from 18 to 86 years. The conceptualization of cultural competence, the view that women in the Hispanic culture are viewed as traditional health educators, and a public health approach were used to design program content and delivery. In addition to risk reduction and skills content included by many of the other studies presented in this review, testing and counseling, information on cleaning needles, free condoms, and referral and advocacy were also incorporated into this intervention. Community health workers matched on gender, ethnicity and language served as individual counselors and led small group discussions. Participants were followed for one year. There was an intervention effect on increasing knowledge, decreasing perception of having and getting AIDS, and decasing the frequency of unprotected sexual acts at 12-month follow-up. Findings revealed only one woman tested positive for HIV and the participants denied illegal injection drug use (100%) and illegal drug use (93%).

The intervention described by Lauby et al. (2000) was implemented among sexually active, low-income African American 15- to 35-year-old women from an urban community (N = 1,836). The Transtheoretical Model of Behavior Change, SLT, and Diffusion of Innovation Theory were used to guide the development of this 2-year community-wide intervention. Risk reduction content was delivered through condom and literature distribution, small group sessions where role-model stories were discussed, safer-sex events, and community workshops led by peers and community organizations. Women from the experimental community were more likely to report using and talking about condoms with their main partners than women from a matched community. No intervention effects on increasing condom use during last sexual act or 100% condom use with main partner, and no impact on any of the behavioral outcomes associated with risky sexual practices with other partners.

The remainder of the studies with samples of adolescents and adults included interventions targeting female and male STD clinic attendees (Bolu et al., 2004; Branson, Peterman, Cannon, Ransom & Zaidi, 1998; Kamb et al., 1998; Pealer et al., 2004). Branson et al. (1998) compared small group counseling developed using the Information-Motivation-Behavioral (IMB) skills model for AIDS risk reduction to standard individual STD counseling among Black males and females between the ages of 13 and 34 (N = 964). The experimental counseling included HIV/STD information as well as motivation and behavioral skills and was delivered in four, 1-hour biweekly sessions and one booster session at two months. There was no intervention effect on the incidence of STDs, intention to use condoms, frequency of intercourse, number of new sex partners, HIV knowledge, or clinic attendance.

The other three studies reported different analyses using data gathered from PROJECT RESPECT. Kamb et al. (1998) described PROJECT RESPECT and the original program evaluation. Heterosexual, HIV negative male and female minority STD clinic attendees (N = 5,758) aged 14 years and older were randomized to one of three groups: enhanced counseling (four 20-minute to 1-hour sessions over 3–4 weeks), brief counseling (two 20-minute sessions over 7–10 days) and standard counseling (two 5-minute sessions over 7–10 days). The TRA and SCT were used to develop the content delivered during the counseling sessions. Goal setting and long-term planning content tailored to individual risks, self-efficacy, STD and condom attitudes and perceived norms were included in both counseling interventions. Both enhanced and brief counseling were effective in reducing the incidence of STDs and increasing 100% condom use at 6 and 12 months. Both groups were also effective in reducing other risky sexual behaviors such as having new and casual sex partners, with brief counseling having more of a treatment effect. There was no treatment effect for frequency of condom use or use during last sexual act.

In a subset analysis (N = 2,239) conducted by Pealer et al. (2004), specific counselor demographics and or the composition of the counselor-client dyad was evaluated. No specific counselor or counselor-client dyads were found to be associated the likelihood of completing the program or the incidence of STDs. Bolu et al. (2004) also conducted a subset analysis (N = 4,328) using data gathered from PROJECT RESPECT to evaluate counseling efficacy among high risk groups. Results showed that both counseling sessions (enhanced and brief) were more effective in preventing STDs among high-risk groups than the control condition. While enhanced counseling was effective in preventing STDs among adolescents, Whites and persons who had an STD at baseline, brief counseling was effective in preventing STDs among adolescents, Blacks, persons who had exchanged sex for money or drugs, and participants of the clinics located in Baltimore.

## Interventions Targeting Adults

Twelve intervention studies included adults over the age of 18, five of which specifically recruited women (Dancy et al., 2000; Kalichman, Rompa, & Coley 1996; Peragallo et al., 2005; Raj et al., 2001; Sikkema et al., 2000) and one of women joined with their sex partners (Nyamathi et al., 2001). Peragallo et al. (2005) targeted sexually active Mexican and Puerto Rican women between the ages of 18 and 44 years from a low-income, urban community (N = 657). The intervention was developed using the SCT of Behavioral Change and included training bilingual Hispanic peers to deliver the program content in six, 2-hour weekly small group sessions. Content included HIV/AIDS and STD knowledge, condom use skills, sexual communication and negotiation, risk awareness and management, as well as violence prevention. Hispanic women who were randomized into the experimental group were more likely to use partner communication skills, had higher HIV knowledge scores, and scored higher on the intention to use condoms and lower on perceived barriers to condom use at 3- and 6-month follow-up periods when compared to women receiving no intervention. There was no intervention effect on 100% condom use and perception of peer norms.

Raj et al. (2001) also focused on adult Hispanic females (N = 162). In this study women between the age of 18 and 35 recruited from a community center and clinic were randomized into the experimental group, a general women's health promotion program or a waiting list. The experimental intervention was developed using the SCT, Freirian Empowerment Adult Education Model, Self-in-Relation Theory, Diffusion of Innovation Theory, and Theory of Gender and Power. Program content included HIV/STD knowledge, substance use, partner violence, body image, and socio-cultural health risk factors information, and was delivered by community health educators during 12, 90–120 minute weekly small group sessions. There was an intervention effect on increasing communication and negotiation skills and HIV testing at 12-weeks and 2-month follow-up periods. However, there was no intervention effect on the frequency of condom use.

Nyamathi et al. (2001) evaluated an intervention developed for African American and Hispanic adult females (N = 325) and their sexual partners (N = 308) from emergency or sober-living facilities. The Comprehensives Health Seeking and Coping Paradigm (CHSCP) was used to develop a culturally sensitive program that was infused into the three treatment groups; a nurse cased managed (NCM) program, a peer-led program, and a standard HIV testing and counseling program; all programs were delivered by different groups of research staff. Both the NCM and peer-led programs focused on HIV/AIDS knowledge, condom use and negotiation skills, and coping strategies, whereas the standard program, focused on the importance of HIV testing and delivered culturally sensitive HIV counseling. Nurse- and peer-led groups of 2 to 3 couples met for 1-hour sessions weekly over 6 weeks. Findings revealed significant changes were found over time for all three groups in life satisfaction, psychological well-being, use of non-injection drugs, sex with multiple partners, and unprotected sex at 6 months. Analysis revealed NCM participants improved significantly in self-esteem compared to their counterparts.

Sikkema et al. (2000) tested an HIV/AIDS intervention developed from models of HIV risk reduction among adult African American and Hispanic females in inner-city housing developments (N = 690). In this study, paired housing developments were randomized into a community-wide intervention or the control condition (mailed AIDS brochures and coupons for free condoms). Throughout a 12-month period, members of the experimental communities participated in four, 90-minute risk reduction workshops and three major community events that delivered AIDS prevention messages. During this same time, they also received safe-sex materials and free condoms, newsletters and participated in women-to-women conversations with popular opinion leaders. There was an intervention effect on decreasing the frequency of unprotected intercourse, increasing condom availability, and increasing HIV knowledge and risk sensitivity. However, there were no intervention effects on the frequency of protected intercourse and AIDS or condom use conversations with partner.

In the study conducted by Kalichman et al. (1996), non-monogamous African American females from an inner-city community (N = 87) were randomized into one of the following groups: (a) HIV education sensitizatior only, (b) HIV education sensitization and sexual communication skills trainin (c) self-management skills instruction, or (d) HIV education sensitization a' sexual communication skills training and self-management skills instruction. T program was developed using the Theory of Behavior Change and was deliv/ in four biweekly small group sessions. The experimental group receiving cor nication skills were more likely to report having discussions about sex and / unprotected sex at 3 months postintervention. There were no interv/

effect differences among the four groups on AIDS-related knowledge and condom use or substance use prior to sexual intercourse.

Dancy et al. (2000) also concentrated on African American females between the ages of 20 and 44 from low-income communities (N = 280). In this study communities were randomized into a HIV/STD prevention program that was developed using a behavioral change approach that included the SCT, TRA, and HBM, or a general health maintenance intervention. In the experimental intervention, peer leaders facilitated six, 90-minute weekly small group sessions and one booster session at each follow-up visit. These sessions covered HIV/STD knowledge, components of sexuality and social norms in relationships, and risk reduction strategies, which included steps in decision making relating to condom use. There was an intervention effect on condom knowledge and HIV protective behaviors (i.e., 100% condom use, having a supply of condoms, asking partner to use condoms) which peaked at 6 months, but dropped at 9 months. There was no intervention effect on self-efficacy, the percent of sexually active women, and community protective behaviors (i.e., talking to friends and neighbors about HIV prevention).

Only two studies were specifically designed for adult males (O'Donnell, O'Donnell, San Doval, Duran, & Labes, 1998; Kalichman, Cherry, & Browne-Sperling, 1999). In the study conducted by O'Donnell et al. (1998), African American and Hispanic males from an STD clinic (N = 1,904) were randomized into one of the following three conditions: (a) video-viewing only (HIV/STD knowledge and condom use), (b) video-viewing with group discussion led by a counselor, or (c) control (regular clinic visit). Participants were followed for 17 months. During this time both the video-only and video and discussion groups had a lower incidence of STDs when compared to the control group. This intervention effect was greatest among subjects reporting multiple sex partners. There was no treatment advantage for the video and discussion intervention over the video-only intervention.

The study conducted by Kalichman et al. (1999) also included males recruited from an STD clinic (N = 117). In this study, African American heterosexual males between the ages of 18 and 50 were randomized into the experimental or control condition. Community-based service providers at a community center delivered an intervention that was developed using the IMB model with enhanced motivational components. The intervention covered motivation skills, risk reduction information, sexual communication skills, condom skills, and group discussions that were delivered in two, 3-hour biweekly small group sessions using video tapes and group discussions. The intervention group was less likely to use drugs and drink alcohol when having sex, and more likely to talk to partners about condoms and plan ahead for sex at the 6-month follow-up when compared to STD participants receiving standard care. Although the intervention group had a higher rate

of condom use, a lower rate of unprotected sex, and was more likely to carry a condom at 3 months, this was not seen during the 6-month follow-up period. There was no intervention effect on AIDS knowledge or behavioral intentions.

The remainder of adult interventions targeted both genders (Boyer, Barret, Peterman, & Bolan, 1997; Harvey et al., 2004; Kalichman, Sikkema, Kelly, & Bulto, 1995; National Institute of Mental Health [NIMH], 1998). Harvey et al. (2004) randomized young Hispanic females between 18 and 25 years of age, recruited from community-based clinics and their male partners (N = 146 couples) to the experimental or control condition. The experimental intervention was developed using Fishbein's Integrated Behavior Change Model and the IMB model for HIV/AIDS risk reduction. Couples in the experimental group participated in three, 2.5, hour weekly small group sessions. Perceived vulnerability, HIV/STD information, strategies for safer sex, condom skill-training, and partner communication was covered through interactive activities. There were no intervention effects on the frequency of unprotected or protected vaginal sexual acts, contraceptive use, or consistent condom use.

The study conducted by Kalichman et al. (1995) was implemented in an inner-city community mental health center. Chronically mentally ill males and females between the ages of 31 and 47 (N = 52) were randomized into the experimental or control condition. The experimental intervention was developed using the Cognitive-Behavioral and Skills Instruction Models and included HIV/AIDS education, risk-reduction skill development, and communication and interpersonal assertiveness skills. This content was delivered in four, 90-minute small group sessions where content was repeated and reinforced by trained counselors. The intervention group scored higher in knowledge of AIDS and condom use, were more likely to report intention to use condoms, use condoms after drinking alcohol, insist on using condoms if partner resisted, and experienced a greater increase in the frequency of condom-protected sex during 1- and 2-month follow-up. Although there was an intervention effect on talking to partners about safer sex and AIDS at 1 month, this was not sustained at the 2-month follow-up.

In the study conducted by Boyer et al. (1997), males and females from racial and ethnic minority groups attending an STD clinic (N = 399) were randomized into the experimental or control condition. While the experimental group received counseling developed from the AIDS-risk reduction model and used a cognitive-behavioral approach, the control group received standard risk-reduction counseling. The individual counseling included HIV/STD knowledge, decision-making and communication, and modification of risk factors, and was delivered in four 60-minute sessions over 4 weeks. There was no intervention effect on the incidence of STDs and HIV/STD knowledge among men and women or the number of sexual partners among women. Although there was an intervention effect on increasing the percentage of protected sexual acts, and decreasing the number of sexual encounters and reasons for not using condoms for men at 3-months, this was not seen at the 5-month follow-up.

In a study conducted by the National Institute of Mental Health (1998), adult African American and Hispanic men and women (N = 1564) were recruited from 37 public health clinics throughout the country and randomized into the experimental or control condition. While the experimental group received an intervention presenting risk-reduction content based on best practices, the control group received standard HIV education. The experimental intervention was developed from behavioral theory and focused on mediating risk factors through content that covered outcome expectancies, skills, and self-efficacy, and was delivered by small group sessions. Those assigned to the experimental group attended seven, 90–120 minute biweekly small group sessions run separately for males and females but coled by both a male and female experienced facilitator. There was an intervention effect on decreasing frequency of self-reported STD symptoms, unprotected acts of vaginal and anal intercourse, increasing 100% condom use, and percent of condom use during intercourse during 3-, 6-, and 12-month follow-up. Although the experimental group had a clinically significant lower incidence of gonorrhea, this difference was not statistically significant.

## OVERVIEW OF CONTEXTUAL ISSUES

### Target Population

All the studies reviewed in this chapter focused on vulnerable populations. Racial and ethnic minority groups were represented in the samples of most of the studies included in the review. Interventions designed to target a single racial or ethnic group were reported in several studies, including five involving African Americans (Dancy et al., 2000; DiClemente et al., 2004; Jemmott et al., 1998; Kalichman et al., 1999; Lauby et al., 2000) and six involving Hispanics (Coyle et al., 2004; Flaskerud et al., 1997; Harvey et al., 2004; Koniak-Griffin, Lesser, Nyamathi, et al., 2003; Lesser et al., 2005; Peragallo et al., 2005; Raj et al., 2001). One intervention described the target group as Black (Branson et al., 1998) without specifying the ethnicity. The remainder of the studies included a combination of minority populations. Although most studies targeted minority ethnic and racial groups, only one reported analysis by ethnic group and found that brief counseling was effective in preventing STDs for Blacks (Bolu et al., 2004). One study looked at the association between race and ethnicity and outcome measures at baseline, and controlled for these, but did not examine intervention effects according to race and ethnicity (NIMH, 1998). Kirby et al. (2004) found a greater intervention effect for Hispanics.

The majority of the interventions described were developed for a female population. Two interventions were specifically developed for males (Kalichman et al., 1999; O'Donnell et al., 1998), and one for females who were paired with their sexual partners (Nyamathi et al., 2001). Thirteen studies included both genders (Bolu, et al., 2004; Boyer et al., 1997; Branson et al., 1998; Coyle et al., 2004; Harvey et al., 2004; Jemmott et al., 1998; Kamb et al., 1998; Kirby et al., 2004; Lesser et al., 2005; NIMH, 1998; Pealer et al., 2004; Rotheram-Borus et al., 1998). All of these examined intervention effects according to gender or controlled for gender in their results. Boyer et al. (1997) reported intervention effects by gender. The number of sexual encounters and reasons for not using a condom decreased and intention to use a condom and encouraging condom use among partners increased in men only. Coyle et al. (2004) found that boys were less likely to report sexual intercourse during the past 12 months but there was no intervention effect for girls. Kirby et al. (2004) found greater intervention effect for males than females.

Various studies targeted populations that have been found to have a higher prevalence of high-risk sexual behaviors. Three studies limited the evaluation analysis to sexually active persons (DiClemente et al., 2004; Lauby et al., 2000; Peragallo et al., 2005). Others included STD clinic attendees, not only providing researchers with a convenience sample but a population with known behavioral risk factors (Bolu et al., 2004; Branson et al., 1998; NIMH, 1998; Kamb et al., 1998; Pealer, et al., 2004). One study targeted the chronically mentally ill from a community mental health clinic (Kalichman et al., 1995). Rotheram-Borus et al. (1998) noted that the positive intervention effects on social-cognitive mediators were found only for individuals with low-vulnerability scores at baseline. Bolu et al. (2004) reported that enhanced counseling intervention was more effective for persons who had an STD at baseline. Kirby et al. (2004) found greater intervention effect for subgroups with high-risk behaviors.

## Intervention Strategies

Intervention strategies varied by setting, dose, content, and method of delivery. The majority of the interventions were implemented in a community, non-clinical setting. Four were based in schools (Coyle et al., 2004; Jemmott et al., 1998; Kirby et al., 2004; Koniak-Griffin, Lesser, Nyamathi, et al., 2003) and three were based in community centers or agencies (Kalichman et al., 1995; Raj et al., 2001; Rotheram-Borus et al., 1998). Five interventions were implemented on a neighborhood level and involved community members from community-based organizations (Dancy et al., 2000; Kalichman et al., 1995; Kalichman et al., 1996; Lauby et al., 2000; Peragallo et al., 2005). One intervention was implemented in emergency and sober-living shelters (Nyamathi et al., 2001). The other interventions were implemented in clinics, the majority of which were STD or community-based clinics or a combination of both. No studies evaluated the impact that the setting of the program had on outcome measures.

Interventions ranged in the number of total sessions, the length of the sessions and the duration of the intervention. The total number of sessions ranged from 2 sessions (Jemmott et al., 1998; Kalichman et al., 1999) to 20 (Coyle et al., 2004). However, the majority of the interventions delivered their content over four sessions. Most sessions were 2 hours or less; however, six sessions ran over 2 hours (DiClemente et al., 2004; Jemmott et al., 1998; Kalichman et al., 1999; Nyamathi et al., 2001; Rotheram-Borus et al., 1998; Shain et al., 1999). Three interventions were implemented over a period lasting for more than a year (Coyle et al., 2004; Kirby et al., 2004; Lauby et al., 2000). The majority of the studies that reported the total length of their intervention ran for one month or less. One intervention had a booster session that was administered 2 months after program completion (Branson et al., 1998). However, only two studies specifically tested for the impact that time of exposure (the number of sessions, length of session, and duration of the intervention) had on their outcomes. Rotheram-Borus et al. (1998) found that longer sessions proved to be more effective in reducing the number of partners and increasing skills assessment scores (only for participants with low baseline scores) but reported mixed results for decreasing acts of risky sexual behaviors. Lauby et al. (2000) stated that there was a greater effect among women who reported exposure to the community intervention. Kamb et al. (1998) found that there was no treatment advantage of enhanced counseling over brief counseling. Although many studies included a control intervention that was delivered over a shorter period of time, the dose could not be compared because of differences in content.

Different content was covered in the interventions included in this review. The vast majority of studies report a risk reduction approach which targeted behavior change. Many of these interventions worked to build upon the participants' condom negotiation and partner communication skills (Boyer et al., 1997; Coyle et al., 2004; DiClemente et al., 2004; Flaskerud et al., 1997; Harvey et al., 2004; Kalichman et al., 1995; Kalichman et al., 1996; Kalichman et al., 1999; Kirby et al., 2004; Lauby et al., 2000; Nyamathi et al., 2001; Peragallo et al., 2005; Rotheram-Borus et al., 1998; Shain et al., 1999; Sikkema et al., 2000). Many studies also report teaching condom use skills (Coyle et al., 2004; DiClemente et al., 2004; Flaskerud et al., 1997; Harvey et al., 2004; Jemmott et al., 1998; Kalichman et al., 1999; Kirby et al., 2004; Koniak-Griffin, Lesser, Nyamathi, et al., 2003; Nyamathi et al., 2001; O'Donnell et al., 1998; Peragallo et al., 2005; Rotheram-Borus et al., 1998; Shain et al., 1999). The majority of interventions also included HIV and STD knowledge and education. In Nyamathi and colleagues' study (2001), having a culturally sensitive couple-approach design in which communication between the partners occurred in all three groups was found to decrease sexual risk behaviors in all groups; however self-esteem was impacted to an even greater extent in the nurse-led group. One study reported abstinence content. However, in this study subjects were randomized to one of three groups, abstinence only, safer sex, and health promotion (Jemmott et al., 1998). Results showed that the safer-sex intervention was more effective for increasing 100% condom use (short-term only) but that both the abstinence and safer-sex interventions increased condom use at 12 months. The safer-sex intervention group had higher scores on safer sex variables.

The content in some of the previously described interventions addressed other, more indirect risk factors that have been associated with HIV/AIDS and STD risk behaviors. Two interventions included violence prevention as a part of the intervention (Peragallo et al., 2005; Raj et al., 2001). Raj et al. (2001) included content relating to body image. Various studies also targeted factors associated with the Theory of Gender and Power and traditional male and female roles (DiClemente et al., 2004; Lesser et al., 2005; Raj et al., 2001). One study taught adolescent pregnant Latinas and African Americans about maternal roles in sex education, about sexual responsibility and accountability, and political awareness of the impact that HIV/AIDS had in their communities (Koniak-Griffin, Lesser, Uman, et al., 2003).

Various methods of delivery, ranging from individuals and small groups to community-wide events were used in the reviewed interventions. School-based interventions used the classroom setting and school-wide promotion programs. The majority of the interventions reported administering either all or some of their content through small group sessions consisting of 5–15 people. The intervention described by Boyer et al. (1997) and PROJECT RESPECT (Bolu et al., 2004; Kamb et al., 1998; Pealer et al., 2004) were the only two interventions that delivered their content through individual counseling alone. Three interventions combined individual and small group activities (Branson et al., 1998; Flaskerud et al., 1997; O'Donnell et al., 1998). Several intervention studies reported taking various approaches to the administration of their content, including neighborhood, community, or school activities, small group sessions, and individual counseling (Coyle et al., 2004; Kirby et al., 2004; Nyamathi et al., 2001; Shain et al., 1999; Sikkema et al., 2000). Only one study evaluated the impact that different methods of delivery had on outcome measures (O'Donnell et al., 1998). This study compared a video-only to a video-and-small-group intervention and found no treatment advantage for the expanded intervention.

The majority of facilitators were matched based on race and ethnicity or gender. Only Pealer et al. (2004) examined specific counselor or counselor-client effects and found that matching was not associated with any outcome measures. Eight of the interventions included peer facilitators (Dancy et al., 2000; DiClemente et al.,

2004; Jemmott et al., 1998; Kirby et al., 2004; Lauby et al., 2000; Nyamathi et al., 2001; Peragallo et al., 2005; Sikkema et al., 2000). The majority of interventions not using peers employed trained facilitators (Boyer et al., 1997; Harvey et al., 2004; Kalichman et al., 1996; Kalichman et al., 1995; Kirby et al., 2004; Sikkema et al., 2000) or health professionals who had formal HIV/STD training. Professional facilitators included nurses (Koniak-Griffin, Lesser, Nyamathi, et al., 2003; Nyamathi et al., 2001), health educators (Coyle et al., 2004), counselors (Bolu et al., 2004; Branson et al., 1998; Kamb et al., 1998; O'Donnell et al., 1998; Pealer et al., 2004; Peragallo et al., 2005; Shain et al., 1999), educators (DiClemente et al., 2004; Kirby et al., 2004) and public health workers or outreach specialists (Flaskerud et al., 1997; Kalichman et al., 1999; Raj et al., 2001). Coyle et al. (2004) used an HIV infected person as a facilitator. Nyamathi et al. (2001) conducted the only study examining the impact of facilitator training on outcomes. Results showed that the intervention implemented by nurse case-managers was more effective in improving AIDS knowledge and decreasing depression and hostility among participants than the peer-managed intervention.

## Design

The studies in this review were all controlled trials except for Flaskerud et al. (1997) which used a prospective longitudinal design. The studies evaluated outcomes for experimental and control conditions. All studies used some way to randomly assign subjects to control and experimental groups either individually or by group. For some studies the recruitment location was the basis of assignment. Assignment was made by school (Coyle et al., 2004; Kirby et al., 2004; Koniak-Griffin, Lesser, Nyamathi, et al., 2003), clinic (Raj et al., 2001), shelter (Nyamathi et al., 2001), small group (Branson et al., 1998), or day of clinic visit (O'Donnell et al., 1998). The remainder of the studies made the assignment on an individual level. PROJECT RESPECT used random assignment at the individual level within geographic location (Bolu et al., 2004; Kamb et al., 1998; Pealer et al., 2004). Two articles reported community intervention evaluations using matched communities (Lauby et al., 2000; Dancy et al., 2000) and another used matched housing developments (Sikkema et al., 2000).

   Most studies were designed to measure outcomes immediately post-intervention and at one or more follow-up times. Eleven studies reported follow-up data for 12 months (Bolu et al., 2004; Branson et al., 1998; DiClemente et al., 2004; Flaskerud et al., 1997; Jemmott et al., 1998; Kamb et al., 1998; Koniak-Griffin, Lesser, Nyamathi, et al., 2003; NIMH, 1998; Pealer et al., 2004; Shain et al., 1999; Sikkema et al., 2000) and one for 9 months (Dancy et al., 2000). Many of these studies also measured outcome variables at interim periods. One community-wide intervention with activities over the course of 2 years measured outcome in two separate surveys, at baseline and at the end of the intervention (Lauby et al., 2000). Two school-wide interventions conducted yearly assessments (Coyle et al., 2004; Kirby et al., 2004). Five studies followed the participants for 6 months (Lesser et al., 2005; Nyamathi et al., 2001; Peragallo et al., 2005; Harvey et al., 2004; Kalichman et al., 1999) and one study (Boyer et al., 1997) concluded the assessment after 5 months. Two shorter studies included 3-month follow-up periods (Kalichman et al., 1996; Rotheram-Borus et al., 1998) and two ended at 2 months (Raj et al., 2001; Kalichman et al., 1995). O'Donnell et al. (1998) tracked subjects for an average of 17 months but ended the follow-up at the time of diagnosis of a new STD infection.

Regression models and generalized estimating equations were most commonly used statistical methods to make inferences about the intervention effect. The regression models allowed the researcher to compare the effect of the intervention while taking into account possible intervening variables such as knowledge, attitudes, prior behavior, gender, race, or age. Other studies reported findings from analysis of covariance and repeated measures analysis of variance. Studies also reported results of t-tests or chi square analysis.

## Outcome Measures

Outcome measures included incidence of new STDs, self-report of behaviors (e.g., condom use, number of partners), skills demonstration (e.g., appropriate condom use), and a variety of variables identified as antecedents of behavior change (e.g., behavioral intentions) collected through interviews and surveys. Ten studies evaluated the interventions by reporting the incidence of STDs post intervention (Bolu et al., 2004; Boyer et al., 1997; Branson et al., 1998; DiClemente et al., 2004; Flaskerud et al., 1997; Kamb et al., 1998; NIMH, 1998; O'Donnell et al., 1998; Pealer et al., 2004; Shain et al., 1999). While the majority of these studies tested for several STDs, Flaskerud et al. (1997) only screened for HIV and the NIMH (1998) multi-site HIV prevention trial tested for gonorrhea. Only three of these interventions were effective in reducing the incidence of STDs (DiClemente et al., 2004; Kamb et al., 1998; Shain et al., 1999).

Although virtually every study included in this review used condom use as one of the primary outcome measures, only nine studies reported an intervention effect to increase condom use (DiClemente et al., 2004; Flaskerud et al., 1997; Kalichman et al., 1999; Kamb et al., 1998; Kirby et al., 2004; Koniak-Griffin, Lesser, Nyamathi, et al., 2003; Lauby et al., 2000; NIMH, 1998; Rotheram-Borus et al., 1998), whereas Nyamathi et al. (2001) reported significant sexual risk reduction behavior (monogamous sex and fewer unprotected sex encounters) at 6 months across all three groups, highlighting the importance of both couple communication and the use of a culturally competent standard approaches to risk behavior modification. Four of these were effective in increasing 100% con-dom use (DiClemente et al., 2004; Lauby et al., 2000; Kamb et al., 1998; NIMH, 1998).

A wide-range of risk and protective outcome measures were used to evalu-ate the effectiveness of the interventions reviewed. Various studies assessed risky behaviors by monitoring the frequency of sexual intercourse (Boyer et al., 1997; Branson et al., 1998; Coyle et al., 2004; Jemmott et al., 1998; Koniak-Griffin, Lesser, Uman et al., 2003; Nyamathi et al., 2001). Only the interven-tion reported by Coyle et al. (2004) was effective in reducing the frequency of sex among its participants (middle school students) for a period longer than 3 months. However, this was only seen among male participants. Some interven-tions targeting middle- and high-school students also assessed for time of first sexual encounter (Kirby et al., 2004) and ever having sexual intercourse or hav-ing sexual intercourse within the last 12 months (Coyle et al., 2004)). There were no intervention effects on these outcomes. Many studies reported the num-ber of lifetime partners (Branson et al., 1998; Coyle et al., 2004; Koniak-Griffin, Lesser, Nyamathi, et al., 2003; Rotheram-Borus et al., 1998) or the number of current partners (Nyamathi et al. 2001; Shain et al., 1999). Kamb et al. (1998) included having a new or casual partner as one of the outcome measures. Shain et al. (1999) included having sexual intercourse with an untreated partner and compliance to medication. Four interventions were effective in reducing these risky sexual practices (Kamb et al., 1998; Koniak-Griffin, Lesser, Nyamathi, et al., 2003; Rotheram-Borus et al., 1998; Shain et al., 1999).

Many studies used skills, knowledge, beliefs and attitudes as well as other psychosocial and theoretical variables that have been identified as precursors to behavioral change to measure the success of their interventions. Condom nego-tiation skills and partner communication skills were measured in many studies. Although the majority of these studies assessed condom negotiation and partner communication skills through questionnaires and interviews, Rotheram-Borus et al. (1998) used role-playing to measure these outcomes. Observed condom appli-cation skills were evaluated in two studies (DiClemente et al., 2004; Rotheram-Borus et al., 1998). The evaluation conducted by Sikkema et al. (2000) was the only study that measured condom negotiation and communication skills found no intervention effect on these outcomes.

Knowledge of condom use and HIV/STDs was also measured by many stud-ies. The interventions described by Boyer et al. (1997), Kalichman et al. (1996), and Nyamathi et al. (2001) were the only treatments that did effect HIV/STD knowledge. Many studies also measured psychosocial and theoretical or concep-tual mediators. Some of these measured perceived peer norms about condom use (Peragallo et al., 2005), psychological well-being and depression, anxiety, and hostility (Nyamathi et al., 2001), perceived vulnerability to STDs and HIV

(Dancy et al., 2000; Flaskerud et al., 1997; Rotheram-Borus et al., 1998; Sikkema et al., 2000) and self esteem and self-efficacy (Dancy et al., 2000; Koniak-Griffin, Lesser, Uman et al., 2003; Nyamathi et al., 2001; Rotheram-Borus et al., 1998). More than half the studies measuring psychosocial and theoretical mediators reported a sustained positive intervention effect (Boyer et al., 1997; Coyle et al., 2004; DiClemente et al., 2004; Jemmott et al., 1998; Koniak-Griffin et al., 2003; Sikkema et al., 2000).

## SUMMARY OF EFFECTIVE STRATEGIES

All of the interventions that had an impact on acquisition of new STDs focused on building skills. Both DiClemente et al. (2004) and Shain et al. (1999) included condom negotiation and partner communication in the interventions, delivered the curriculum in small groups and matched the facilitators based on ethnicity or race and gender. Project Respect's content focused on goal setting and risk reduction planning and delivered the content through individual risk reduction counseling (Bolu et al., 2004; Kamb et al., 1998; Pealer et al., 2004).

Only four intervention studies were successful in increasing condom use. The intervention described by Lauby et al. (2000) was implemented community-wide through safer-sex events and community workshops on risk reduction. Other effective interventions were implemented in community clinics. DiClemente et al. (2004) focused on communication and negotiation skills, Kamb et al. (1998) focused on content tailored to the individual's risk through counseling, and NIMH (1998) focused on risk reduction strategies that were based on best practices such as delivering content in small group sessions and including outcome expectancies, skills, and self-efficacy.

Almost all the studies that measured partner communication and condom negotiation content were effective in increasing these skills. However, none of these studies reported both a positive intervention effect on skills and a sustained impact on sexual risk behaviors. Various interventions that reported an increase in HIV/STD knowledge and a positive treatment effect on psychosocial mediators also reported behavior change (Coyle et al., 2004; DiClemente et al., 2004; Jemmott et al., 1998; Koniak-Griffin, Lesser, Nyamathi, et al., 2003; Nyamathi et al., 2001; Sikkema et al., 2000; Dancy et al., 2000). All of these interventions were delivered in a non-clinical community setting and used group sessions as one of their methods of program delivery. Other methods included women to women conversations and community events (Sikkema et al., 2000). In addition to condom negotiation and partner communication training, other interventions also included condom demonstration (Coyle et al., 2004; DiClemente et al., 2004) and self-efficacy (Jemmott et al., 1998).

## DESIGN AND METHODOLOGY LIMITATIONS

Many design and methodological limitations need to be considered when comparing the samples, settings, intervention strategies, outcome variables, and results in the articles included in this review. Most studies used convenience samples recruited from STD clinics, schools, and community agencies. These recruitment strategies along with high attrition rates limit the generalizability of the results reported by these studies. Interventions were developed for various populations targeting specific age, race and ethnicity, gender, and other demographic factors. Lack of uniformity in methods for program implementation and content make it difficult to compare interventions. Additionally, few researchers assessed how program implementation methods, such as counselor-client dynamic, dose and intensity of the intervention, and intervention strategies, impacted the outcome measures. Therefore, it is not possible to identify which strategies are most effective for the different target populations.

Another limitation in comparing across studies is the lack of uniformity in the outcome variables used to evaluate intervention strategies. Studies have shown that clinical tests for STDs provide the most reliable indication of the final intervention effectiveness (Harrington et al., 2001). However, the majority of the studies used self-reported behaviors such as condom use to predict likely exposure and incidence of STDs in the future. Self-reported behaviors may not reflect the true intervention effect of prevention programs. Additionally, condom use was measured differently by the researchers. While some used self-reported 100% condom use, many used other measures such as behavioral intention or frequency of use. Consistent or 100% condom use should be the behavioral outcome of interest because inconsistent condom use does not protect against STDs (The Medical Institute, 2005). Many studies also included skills, knowledge, attitudes, and beliefs as outcome measures. However, positive intervention effects on these outcomes do not necessarily translate into behavior change and risk reduction. Lastly, follow-up periods were short, making it difficult to assess long-term program effects.

It is also important to consider the limitations of the data collection methods. While some studies used surveys, others used face-to-face interviews. Different data collection techniques were used, few of which were blinded to the assignment of the individual being interviewed. Little is known about how data collectors were trained and whether data collections tools and scales had been validated among the target populations. All of these factors introduce bias relating to the literacy, language, and reporting of behaviors, affecting the quality of the data that were collected and the interpretation of results.

## TRANSLATING FINDINGS INTO PRACTICE

HIV and STD prevention programs can be separated between risk-avoidance and risk-reduction strategies. In response to the U.S. HIV epidemic of the 1980s among men who have sex with men and injection drug users, an HIV prevention model was developed to target risk behaviors which focused on condom promotion, screening and treatment, and providing clean needles (The Medical Institute, 2005). This risk reduction model has been adapted and implemented among the other high risk populations in the United States. Although most of the interventions summarized in this review used risk reduction strategies, the more effective intervention strategies appear to be programs that address the risk factors and socioeconomic and cultural factors that were specific to their target population. Because the majority of the studies targeted females, the more effective strategies included not just education and condom availability, but also skills training in safer sex negotiation and partner communication. However, not many of these studies reported a positive intervention effect on these outcome measures. Tailoring program content to the risk factors associated with the target population may lead to more promising program effects. This strategy has also been supported by other experts in the field of HIV prevention (Ellen, 2003; The Medical Institute, 2005). Ellen (2003) conducted a review on effective primary HIV prevention interventions for female adolescents and suggested that there is epidemiological evidence that future interventions need to focus on social cohesion and parenting skills, other risk factors such as lack of control over sexual behaviors and condom use, and sexual risk networks that traditional risk-reduction interventions have not addressed in the past.

## IMPLICATIONS FOR FUTURE RESEARCH AND POLICY

Although a great deal of nursing research has focused on assessing STD risk factors among vulnerable groups, there are only a few published articles describing primary prevention nursing interventions developed and implemented among these populations. While it is important to first understand risk factors among vulnerable groups in the United States in order to develop effective strategies, nurses need to start moving toward action. By working more closely with other disciplines that have contributed to prevention research, nurses can become an increasingly important agent in the prevention of STDs and HIV. However, in order to move forward, greater caution is needed when research methods are being developed. By more carefully designing the recruitment process, selecting more reliable outcome measures that are consistent across studies, evaluating long-term program effects, and evaluating results according to differences in demographic and risk factors among participants, more can be learned about effective primary prevention strategies.

## REFERENCES

Bolu, O. O., Lindsey, C., Kamb, M. L., Kent, C., Zenilman, J., & Douglas, J. M., et al. (2004). Is HIV/sexually transmitted disease prevention counseling effective among vulnerable populations?: A subset analysis of data collected for a randomized, controlled trial evaluating counseling efficacy (PROJECT RESPECT). *Sexually Transmitted Diseases, 31*(8), 469–474.

Boyer, C. B., Barret, D. C., Peterman, T. A., & Bolan, G. (1997). Sexually transmitted disease (STD) and HIV risk in heterosexual adults attending a public STD clinic: Evaluation of a randomized controlled behavioral risk-reduction intervention trial. *AIDS, 11*(3), 359–367.

Branson, B. M., Peterman, T. A., Cannon, R. O., Ransom, R., & Zaidi, A. A. (1998). Group counseling to prevent sexually transmitted disease and HIV: A randomized controlled trial. *Sexually Transmitted Diseases, 25*(10), 553–560.

Centers for Disease Control. (2002). *Fact sheet—Young people at risk: HIV/AIDS among America's youth.* Retrieved April 12, 2005, from http://www.cdc.gov/hiv/pubs/facts/youth.htm

Centers for Disease Control. (2003). *STD surveillance: Special focus profile.* Retrieved April 13, 2005, from http://www.cdc.gov/std/stats/toc2003.htm

Centers for Disease Control. (2004). *Fact sheet—HIV/AIDS among women.* Retrieved April 12, 2005, from http://www.cdc.gov/hiv/pubs/facts/women.htm

Centers for Disease Control. (2005a). *Fact sheet—HIV/AIDS among African Americans.* Retrieved April 12, 2005, from http://www.cdc.gov/hiv/pubs/Facts/afam.htm

Centers for Disease Control. (2005b). *Fact sheet—HIV/AIDS among Hispanics.* Retrieved April 12, 2005, from http://www.cdc.gov/hiv/pubs/Facts/hispanic.htm

Chou, F. Y., Holzemer, W. L., Portillo, C. J., & Slaughter, R. (2004). Self-care strategies and sources of information for HIV/AIDS symptom management. *Nursing Research, 53*(5), 332–339.

Coverdale, J. H., & Turbott, S. H. (2000). Risk behaviors for sexually transmitted diseases among men with mental disorders. *Psychiatric Services, 51*(2), 234–238.

Coyle, K. K., Kirby, D. B., Marin, B. V., Gomez, C. A., & Gregorich, S. E. (2004). Draw the line/respect the line: A randomized trial of a middle school intervention to reduce sexual risk behaviors. *Research & Practice, 94*(5), 849–851.

Crespo-Fierro, M. (1997). Compliance/adherence and care management in HIV disease. *Journal of the Association of Nurses in AIDS Care, 8*(4), 43–54.

Dancy, B. L., Marcantiono, R., & Norr, K. (2000). The long-term effectiveness of an HIV prevention intervention for low-income African American women. *AIDS Education & Prevention, 12*(2), 113–125.

Department of Health and Human Services. (2004). *What is Healthy People 2010?* Retrieved April 20, 2005, from http://www.healthypeople.gov/About/hpfact.htm

DiClemente, R. J., Wingood, G. M., Harrington, K. F., Lang, D. L., Davies, S. L., & Hook, E. W., et al. (2004). Efficacy of an HIV prevention intervention for African-American adolescent girls: A randomized controlled trial. *JAMA: Journal of the American Medical Association, 292*(2), 171–179.

Duffy, L. (2005). Suffering, shame and silence: The stigma of HIV/AIDS. *Journal of the Association of Nurses in AIDS Care, 16*(1), 13–20.

Ellen, J. M. (2003). The next generation of HIV prevention for adolescent females in the United States: Linking behavioral and epidemiologic sciences to reduce incidence of HIV. *Journal of Urban Health, 80*(4; Supplement 3), iii40-iii49.

Flaskerud, J. H., Nyamathi, A. M., & Uman, G. C. (1997). Longitudinal effect of an HIV testing and counseling program for low-income Latina women. *Ethnicity and Health, 2*(1/2), 89–103.

Guenter, D., Majumdar, B., & Williams, D. (2005). Community-based HIV education and prevention workers respond to a changing environment. *Journal of the Association of Nurses in AIDS Care, 16*(1), 29–36.

Harrington, K. F., DiClemente, R. J., Wingood, G. M, Crosby, R. A., Person, S., Oh, M. K., & Hook, E. W. (2001). Validity of self-reported sexually transmitted diseases among African American female adolescents participating in an HIV/STD prevention intervention trial. *Sexually Transmitted Disease, 28*(8), 468–471.

Harvey, S. M., Henderson, J. T., Thorburn, S., Beckman, L. J., Casillas, A., & Mendez, L., et al. (2004). A randomized study of a pregnancy and disease prevention intervention for Hispanic couples. *Perspectives on Sexual and Reproductive Health, 36*(4), 162–169.

Jemmott J. B., Jemmott, L. S., & Fong, G. T. (1998). Abstinence and safer sex HIV risk-reduction interventions for African-American adolescents: A randomized controlled trial. *JAMA: Journal of the American Medical Association, 279*(19), 1529–1536.

Kalichman, S. C., Cherry, C., & Browne-Sperling, F. (1999). Effectiveness of a video-based motivational skills-building HIV risk-reduction intervention for inner-city African-American men. *Journal of Consulting & Clinical Psychology, 67*(6), 959–966.

Kalichman, S. C., Rompa, D., & Coley, B. (1996). Experimental component analysis of a behavioral HIV-AIDS prevention intervention for inner-city women. *Journal of Consulting & Clinical Psychology, 64*(4), 687–693.

Kalichman, S. C., Sikkema, K. J., Kelly, J. A., & Bulto, M. (1995). Use of a brief behavioral skills intervention to prevent HIV infection among chronic mentally ill adults. *Psychiatric Services, 46*(3), 275–280.

Kamb, M. L., Fishbein, M., Douglas, J. M., Rhodes, F., Rogers, J., Bolan, G., et al. (1998). Efficacy of risk-reduction counseling to prevent human immunodeficiency virus and sexually transmitted diseases: A randomized controlled trial. PROJECT RESPECT study group. *Journal of American Medical Association, 280*(13), 1161–1167.

Kirby, D. B., Baumler, E., Coyle, K. K., Basen-Engquist, K., Parcel, G. S., Harrist, R., et al. (2004). The "safer choices" intervention: Its impact on the sexual behaviors of different subgroups of high school students. *Journal of Adolescent Health, 35*(6), 442–452.

Koniak-Griffin, D., & Brecht, M. L. (1995). Linkages between sexual risk-taking, substance use, and AIDS knowledge among pregnant adolescents and young mothers. *Nursing Research, 44*, 340–346.

Koniak-Griffin, D., Lesser, J., Nyamathi, A., Uman, G., Stein, J. A., & Cumberland, W. G. (2003). Project CHARM: An HIV prevention program for adolescent mothers. *Family Community Health, 26*(2), 94–107.

Koniak-Griffin, D., Lesser, J., Uman, G., & Nyamathi, A. (2003). Teen pregnancy, motherhood, and unprotected sexual activity. *Research in Nursing & Health, 26,* 4–19.

Lauby, J. L., Smith, P. J., Stark, M., Person, B., & Adams, J. (2000). A community-level HIV prevention intervention for inner-city women: Results of the women and infants demonstration projects. *American Journal of Public Health, 90*(2), 216–222.

Lesser, J., Verdugo, R. L., Koniak-Griffin, D., Tello, J., Kappos, B., & Cumberland, W. G. (2005). Respecting and protecting our relationships: A community research HIV prevention program for teen fathers and mothers. *AIDS Education and Prevention, 17,* 347–360.

Mayo, K., White, S., Oates, S. K., & Franklin, F. (1996). Community-collaboration: Prevention and control of tuberculosis in a homeless shelter. *Public Health Nursing, 13*(2), 120–127.

McCusker, J., Goldstein, R., Bigelow, C., & Zorn, M. (1995). Psychiatric status and HIV risk reduction among residential drug abuse treatment clients. *Addiction (90),* 1377–1387.

National Institute of Mental Health. (1998). The NIMH Multisite HIV prevention trial: Reducing HIV sexual risk behavior. *Science, 280*(5371), 1889–94.

National Institute of Nursing Research. (2005). *Mission statement.* Retrieved April 20, 2005, from http://ninr.nih.gov/ninr/research/diversity/mission.html

Nyamathi, A., Flaskerud, J. H., Leake, B., Dixon, E. L., & Lu, A. (2001). Evaluating the impact of peer, nurse case-managed, and standard HIV risk-reduction programs on psychosocial and health-promoting behavioral outcomes among homeless women. *Research in Nursing & Health, 24*(5), 410–422.

O'Donnell, C. R., O'Donnell, L., San Doval, A., Duran, R., & Labes, K. (1998). Reductions in STD infections subsequent to an STD clinic visit: Using video-based patient education to supplement provider interactions. *Sexually Transmitted Diseases, 25*(3), 161–168.

Pealer, L. N., Peterman, T. A., Newman, D. R., Kamb, M. L., Dillon, B., & Malotte, C. K., et al. (2004). Are counselor demographics associated with successful human immunodeficiency virus/sexually transmitted disease prevention counseling? *Sexually Transmitted Diseases, 31*(1), 52–56.

Peragallo, N., DeForge, B., O'Campo, P, Lee, S. M., Kim, Y. J., Cianelli, R. et al. (2005). A randomized clinical trial of an HIV-risk-reduction intervention among low-income Latina women. *Nursing Research, 54* (2), 108–118.

Plowden, K. O., Fletcher, A. & Miller, J. L. (2005). Factors influencing HIV-risk behaviors among HIV-positive urban African Americans. *Journal of the Association of Nurses in AIDS care, 16,* (1), 21–28.

Rahav, M., Nuttbrock, L., Rivera, J. J., & Link, B. G. (1998). HIV infection risks among homeless, mentally ill, chemical misusing men. *Substance Use Misuse, 33*(6), 1407–1426.

Raj, A., Amaro, H., Cranston, K., Martin, B., Cabral, H., Navarro, A., et al. (2001). Is a general women's health promotion program as effective as an HIV-intensive prevention program in reducing HIV risk among Hispanic women? *Public Health Reports, 116*(6), 599–607.

Rotheram-Borus, M. J., Gwadz, M., Fernandez, M. I., & Srinivasan, S. (1998). Timing of HIV interventions on reductions in sexual risks among adolescents. *American Journal of Community Psychology, 26* (1), 73–98.

Shain, R. N., Piper, J. M., Newton, E. R., Perdue, S. T., Ramos, R., Champion, J. D., et al. (1999). A randomized, controlled trial of a behavioral intervention to prevent sexually transmitted disease among minority women. *The New England Journal of Medicine, 340*(2), 93–100.

Sikkema, K. J., Kelly, J. A., Winett, R. A., Solomon, L. J., Cargill, V. A., Roffman, R. A., et al. (2000). Outcomes of a randomized community-level HIV prevention intervention for women living in 18 low-income housing developments. *American Journal of Public Health, 90*(1), 57–63.

The Medical Institute. (2005). *Evidence that demands action: Comparing risk avoidance and risk reduction strategies for HIV preventions.* Austin, TX: The Medical Institute.

Villarruel, A. M., Jemmott, J. B., 3rd, Jemmott, L. S., & Ronis, D. L. (2004). Predictors of sexual intercourse and condom use intentions among Spanish-dominant Latino youth: A test of the planned behavior theory. *Nursing Research, 53*(3), 172–181.

Williams, A. B., Burgesess, J. D., Danvers, K., Malone, J., Winfield, S. D., & Saunders, L. (2005). Kitchen table wisdom: A Freirian approach to medication adherence. *Journal of the Association of Nurses in AIDS Care, 16*(1), 3–12.

# Chapter 5

## Promoting Research Partnerships to Reduce Health Disparities Among Vulnerable Populations: Sharing Expertise Between Majority Institutions and Historically Black Universities

M. Katherine Hutchinson, Bertha Davis, Loretta Sweet Jemmott, Susan Gennaro, Lorraine Tulman, Esther H. Condon, Arlene J. Montgomery, and E. Jane Servonsky

### ABSTRACT

*This chapter focuses on promoting cultural competence in research and the care of vulnerable populations by establishing inter-university nursing partnership centers for health disparities research between historically Black universities and minority-serving*

*institutions and research-intensive majority institutions. The Hampton-Penn Center to Reduce Health Disparities (HPC), an inter-university collaborative center funded through the National Institutes of Health (NIH) National Institute of Nursing Research (NINR) P20 funding mechanism, is discussed as the exemplar. The mission of the Hampton-Penn Center is to promote culturally competent research on health promotion and disease prevention and the examination of how culture, race and ethnicity and their interactions with the health care system and the larger society influence health outcomes and the occurrence of health disparities. The history, goals, and conceptual model underlying this collaborative effort between the University of Pennsylvania and Hampton University Schools of Nursing are described as are the accomplishments and lessons learned to date. Based upon the Hampton-Penn experience, recommendations for similar collaborations to reduce health disparities among vulnerable populations are made in three major areas: (a) increasing the study of the multi-system level factors that contribute to health disparities among vulnerable populations, (b) promoting the development of culturally competent research on health disparities, and (c) promoting the recruitment and training of health researchers who are themselves members of vulnerable populations.*

Keywords: nursing research; cultural diversity; health disparities

## INTRODUCTION

In late 2001, the National Institutes of Health (NIH), the National Institute of Nursing Research (NINR), and the National Center on Minority Health and Health Disparities (NCMHD) issued a request for proposals, "Nursing Partnership Centers on Health Disparities" (RFA-NR-02–004), which called for the development of collaborative research centers to "foster development of nursing partnerships between researchers, faculty and students at minority serving institutions (MSIs) and institutions with established health disparity research programs" (NINR, 2001, p. 1). In response to this call, the University of Pennsylvania and Hampton University Schools of Nursing, building upon a long-standing history of collaboration, submitted a proposal to establish the Hampton-Penn Center to Reduce Health Disparities (HPC) (P20 NR008361) (Jemmott et al., 2002). A cornerstone of the HPC has been the emphasis on fostering inter-university collegiality and collaboration between research-intensive institutions and historically minority-serving, educationally focused institutions. The HPC experience to date has shown that this type of collaborative effort can be both productive and mutually beneficial. This chapter focuses on the resultant HPC, its conceptual framework, goals, accomplishments, and lessons learned through its first 3 years of funding.

Diversity is increasing in the United States, and according to the 2000 U.S. Census, approximately 30% of the population belongs to a racial or ethnic minority group. African Americans constitute approximately 13% of the population, almost 35 million individuals. The Census Bureau projects that by the year 2035, African Americans will constitute approximately 14.3% of the U.S. population, more than 50 million African Americans. The Bureau further projects that by the year 2100, non-Hispanic Whites will make up only 40% of the U.S. population.

Racial and ethnic minorities are less likely to have health insurance and more likely to experience adverse health outcomes and conditions than Whites. In 2003, 20% of African Americans, 33% of Hispanics, and 19% of Asians were without health insurance year round compared to 11% of Whites (Rockeymoore, 2005). According to the National Center for Health Statistics, the age-adjusted death rate for African Americans was higher than that of Whites by 41% for stroke, 30% for heart disease, 25% for cancer, and more than 750% for HIV disease in 2002 (National Center for Health Statistics, 2002; Rockeymoore, 2005). Other disparities in health outcomes experienced by racial and ethnic minorities include shorter life expectancies, higher rates of cancer, birth defects, infant mortality, asthma, diabetes, and HIV/AIDS (Smedley, Stith, & Nelson, 2002). Without comprehensive strategies that address the multiplicity of factors that contribute to these health disparities, the gap will only continue to widen. Hence, programs and strategies are urgently needed to reduce health disparities that currently exist among Americans who are members of racial and ethnic minority groups. The HPC was proposed and funded to foster health promotion and disease prevention research that considers cultural, ethnic and health care system factors as contributors to the health and illness of vulnerable minority populations (Jemmott et al., 2002).

Vulnerable populations are those persons who are at risk for poor physical, psychological, or social health (Aday, 2001). Although exact definitions vary by author, most agree that vulnerable populations are those groups who possess fewer resources and experience greater exposure to risk with resultant increases in morbidity, mortality, and decreases in life expectancy and quality of life (Dixon, et al., in press; Flaskerud & Winslow, 1998). Vulnerable populations can best be studied from a theoretical perspective that addresses caring within a cultural context (de Chesnay, 2005). De Chesnay proposes taking a systems approach and aggregate view to understand vulnerability in context. This approach requires that health care professionals must address issues related to both groups, clients, and health care providers, as contributors to vulnerability.

The elimination of health disparities among vulnerable populations was identified as one of the Department of Health and Human Services' (DHHS) two overarching goals for Healthy People 2010 (DHHS, 2001). NINR has designated minority health and health disparities research as an institutional priority and has followed through in both word and action in its mission statement, strategic plan, and allocation of resources. As Dixon and her associates (in press) point out, NINR allocated a significant portion of its 1999 budget of $138 million to addressing minority health and health disparities among vulnerable populations. As part of this effort to alleviate health disparities, NINR has convened task forces, set aside funding, and issued specific requests for proposals and the establishment of research centers to address minority health issues and health disparities.

## Establishment of Nursing Partnership Centers on Health Disparities

In late 2001, in collaboration with the National Center on Minority Health and Health Disparities (NCMHD), the NINR undertook further action to eradicate health disparities by issuing a request for proposal (RFA) calling for the establishment of inter-university partnerships and centers for health disparities research. RFA-NR-02–004, "Nursing Partnership Centers on Health Disparities," was intended to "increase the capacity for health disparities research and increase the support of research aimed at elucidating the etiology of health disparities" (NINR, 2001, p. 3). The purpose was to increase the capacity for nursing research in health disparities by encouraging the formation of partnerships between minority and majority institutions and increasing the number of researchers in minority health and health disparities (NINR, 2001, p. 3). The specific aims for these Nursing Partnership Centers were to: "(1) expand the cadre of nurse researchers in minority health or health disparities research, (2) increase the number of research projects aimed at eliminating health disparities, and (3) enhance the career development of potential minority nurse investigators." (NINR, 2001, p. 1).

This request for proposal provided the funding for the establishment of a 5-year program to develop more intensive research programs by creating partnerships between schools of nursing with established track records in health disparities research and schools of nursing with significant numbers of minority students (Grady, 2001). Centers were to be funded through the P20 Exploratory Center Grant mechanism, the purpose of which is to "support planning for new programs, expansion or modification of existing resources, and feasibility studies to explore various approaches to developing minority health/health disparities research programs that address areas consistent with the missions of NINR and NCMHD" (NINR, 2001, p. 2).

## Funded Centers

In 2002, NINR funded eight P20 inter-university nursing research centers focusing on health disparities (National Institute of Health [NIH], 2002; National

Institute of Nursing Research [NINR], n.d.). The funded centers, shown in Table 5.1, represent both geographical and cultural diversity. Each partnership includes at least one partner designated as a traditionally so-called minority-serving institution, and a partner with an established record in health disparities research, designated as the so-called majority institution. Some of these exploratory centers include partners that are in geographic proximity (e.g., University of North Carolina-Chapel Hill, Winston-Salem State University, and North Carolina Central University), whereas others are quite distant (e.g., University of Washington and University of Hawaii; University of California San Francisco and University of Puerto Rico).

Each of these partnership centers has its own specific focus, including the health needs of Asians and Pacific Islanders, health promotion and restoration in the Hispanic population, patient access to care and processes of care, minority groups living with HIV disease, culturally competent nursing research, and the health needs of rural, low-income Mexican American and American Indian populations (Grady, 2003). The eight partnership centers funded by NINR, their university partners, principal investigators, and primary foci are shown in Table 5.1.

Each of the centers have funded pilot studies within their specific areas of focus. For example, the University of California San Francisco-University of Puerto Rico partnership has funded pilot studies examining the symptom experience of Latina women with HIV; the providers perception of adherence of women to HIV medication protocols; the validation of a stigma scale among an HIV Puerto Rican population; and self-care management in HIV/AIDS. The Yale-Howard partnership has funded pilot studies examining Black women's views on menopause and midlife health risks; colorectal cancer knowledge, perceptions, and behaviors in African Americans; and nurses' impact on the quality life outcomes in minority family caregivers.

One of these P20-funded centers, the HPC is the focus of the remainder of this chapter. Below we describe and discuss the HPC, its history, focus, goals, accomplishments, and lessons learned to date.

## THE HAMPTON-PENN CENTER TO REDUCE HEALTH DISPARITIES

### History of the Partnership

Faculty at the University of Pennsylvania and Hampton University Schools of Nursing have a long history of collaboration and expertise in health disparities research that made them uniquely qualified to establish a formal partnership research center on health disparities. The resultant HPC thus represents a mutually beneficial, natural progression of the historical relationship that builds on

**TABLE 5.1** P20 Nursing Partnership Centers on Health Disparities Funded by NINR 2002–2007 (NIH, n.d.). Italics indicates the university designated as the Minority Serving Institution (MSI)

| Center | University Partners | Principal Investigators | Focus (Grady, 2003) |
|---|---|---|---|
| Center for Innovation in Health Disparities Research | Univ. of North Carolina-Chapel Hill *North Carolina Central University Winston-Salem State University* | C. McQuiston (UNC-CH) *J. Roland (NCCU)* *S. Flack (WSSU)* | Culturally competent nursing research |
| Center for Reducing Health Disparities by Self and Family Management | Yale University *Howard University* | M. Funk (YU) *D. Powell (HU)* | Self-management and self-assessment strategies in minority families |
| Center on Health Disparities Research | Johns Hopkins University *North Carolina A&T University* | F. Gaston-Johnson (JHU) *V. Whitaker (NCA&T)* | Access to care, process of care, and health outcomes |
| Hampton-Penn Center to Reduce Health Disparities | University of Pennsylvania *Hampton University* | L. Jemmott and S. Gennaro (UP) *B. Davis (HU)* | Influence of culture, race, and ethnicity on health promotion and prevention |
| MESA Center for Health Disparities | University of Michigan *University of Texas Health Science Center* | A. Villarruel (UM) *C. Braden (UTHSC)* | Health promotion and restoration among Hispanics |
| Nursing Research Center on HIV/AIDS Health Disparities | Univ. of California at San Francisco *University of Puerto Rico* | W. Holzemer (UCSF) *M. Rivero (UPRMS)* | Needs of minority groups living with HIV disease |
| Southwest Center: Partners in Health Disparities Research | University of Texas at Austin *New Mexico State University* | D. Rew (UTA) *M. Hoke (NMSU)* | Health needs of rural Mexican-Americans and American Indians |
| Center for Health Disparities Research | University of Washington *University of Hawaii, Manoa* | B. Berkowitz (UW) *M. McCubbin (UHM)* | Health needs of Asians and Pacific Islanders |

124

the acknowledged strengths of each school. The selected focus of this center concentrates on advancing culturally competent research that promotes health and prevents illness in diverse patient populations.

From the mid-1990s through 2002, faculty members from Hampton and Penn worked together on initiatives funded by both the Teagle Foundation and NINR. Faculty from Hampton have been postdoctoral fellows at Penn. Faculty from Penn have conducted seminars on the development of doctoral programs at Hampton and research training workshops on strategies for translating clinical practice into research and strategies for building a program of research. Faculties from both schools have worked together in the Summer Nursing Research Institute at Penn. This ongoing collaboration has been facilitated by Dr. Loretta Sweet Jemmott, who is an alumna of both Hampton (BSN, 1978) and Penn (MSN, 1982; PhD, 1987), was elected to the Hampton School of Nursing Hall of Fame in 1994, and named an outstanding alumna in 2000.

## Hampton University School of Nursing

Hampton is a historically Black university with linkages throughout the contiguous areas of Southeast Virginia and beyond. The 110-year-old School of Nursing has provided care for underserved communities since its inception. In 1985, the Hampton University Nursing Center and Health Mobile were established to insure accessibility to health care for impoverished communities; these have resulted in the development of trusting relationships with community leaders and members, who are necessary in the recruitment of participants for research. These relationships are invaluable to faculty and researchers as they seek to identify community needs and priorities and develop community-based participatory research projects.

Hampton's Center for Minority Family Health is a focal point for research on people of color and a repository for information on families, with an emphasis on minority families. The primary goal of the Center is to provide opportunities for faculty and students to collaborate with global researchers on family health issues, such as the family's response to illness, social factors affecting family health, family factors in health promotion and disease prevention, and models for delivering primary and community-based health care to families in crisis. The Center for Minority Family Health cooperates with the Hampton University Nursing Center, the Hampton Behavioral Sciences Research Center, Hampton School of Pharmacy, and professional schools at other institutions where an emphasis on health disparities forms a common denominator. These collaborations are leading to greater access to care for the medically underserved and assisting in providing a more global perspective for students from each participating institution. The center convenes an annual health summit in conjunction with Hampton

University's Conference on the Black Family, a 25-year-old international event bringing in experts with innovative approaches to issues on and about the Black family's experience in America.

Ongoing research at Hampton University occurs around a broad range of ages and conditions. Earlier studies at Hampton's School of Nursing revolved around adolescents and elderly populations and the maladies that affect them. Through the Nursing Center, a faculty-student practice model was used, which led to increased interest in children and parents. Nursing faculty members have received funding from the National Institute for Mental Health, which broadened the school's research base to include behavioral studies underlying physical and mental pathology in families. All of this previous work strengthened the school's research framework around family and family-related research. The establishment of the Center for Minority Family Health in 2002, under the direction of Dr. Cheryl Killion, served as the umbrella for bringing all research interests in the school into focus. Because of the historical mission of minority serving institutions, Hampton's faculty has had heavy teaching and clinical emphasis that has resulted in the development of expertise in clinical issues and the provision of culturally competent care to diverse populations. This expertise serves both institutions well as they plan and conduct research supported by the HPC.

During the 1990s, the Hampton University School of Nursing administration and faculty strategically made a decision to increase a focus on the research arm of the academic triad (research, practice, and education). With that in mind, the school planned its research trajectory in two approaches: faculty development in research training and grant funding for faculty members with PhDs and faculty development in planning, creating, and implementing a doctoral program in nursing through collaboration with nursing colleagues experienced in developing doctoral programs, curricula, and associated requirements. Through the Hampton-Penn Initiative, funded by the Teagle Foundation, the doctoral program was begun in 1999 under the capable leadership of Dean Pamela Hammond. Hampton's rationale for investing in a doctoral program included its leadership in nursing among historically Black colleges and universities, its mission to insure the fullest range of high-quality education for its students, and a commitment from other historically Black colleges and universities to support the program.

The HPC is a perfect complement to the work already being done at Hampton. The HPC provides additional expertise for mentoring students and junior faculty as they develop needed skills in minority health and health disparities research. The HPC also provides additional support for faculty development and the development of Hampton's School of Nursing as an incubator for current and future minority research scholars. There is a diverse faculty at Hampton, making the programs of research relevant to both local communities and the global community as a whole. Hampton's expertise in the conduct of culturally competent care using a multi-system approach is complementary to and informs the research agenda at Penn, and strengthens the research capabilities at both universities.

The funding of the HPC has allowed researchers in the Hampton University School of Nursing to be included in the infrastructure that Hampton University has planned for the establishment of a new biomedical and biobehavioral facility. Researchers in the HPC will be housed with investigators engaging in leading-edge research from throughout the university. Included in the planning for this state-of-the-art facility are formalized partnerships among the Departments of Nursing, Science, Pharmacy, and Physical Therapy on the Hampton campus. These partnerships will build a multidisciplinary approach that will permit the development of new biological insights into the underlying causes of cancer, cardiovascular disease, and other illnesses, and the ways in which these diseases interfere with normal cellular processes. HPC's research will also provide insights into the role of genetic and environmental factors, and their interactions in the manifestation of disease, and support the science necessary to develop new approaches to prevention, detection, and treatment.

## University of Pennsylvania School of Nursing

The University of Pennsylvania School of Nursing brings to the partnership its expertise and infrastructure as a research intensive university and as a leading procurer of extramural research funding from both federal and private sources. Within the School of Nursing, there are five specialized research centers; each is a leader in nursing research in its substantive area. The five centers include the Center for Health Disparities Research (codirected by Loretta Sweet Jemmott and Susan Gennaro), the Hartford Center for Gerontologic Nursing Science (directed by Neville Strumpf), the Center for Health Outcomes and Policy Research (directed by Linda Aiken), the Center for Nursing History (directed by Karen Buhler Wilkerson), and the Center for Biobehavioral Research (directed by Barbara Medoff-Cooper). The activities of all of these centers are coordinated by the Center for Nursing Research (directed by Linda McCauley). Penn has a strong research agenda in addressing disparities in health status, access and utilization of appropriate care, health behaviors, issues related to client-provider relationships, and disparities in condition-specific outcomes.

Additionally, Penn has a strong history in providing mentorship and training in the conduct of culturally competent research. Penn's research agenda is strengthened by its large and well-established doctoral program (60 doctoral students currently, 10–12 new students admitted per year) and a large postdoctoral program (15 current postdoctoral fellows). Predoctoral and postdoctoral fellows are currently funded by NIH and a private foundation (Hartford Foundation). NIH funding occurs through two T32 institutional training programs located within the School of Nursing. The first of these, the Center for Health Outcomes and Policy Research (CHOPR) (Linda Aiken, PI and Director, T32 NR07104), was first funded in 1999; its current funding continues into 2009. The second T32 training program centers around Research on Vulnerable Women, Children, and Families (Susan Gennaro, PI and Director, T32 NR07100). This T32 is currently funded through 2008. Each year, the T32 headed by Dr. Aiken funds two predoctoral fellows and two postdoctoral fellows and the T32 headed by Dr. Gennaro funds four predoctoral fellows and four postdoctoral fellows. The purpose of the T32 "Research on Vulnerable Women, Children, and Families," headed by Dr. Gennaro, is to increase the ability of majority and minority researchers to conduct culturally competent research and to develop a knowledge base that will enable health care providers to improve the health of vulnerable populations. The T32 was begun in 1998 and has had many positive outcomes. Approximately 40% of predoctorates in this program and 44% of postdoctorates have been from minority backgrounds. This year, four of the graduates of the "Research on Vulnerable Women, Children, and Families" training program have received federal funding from NIH.

The Penn School of Nursing is situated on an urban campus and is the only Ivy League university with professional and health schools on the same campus as the rest of the university. Therefore, there is a rich interdisciplinary environment that is supported by the geography and the administrative infrastructure of the university. The Penn School of Nursing is uniquely positioned to move to the next level of scholarship, which includes the conduct of methodologically rigorous research that is sensitive to culture, ethnicity and race, and takes into consideration the effect that culture has on individuals' health behaviors. In this new century, the challenge to clinicians will be to work with clients to promote healthy behaviors that decrease the risk of disease (including HIV/AIDS, sexually transmitted infections, cancer, diabetes, stroke, and cardiac disease) and increase well-being through diet, exercise, weight management, stress management, and responsible sexual behavior, and so forth. Many of these key behaviors are being studied by HPC members at the University of Pennsylvania School of Nursing. By working together, nurse researchers at Hampton and Penn are better able to undertake culturally competent studies of health disparities among vulnerable minority populations as well as to train the next generation of health disparity nurse researchers.

## Background and Focus of HPC

The HPC represents a natural extension of an ongoing collaboration that takes full advantage of the strengths of each institution and its respective faculty for the mutual benefit of all and the enhancement of culturally competent research and programming to reduce health disparities. The HPC focuses specifically on health promotion and disease prevention with vulnerable populations and the influence that culture, race, and ethnicity exert within the client system, health care system, and the larger society that impact health and illness.

Vulnerable populations are defined by the HPC as those who are members of racial or ethnic minorities, poor, marginalized, or underserved populations. Although the HPC employs an inclusive definition of vulnerable populations, its primary focus is on racial/ethnic minorities and the multi-system level factors that contribute to their experiences with health disparities. The HPC focus builds on the previous research and expertise of HPC faculty, in which culturally appropriate interventions have been designed to promote health and to reduce the risk of disease among vulnerable minority populations, particularly African American populations.

## HPC Goals

The specific goals of the HPC are to: (a) foster the development of nursing partnerships between researchers, faculty, and students at Hampton University and the University of Pennsylvania to develop health disparities research at both institutions; (b) promote a broad ecological conceptualization of contributors to health disparities; (c) further the development and dissemination of culturally competent research and interventions related to health disparities among vulnerable and underserved populations; and (d) enhance the recruitment, retention, and education for research careers of nurses who are themselves members of racial or ethnic minorities and who will be able to build the science that will reduce health disparities among vulnerable populations (Jemmott et al., 2002; Powell & Gilliss, 2005; Wallen, Rivera-Goba, Hastings, Peragallo, & De Leon Siantz, 2005).

## HPC Organization

The HPC meets these aims through its three cores: (a) an administrative core that fosters relationships between the two institutions and provides infrastructure support such as Web site development, advertisement of HPC activities and research opportunities, communication between cores and across institutions, Listserv maintenance, budget management, and procurement of services and resources for HPC activities, programs, and meetings; (b) a pilot core that provides funding to foster the conduct of research designed to reduce health disparities; and (c) a mentorship core in which undergraduate, graduate students, doctoral students, postdoctoral fellows, and faculty who are themselves members of racial or ethnic minority groups are encouraged to pursue careers in health disparities research and are mentored to acquire the skills necessary to enhance their research career trajectories. The mentorship core also provides support for students, fellows, and faculty who are from majority populations who wish to increase their skills in conducting culturally competent research or in conducting research to reduce health disparities. Dissemination of research and community outreach is critically important to the HPC; therefore these activities occur across both the pilot and mentorship cores. The HPC organizational chart is presented in Figure 5.1; Table 5.2 summarizes the aims and activities of each of the HPC's cores.

## The Conceptual Approach: Multi-System Level Influences of Health Disparities Among Vulnerable Minority Populations

The HPC conceptualizes factors within both the client-family-community systems and the health care provider-health care systems as contributing to disparities in health outcomes among members of racial or ethnic minorities, and vulnerable and marginalized populations. This type of multi-system conceptualization is consistent with the Bronfenbrenner's (1979, 1989) ecological perspective and a multisystem-level ecological model of health behavior and disparities (Hutchinson, 2000; Hutchinson & Vasas, under review). Figure 5.2 displays this multi-system level ecological view of health outcomes and disparities. Within this model, both the client system and health care system are viewed as nested multi-level systems, existing within the larger society or macrosystem. These systems may or may not be synchronous with one another. On the right side of Figure 5.2, the client-family-community component of the model consists of the characteristics of the individual, his or her family, culture, and community, which may contribute to disparities in health outcomes.

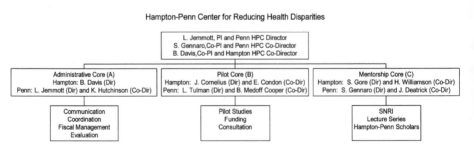

FIGURE 5.1    Hampton-Penn Center to Reduce Health Disparities: Organizational chart.

**TABLE 5.2** Specific Aims and Selected Activities of Hampton-Penn Center (HPC) Cores

| Core | Specific Aims | Selected Activities |
|------|---------------|---------------------|
| Administrative core A | 1. Ensure that an interactive environment among HPC investigators at PENN and at Hampton is established.<br>2. Strengthen and build, where absent, interdisciplinary ties to researchers, research centers, and research laboratories throughout and between both universities.<br>3. Foster communication and interaction between researchers interested in conducting culturally competent research.<br>4. Ensure sound fiscal management and accountability of HPC administrative activities; enhance the recruitment, retention, and training of nurses from racial/ethnic minority groups and marginalized populations into research careers.<br>5. Facilitate the development of new knowledge and scientific rigor in the conduct of culturally competent research related to health disparities.<br>6. Conduct formative and summative evaluations of the extent to which the HPC and each of the three cores meet their stated specific aims. | Communication and coordination for cores in the HPC, maintaining directory of Center Directors, Codirectors, and other health disparities centers; updating Listservs and Web site; following conference call protocol; sending out formal notices regarding HPC activities; identifying interdisciplinary conferences and publications of interest, calls for pilot proposals, calls for nominations, and monitoring applications for Hampton-Penn fellows and scholars for applying for research opportunities in bulletins and applications concerning the upcoming Summer Nursing Research Institutes (SNRI); cosponsoring a session within the Annual Conference on the Black Family; planning travel and meetings between HPC Core Directors and faculty for the yearly P20 Executive Committee Board members; providing fiscal management, accountability, and reporting with university's Business Affairs and Treasurer. |
| Pilot core B | 1. Increase the knowledge base by which health disparities are understood by identifying and evaluating client, family, community, and health care system factors and testing interventions to reduce health disparities by fostering health promotion and disease prevention | Reviewing efforts of faculty and graduate students interested in submitting pilot study proposals; promoting the visibility of the HPC; developing and strengthening networks with health disparities researchers; providing funds and services for the development and professional |

*(Continued)*

131

**TABLE 5.2** Specific Aims and Selected Activities of Hampton-Penn Center (HPC) Cores (*Continued*)

| Core | Specific Aims | Selected Activities |
|---|---|---|
| | 2. Develop methodologies that are sensitive to answering research questions from diverse communities.<br>3. Provide feasibility data and preliminary findings that will enable investigators funded by this pilot core to successfully compete for full scale extramural funding.<br>4. Increase the pool of new investigators from both Hampton and Penn in the conduct of culturally competent health disparity research.<br>5. Encourage innovative research from established investigators with no previous connection to health disparities research.<br>6. Disseminate the findings of the funded pilot studies to the professional and lay communities. | printing of posters for presentations, software for data analysis for those fellows and investigators; facilitating the number of viable proposals for a preliminary review with feedback given prior to final submission; connecting established investigators with investigators who are beginning to build a program of research or changing research focus or accessing communities to involve them in research for and about them. |
| Mentoring core C | 1. Train a cadre of minority nurse researchers who will be able to build the science to reduce health disparities through mentorship, including mentorship that will begin in the Summer Nursing Research Institute through a Hampton/Penn Penn/Hampton scholar program and through education that will occur through a lectureship series held at Penn and at Hampton. | Support SNRI and other training opportunities to meet the needs participants by increasing the number of mentorship services available to faculty and student to include supplemental funding for qualitative and quantitative consultants; assistance, and research training including use of secondary data to access issues of concern to vulnerable populations; developing culturally competent skills, culturally sensitive language and methodologies to recruit participants for research; maintaining the Hampton-Penn Scholars Program to build a cadre of minority scholars skilled in research, especially concerning vulnerable racial and ethnic minority populations experiencing disparities in access and care. |

2. Build partnerships between Hampton University and the University of Pennsylvania that will facilitate the conduct of culturally competent research with the ultimate goal of reducing health disparities.

3. Improve the ability of all nurse researchers to conduct culturally competent research through mentorship, including mentorship that will occur through a Hampton/Penn Penn/Hampton scholar program and through education that will occur through a lectureship series held at Penn and at Hampton.

4. Improve health care as it relates to health disparities through effective dissemination of research designed to reduce health disparities.

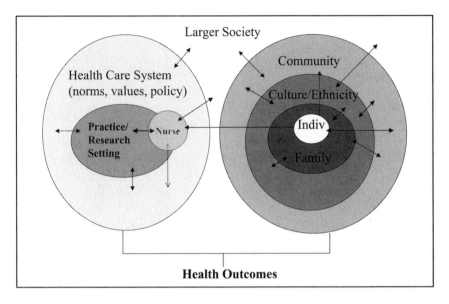

**FIGURE 5.2**   Hampton-Penn Center to Reduce Health Disparities Conceptual Model: Multi-system ecological influences on health disparities.

At the individual level, such factors include genetic predispositions, health-related behaviors (e.g., diet, exercise, tobacco and other substance use, sexual behaviors, condom use), and health-care-seeking behaviors. Family-level factors that are potentially important influences of health behaviors and outcomes include parental modeling of health-related behaviors, parental monitoring of child and adolescent activities and behaviors, family environment and cohesion, parent-child relationships, and communication concerning substance use and sexual behaviors. Cultural or ethnic influences include language differences and barriers, health-related beliefs and traditions of the cultural subgroup, acculturation, and historical interactions with the health care system. Community factors include environmental quality, resources, availability of services, transportation, and community infrastructure.

On the left-hand side of Figure 5.2, the health care system component of the model includes individual practitioners (nurses, physicians, and others), the research or practice setting, and the larger health care system, including norms, values, and policies. Because individual health care practitioners are trained within the existing health care system, Euro-American norms, values, ethnocentrism, and assumptions are major influences across all levels.

When considering the health behaviors and health disparities of clients from racial or ethnic minorities and other vulnerable populations, one must recognize that the norms, values, and beliefs at the individual, family, and community levels that influence health beliefs and behaviors may be significantly different than those of health care providers within the health care system level (Horowitz, Davis, Palermo, & Vladeck, 2000). These differences and providers' lack of understanding of the needs of minority and marginalized clients, and institutionalized biases at the macrosocial and health care system levels may create communication and access barriers that inhibit clients from accessing and receiving timely and appropriate health promotion and preventive care services and treatment at all levels, thus contributing further to health disparities among racial and ethnic minorities (Horowitz et al., 2000). Because factors which contribute to disparities exist across and between all levels, multiple potential targets for research, clinical practice, and mentorship occur within and between all levels (Hutchinson, 2000; Hutchinson & Vasas, under review; Jemmott et al., 2002).

## Client Systems

Individual health behaviors play a major role in an individual's health and well-being over the course of a lifetime. Poor nutrition, sedentary lifestyle, tobacco, alcohol and other substance use, and unprotected sexual intercourse are health behaviors that contribute to many of the leading causes of morbidity and mortality within the United States. Although the behaviors themselves may involve individual actors, these behaviors are, nonetheless, influenced by a variety of factors within the individual's ecological network, including family, peers, other social referents, media influences, social norms, educational and employment opportunities, and community resources. Examples of behavior-mediated adverse health outcomes include obesity, diabetes, hypertension, many cancers, and sexually transmitted infections (STIs), including HIV and AIDS. African Americans, particularly females, are more likely than their White counterparts to be obese (DHHS, 2001), and 1.6 times more likely than non-Hispanic Whites to have diabetes (American Diabetes Association [ADA], 2004). African Americans are also disproportionately represented among those with HIV/AIDS (Centers for Disease Control [CDC], 2004).

Some of the health behaviors that are known to contribute to these adverse outcomes occur at higher rates among racial and ethnic minority group members. For example, regular exercise has been associated with decreased rates of obesity, diabetes, and heart disease (DHHS, 2001). African Americans and Hispanics report less physical activity than Whites, and that may in part, contribute to their higher rates of obesity, diabetes, and heart disease (DHHS).

However, it must be noted that patterns and rates of individual behaviors do not occur in isolation. There are a multitude of factors that contribute to group differences in patterns of individual health behaviors (DHHS, 2001). For example, diet and exercise patterns vary with the availability of playgrounds, recreational facilities, and organized physical and recreational activities for children and adolescents. The availability of these resources varies by the socioeconomic status and resources of the community. Another factor influencing the pattern of individual health behavior is the level of household responsibilities. All these factors are equally important to consider as contributors to health disparities and as potential targets for intervention.

It is essential to move beyond the individual level and consider the underlying multi-system level factors that influence health behaviors and health disparities (DiClemente & Wingood, 2000). More and more, cutting-edge research and interventions are taking multi-targeted approaches that include individual, family-, school-, and community-level factors in their designs. For example, the National Institute of Mental Health formulated a consortium on family and HIV/AIDS that promotes research on family strategies in the prevention and adaptation to HIV and AIDS (Pequegnat & Szapocznik, 2000), and the development of multi-targeted interventions with community partners. Examples from the consortium include defining the role of parents in preventing HIV infection in their children (DiIorio, 2000), designing support systems for HIV-infected parents and their children (Bauman, 2000), and helping women to adapt to HIV/AIDS by improving family relationships and other community support systems (Wingood & DiClemente, 2000). Given the wide range of factors at the family, community, policy, and cultural levels that influence sexual risk behaviors and that fuel the HIV epidemic, multi-level interventions are needed to reach broader audiences and sustain meaningful behavior change (DiClemente & Wingood, 2000).

## Health Care System and Societal Factors

In addition to the individual, family, cultural, and community influences of individual health behaviors and risk, there are also factors at the society, policy, health care system, and health care provider levels that contribute to the disparities in health outcomes experienced by vulnerable minority populations. Some of these factors include disparities in access to consistent care providers, barriers to effective utilization, and difficulties in effective provider-client interactions. These barriers to effective care are important to consider as access to appropriate care has been associated with more positive health outcomes (Powell & Gilliss, 2005).

In 2001, the NIH Office of Minority Health (OMH) reported that the number of uninsured children declined between 1998 and 1999 from 11.9 million to 10.8 million. However, the number of uninsured children declined 15% among Whites, compared to 9% among Blacks and 6% among Hispanics. Furthermore, children from minority groups had less access to primary care than White children and received less primary care, even when differences in insurance coverage and income were taken into account. More than half of the children who were uninsured in 1999 were Black or Hispanic (5.5 million) (Office of Minority Health [OMH], 2000). In 1996, over 20% of Blacks and 30% of Hispanics did not have a usual source of health care (Braithwaite, 2001; OMH, 2000).

Even when care is accessed, studies on health care utilization have found racial inequalities in the use of procedures in patients with ischemic heart disease, with Whites undergoing more procedures than Black patients (Wenneker & Epstein, 1989). Recently, Shapiro (1999) reported that between 1996 and 1998, patterns of care in different groups of HIV patients and others with chronic diseases tended to be unequal. Using a variety of indicators, the researchers found deficiencies in care for women, minorities, and the uninsured. Treatment costs have also been shown to impact care and clients' abilities to adhere to a treatment regimen. In the Commonwealth Fund's 2001 Health Care Quality Survey, 41% of Hispanics and 30% of African Americans who did not follow a physician's advice reported that high cost was the reason for their noncompliance (Commonwealth Fund, 2002).

African American patients report less participatory interactions with White physicians than White patients. Further, they report that seeing physicians of their own race usually resulted in greater participation in the process (Cooper-Patrick et al., 1999). Therefore, it is imperative that the numbers of ethnically diverse and culturally competent health care providers be increased (Fawcett & McCorkle, 1995; Flaskerud, 2000; Powell & Gilliss, 2005). Moreover, the need for culturally competent researcher and practitioners becomes evident in order to efficiently and effectively work with diverse groups of clients to eliminate health disparities (Flaskerud, 2000; Flaskerud & Winslow, 1998; Meleis, 1996).

During its first 3 years, the HPC has sought to address these issues by promoting the use of a multi-system ecological approach to understanding health disparities, promoting the conduct of culturally competent research in health disparities, increasing the recruitment and training of health disparities researchers, and promoting the career trajectories of nurse researchers who are members of racial and ethnic minorities. The HPC's activities and outcomes to date have been encouraging and are discussed in the next sections.

## HPC Mentorship Core Activities and Outcomes: Promoting Culturally Competent Research and Enhancing the Career Trajectories of Health Disparities Researchers

The HPC mentorship core accomplishes its mission to promote culturally competent health disparities research and enhance the training and career trajectories of health disparities researchers through three primary activities:

(a) hosting the Summer Nursing Research Institute (SNRI); (b) recruiting and launching the career trajectories of Hampton-Penn Student Scholars, and undergraduate and graduate students with interests in health disparities research, particularly those who are themselves members of racial and ethnic minorities; and (c) sponsoring conferences, workshops, and lectures on cultural competence in health disparities research and practice. SNRI and similar workshops offered by the HPC and its faculty introduce graduate students, postdoctoral fellows, and colleagues to interdisciplinary ecological perspectives and the ecological modeling of health behaviors. Participants are assisted to move beyond the individual level in how they conceptualize health disparities. These types of workshops have been well received by nurse researchers, who are then better able to communicate, collaborate, and contribute with colleagues from a variety of disciplines. The broader perspective allows for the identification of multiple potential targets for intervention and the development and implementation of health promotion and risk reduction interventions, which are designed to address multiple influences of health and risk behaviors. This approach is consistent with the calls from many health behavior experts to move beyond the individual level of intervention to more effective multiple-targeted intervention approaches (DiClemente & Wingood, 2000).

Workshops and seminars generally rely upon didactic content, review, and critique of leading health behavior models, and presentation and discussion of ecological expansions of existing health behavior models that have been used as the theoretical frameworks for current studies. Participants then engage in detailed examinations and discussions of case study examples of ongoing HPC studies which utilize ecological frameworks to conceptualize the multiple influences of health behavior and health disparities. Through SNRI, workshops and training programs, the HPC has promoted the use of ecological multi-system approaches to conceptualize and conduct research and interventions to reduce health disparities.

## Summer Nursing Research Institute

In May of each year, the HPC holds a 2-week SNRI to enable minority and majority nurse researchers to hone their skills in conducting culturally competent research. SNRI fellows apply and attend the 2-week institute for 2 consecutive years. The SNRI provides a forum to explore the state of the science on nursing care of vulnerable and minority populations, including building collaborative partnerships, improving cultural competency strategies, understanding methodological issues, and identifying gaps in knowledge that need to be filled in order to reduce disparities in health outcomes. The goal of the institute is to develop studies in which nursing research can make a greater contribution to improving the health of vulnerable individuals and families. After participating in the 2-year SNRI program, fellows will be able to:

1. Plan a research trajectory that will help decrease disparities between different ethnic and racial groups
2. Develop a publication plan
3. Develop a research proposal
4. Evaluate a proposal's ethical considerations
5. Apply for extramural funds to the most appropriate agencies and foundations
6. Submit manuscripts for publication
7. Develop a network of research colleagues.

Each SNRI fellow attends sessions, participates in workshops, and works with mentors from the HPC during the year between the annual sessions. Fellows focus on building skills, identifying timelines, and developing and implementing strategies to use at SNRI and at their own institutions to conduct research designed to lessen health disparities and facilitate their own individual research trajectory. Many of the fellows who attend the institute are from institutions where there are limited resources available to facilitate the conduct of research. For those SNRI fellows unable to undertake formal postdoctoral training because of institutional policies, work, and other obligations, SNRI serves as an alternative experience to formal postdoctoral training, particularly for promising researchers who are motivated to increase their individual research productivity and are committed to improving the health of vulnerable populations. However, an exciting outcome of SNRI is that eight of its fellows have gone on to undertake formal postdoctoral training at the University of Pennsylvania. Four of these fellows have been African American; thus the institute has served as an excellent mechanism to increase the number of minority fellows who are engaged in formal postdoctoral training. SNRI has also been successful in furthering the research skills and facilitating the career trajectories of minority fellows who forego formal postdoctoral training but who increase their research productivity in health disparities while remaining at their home institutions.

Each year, more than 20 fellows are selected from around the country to attend the institute. The 2003–2004 cohort of 23 fellows who attended included: 11 African Americans, 1 Native American, 1 Pakistani, 1 Australian, and 9 Whites. The 2005–2006 cohort of 26 attendees was comprised of 11 African Americans, 2 Nigerians, and 13 Whites. Fellows come from a wide geographic area and were able to share their expertise about the health needs of specific segments of the population. Thus, all participants serve as consultants to one another and to HPC members in helping each other to develop more generalizable culturally competent research. It has been extremely helpful to have fellows from rural and urban areas discuss interventions to improve minority health and to compare strategies that may be more culturally appropriate in some areas of the country than in other areas.

Examples of the kinds of studies proposed by SNRI fellows include:

- interventions to increase breast-feeding in African American communities
- interventions to improve screening in African American women for breast cancer
- strategies to improve screening in African American men for prostate cancer
- studies to understand cultural beliefs surrounding health decision making for Native Americans
- interventions to improve exercise in elderly African Americans
- interventions to improve health promotion in Filipinos
- research to evaluate family support for chronically mentally ill Koreans

## Hampton-Penn Student Scholars

The mentorship core also conducts a very active training program for students. Penn and Hampton undergraduate and graduate students can apply to be designated as Hampton-Penn Student Scholars. Student scholars work with faculty to stimulate student interest in health disparities research, increase their understanding of issues surrounding health disparities, and begin to develop a research trajectory of their own designed to improve the health of vulnerable populations. Hampton-Penn Student Scholars are invited to attend the 2-week SNRI and participate in sessions with fellows and attend separate sessions designed especially for students. The Hampton-Penn Student Scholars program was highlighted in the National Black Nurses Newsletter in 2005. The activities and accomplishments of these very productive young scholars are listed in Table 5.3. Selected activities include:

- participating in research on racial disparities in the delivery of health care in Pennsylvania and Virginia
- preparing a paper on strategies used by African American men to prevent STIs
- preparing a paper on sexual risk factors among Caribbean adolescents

**TABLE 5.3** HPC Student Scholars' Activities

| HPC Scholar | Interest in Health Disparities | Current Research, Scholarly, or Educational Activities | Mentor |
|---|---|---|---|
| Karen Celestine | Risky sexual behaviors in Black adolescents of Caribbean (Jamaica and Barbados) descent | Paper (State of the science review) to submit for publication regarding risk factors in these adolescents<br>Completed:<br>• 10-week course on HIV/AIDS prevention and nursing management<br>• 16-week course on addressing health disparities in vulnerable urban communities | Loretta Jemmott, PhD, FAAN (Penn) |
| Kennedy Gachiri | Developing health systems for developing countries especially in Africa | Research on racial disparities in the delivery of health care in Pennsylvania and Virginia (funded by P20)<br>Research to identify which provinces in South Africa are most suited for an HIV/AIDS intervention at the firm/industry level (funded by the Wharton Research Scholars Program)<br>Research Assistant, Center for Health Outcomes and Policy<br>Student in Nursing and Health Care Management Program: BS in Nursing and BS in Economics; French Minor | Sean Clarke, PhD, RN (Penn)<br>Ian MacMillan, PhD (Wharton) |

*(Continued)*

**TABLE 5.3** HPC Student Scholars' Activities (*Continued*)

| HPC Scholar | Interest in Health Disparities | Current Research, Scholarly, or Educational Activities | Mentor |
|---|---|---|---|
| Trina L. Gipson-Jones | 23 African American or Black nurses participated in focus groups 51 participated in quantitative phase | Dissertation; mixed methods research to examine the spillover between work and family, family and work, job satisfaction, and psychological well-being among African American nurses. Participants viewed their well-being as something that was affected by multiple factors such as work to family spillover, family to work spillover, work-family balance spirituality and school-to-family spillover. Findings presented at conference | Bertha Davis, PhD, FAAN (Hampton) |
| Salimah Maghani | Factors that affect negotiation of treatment for cancer pain among African Americans Issues related to disparities in the provision of palliative care and end-of-life care | Dissertation: mixed methods research to understand social, cultural, and political factors related to pain treatment disparities among African Americans 2-week Palliative Care Education and Practice Program at Harvard Medical School Member of End-of-Life Care Taskforce, Dept of Aging, Commonwealth of Pennsylvania | Anne Keane, PhD, FAAN Janet A. Deatrick, PhD, FAAN, Arlene Houldin, PhD, RN (Penn) |
| Abayomi Walker | African American women pregnancy and reproduction; prevention of STDs | Paper to submit for publication concerning efforts by African American men to prevent contracting or transmitting STDs | Katherine Hutchinson, PhD, RN (Penn) |

- completing a dissertation study on conflicts between work and family, job satisfaction, and well-being among African American nurses
- completing a dissertation study to understand social, cultural, and political factors related pain treatment disparities among African Americans
- presenting dissertation research findings at the 7th International Family Nursing Conference, the 2004 National Conference to End Health Disparities, and the Sigma Theta Tau 38th Biennial Convention-Scientific Sessions
- submitting a doctoral dissertation for publication

## Sponsored Conferences and Lecture Series

In addition to the SNRI, the HPC sponsors, contributes to, and participates in a number of conferences, lecture series, and workshops to promote the conduct of culturally competent health disparities research, and to promote the training and career trajectories of health disparities colleagues nationally and internationally. The Hampton University School of Nursing cohosts the annual Conference on the Black Family at Hampton University. This interdisciplinary conference focuses on "finding solutions to the problems that affect African-Americans and minority communities" (Hampton University, 2003, p. 1). Dr. Loretta Sweet Jemmott spoke as the keynote speaker at the 27th annual conference in March, 2005. In addition, from 2003–2005, the HPC cosponsored several interdisciplinary conferences at the University of Pennsylvania, including a Conference on Cultural Competence an International Conference on Women's Health, and a Conference on Native American Health. All three events were well attended by national audiences of faculty, researchers, practitioners, and students.

The HPC Lectureship Series hosts nationally known expert speakers on both the Penn and Hampton campuses to discuss key and emerging issues in health disparities and cultural competence. Always well attended, these events draw regional audiences from the Middle Atlantic and Southern states. Hampton University launched the lectureship series with a legislative- and community-action presentation. The Health Consortium Seminar, entitled "Health and Well-Being: Lifelong Choices," was held during the 2004 Virginia Legislative Black Caucus, Norfolk, VA. The session was moderated by Delegate Algie T. Howell, Jr., from the 90th District and consisted of a panel of faculty scholars and presentations including: "Overview-School of Nursing for Caring of Families," Constance Smith Hendricks, PhD, RN, Dean; "Nursing Center and Health Mobiles: Deserving to Be Served," Darylnet Lyttle, APRN, BC; "Health Disparities Reduction Project: Joining Hands for

Service," Cheryl Killion, PhD, RN; "Removing the Despair from Disparities: The Tie That Binds," Bertha L. Davis, PhD, RN, FAAN; and "The Heart of Caring-Love Mom!" Shelia Cannon, PhD, APRN, PMH, BC. A number of other speakers have participated in the lectureship series held at Hampton University. Eva Gustafsson, qualitative researcher and lecturer, presented on "The Nursing Program at the University of Kalmar, Sweden." Students Emma Jiveland and Therese Thorstensson presented "What it's like to be a Nurse in Kalmar." They also focused on the research conducted currently at their university and in Sweden and dialogued with faculty and students about research in the School of Nursing at Hampton and in America. Past speakers at the Penn campus have included Drs. Nathan Stinson, Adeline Nyamathi, Loretta Sweet Jemmott, and others.

Many HPC members conduct workshops in their area of expertise. Drs. Lorraine Tulman and Barbara Medoff-Cooper from Penn conduct annual workshops at both Hampton and Penn on how to write a fundable pilot study application. Dr. Bertha Davis and other faculty from Hampton have presented seminars on the conduct of culturally competent research. Dr. M. Katherine Hutchinson has presented a series of workshops on the use of ecological multi-system level modeling and secondary analysis in health disparities research both at Penn and various sites across the country. Dr. Janet Deatrick has done numerous presentations on the design and conduct of qualitative research, and Dr. Susan Gennaro is a much sought-after speaker on topics including cultural competence, international research, and developing research proposals.

## HPC Pilot Core Activities and Outcomes: Increasing Research on Health Disparities Among Vulnerable Minority Populations

In the first 3 years, the HPC Pilot Core has funded nine pilot studies addressing a diverse array of topics on health disparities within the client-family community and the health care provider-health care systems. Each pilot study was awarded $10,000 in direct costs; many were also provided with additional funding for dissemination of results through conference podium presentations and poster sessions. Each pilot study was required to include investigators from both institutional partners. Some pilot studies have had doctoral students as investigators; some have also included undergraduate and graduate students as research assistants. The pilot studies have contributed to HPC objectives of promoting institutional collaboration; enhancing research trajectories of investigators in health disparities research; recruiting, training, and developing interest among undergraduate and graduate students in health disparities research; and increasing the knowledge about health disparities.

As is shown in Table 5.4, several of the pilot studies funded through the HPC have examined health disparities within the client-family-community system. For example, Hutchinson and Montgomery (July, 2005) examined the family influences of sexual risk attitudes and behaviors among African American college students and assessed the reliability of the Parent-Teen Sexual Risk Communication Scale (PTSRC) when used with African American families. The PTSRC was found to have high levels of internal reliability for reports of communication with both mothers and fathers (alpha = .91 and .93, respectively); PTSRC scores were significantly correlated with students' reports of condom use self-efficacy (r = .18, p < .01), which was itself strongly associated with intentions to use condoms (r = .30, p < .001).

Cornelius and Jemmott (July, 2005) conducted a qualitative study of African American custodial grandparents' perceived needs about communicating with grandchildren about HIV and STIs. Preliminary analyses indicate that there were significant differences between grandparents and their grandchildren in attitudes about HIV risk reduction communication, with grandparents interestingly having more favorable attitudes than grandchildren about discussing sexuality issues. These preliminary findings were presented at the Sigma Theta Tau research conference in Hawaii in July, 2005.

Spruill and Riegel (October, 2005) examined beliefs about obesity and exercise among the diabetic and non-diabetic adults in the Gullah population of South Carolina. Preliminary findings reveal no difference in exercise patterns between those who believed that diabetes could be prevented or controlled and those not possessing this belief. They also found no difference in the incidence of obesity among those genetically predisposed to diabetes compared to those not at genetic risk for this disease.

Other pilot studies have examined health disparities in health care providers and health care systems. For example, Clarke and Davis (unpublished data) undertook a study of racial differences in risk-adjusted mortality in Pennsylvania and Virginia by examining hospital discharge records, segregation, and distances between residence and hospitals. Preliminary analyses indicate that the distances between Black patients' home addresses and the hospital where they are treated tend to be shorter than those of non-Black patients in these sites. Moreover, unexplained differences in inpatient mortality were observed between African Americans and other patients at these sites. Stringer, Gennaro, Slade, and Davis (unpublished data) have been studying the validity and reliability of stress assessment tools and language used by African American women to report signs of premature labor and ways they identify stressors in their lives. Preliminary analysis of their data indicates that almost half of the women were currently experiencing stress and of these, only slightly more than half could identify a specific stressor. Furthermore, only about half tried to decrease stress with self-management strategies such

**TABLE 5.4** Pilot Studies Funded by the Hampton-Penn Center to Reduce Health Disparities

| Sample | Ethnicity/Race | Design | Intervention/Aim | Outcome Variables | Results |
|---|---|---|---|---|---|
| Pilot study 1 | Clarke, S., & Davis, B. (2002–2004). *Racial differentials in hospital outcomes across two states.* | | | | |
| 763,271 hospital discharge records | Approximately 20% Black or African American; 80% White or other | Secondary data analysis | To examine racial segregation in hospital care in Virginia and to examine whether racial differentials in risk-adjusted mortality exist in Virginia | Risk-adjusted mortality rates; distances between residence and hospital | Analyses ongoing. Preliminary results: In Pennsylvania, segregation of care was most prominent in the Philadelphia area and considerably lower outside. In Virginia, it was considerably lower and was most prominent in one urban and in the rural regions of the state. In both states, there were unexplained inpatient mortality differences between African Americans and others. Geographic and demographic differences in the two states appear to produce unique patterns of hospital care utilization and outcomes that deserve further study. |

| | | | | | |
|---|---|---|---|---|---|
| Pilot study 2 | Montgomery, A., & Hutchinson, M. K. (2003–2005). *Family influences of sexual risk behaviors among African American college students* | | | | |
| 518 | African American college students | Longitudinal, 2 wave survey | To examine the influence of parents' attitudes and sexual communication on college students' sexual risk attitudes and behaviors | Students' reports of sexual risk behaviors and STIs at Wave 2 | Analyses ongoing. Preliminary results presented at conference |
| Pilot study 3 | Cornelius, J., & Jemmott, L. S. (2002–2004). *African American grand family HIV prevention—Identifying needs, barriers and concerns* | | | | |
| 80 total 40 children 40 grandparents | African American dyads | Focus Groups and Brief Questionnaires | To identify needs, barriers and concerns that Black Baptist grandparents have about communicating with grandchildren about HIV and STIs | Reports from both grandparents | Grandparents reported discussing STI/HIV prevention and postponing sexual activity with their adolescent grandchildren. They also reported that the church should play a greater role in promoting abstinence and safer sex and that younger people should teach church-based sexuality classes so the youth can better relate. Presented at conferences. |

*(Continued)*

**TABLE 5.4** Pilot Studies Funded by the Hampton-Penn Center to Reduce Health Disparities (*Continued*)

| Sample | Ethnicity/Race | Design | Intervention/Aim | Outcome Variables | Results |
|---|---|---|---|---|---|
| Pilot study 4 | Stringer, M., Gennaro, S., Slade, S., & Davis, B. (2002–2005). *Cultural sensitivity of instruments used in women experiencing preterm labor.* | | | | |
| 60 women | 30 African American and 30 White women admitted to hospital with diagnosis of "rule-out preterm labor" | Cross-sectional | To assess for differences in the validity and reliability of stress assessment tools and descriptions of preterm labor warning signs between African American and White women. | Interview reports and self-reported data on three question-naires/instruments: Signs and Symptoms of Labor; Perceived Stress Scale and Prenatal Distress Scale | Data collection ongoing |
| Pilot study 5 | Simpson, E., Medoff-Cooper, B., & Daniels, L. (2003–2005). *Parents' seat belt use, race and SES* | | | | |
| 16 women | 8 White; 4 Black/African American; 4 Hispanic/Latina | Focus groups | To explore factors that contribute to mothers' use of | Mothers' reports of factors that promote and in-hibit their use of | Data analysis ongoing |

| | | | | | |
|---|---|---|---|---|---|
| Pilot study 5 | Simpson, E., Medoff-Cooper, B., & Daniels, L. (2003–2005). *Parents' seat belt use, race and SES* | | appropriate child safety restraints in automobiles for their 3- to 8-year-old children | child safety restraints in automobiles | |
| Pilot study 6 | Lipman, T., & Servonsky, J. (2003–2005). *Racial disparities in the epidemiology of pediatric type 2 diabetes in Philadelphia, PA and Hampton Roads, VA* | | | | |
| 492 cases reported in Philadelphia, PA schools; data collection ongoing in VA | Data not yet analyzed | Survey of school nurses | To examine the prevalence of Type 2 Diabetes in Hampton Roads, VA and compare it with Philadelphia, PA; To examine racial disparities in the prevalence | Case reports on children with type 2 diabetes completed by school nurses | Data collection ongoing |

*(Continued)*

**TABLE 5.4** Pilot Studies Funded by the Hampton-Penn Center to Reduce Health Disparities (*Continued*)

| Sample | Ethnicity/Race | Design | Intervention/Aim | Outcome Variables | Results |
|---|---|---|---|---|---|
| Pilot study 7 | Sochalski, J., & Condon, E. (2005). *Racial disparities in palliative care.* | | | | |
| The 2002 California Hospital Discharge Data Base and the American Hospital Association Annual Surveys 1998–2002 | Not yet determined | Secondary Data Analysis | To identify characteristics of patients who use inpatient palliative care services; To identify characteristics of hospitals that offer palliative care; to evaluate whether the racial/ethnic gap in palliative care use narrows with service availability | Link data from CA hospitals and the AHA annual surveys to the patient discharge data files to describe patients who use the palliative care services | Data analysis ongoing |
| Pilot study 8 | Spruill, I., & Riegel, B. (2005). *Linking genetics and obesity to diabetes.* | | | | |
| 1322 | Black or African American | Secondary Data Analysis | To examine the relative influence and interrelationships between | A model of 11 variables was tested with linear regression analysis | Eight of the 11 variables were significant (F (8,865) = 25.4, p < .0001), explaining 19% of the |

| | | | | |
|---|---|---|---|---|
| | | | genetics and exercise on obesity and diabetes complications among rural Gullahs in South Carolina | to identify significant predictors of complications | variance in diabetic complications: higher HbA1c, presence of hypertension, older age, female gender, health insurance, beliefs being given a diabetic diet and a class on diabetes |

Sumpter, D., Medoff-Cooper, B., & Barnes, S. (2005). *Minority families of vulnerable infants and their perceptions of research.*

Pilot study 9

| Parents of infants who were hospitalized with a congenital heart defect | African American and White | Qualitative study | To identify the perceptions of and motivations for participation in a (minimal risk) research study | Parents' descriptions of their perceptions of research and their motivations to participate or not participate in minimal risk research studies | Subject recruitment is just beginning |

as praying, resting, keeping active, or walking. Their study directly addresses issues related to differences in communication that may exist between majority providers and minority clients and contribute to disparities in African American birth outcomes.

These pilot studies capitalize on the HPC's ecological, multi-system level framework to further our understanding of health disparities influences and potential targets for intervention. By having both minority and majority researchers serving as principal investigators on each project, the pilot studies benefit from having both internal and external perspectives applied to the health issues affecting vulnerable African American populations.

The HPC Pilot Core directors and codirectors were instrumental in facilitating the partnerships necessary for the development of these pilot studies. These pilot studies have all included collaborations between investigators, both faculty and doctoral students, from both Hampton University and the University of Pennsylvania. Because of the geographic distance between collaborators, research teams have relied upon electronic forms of communication to supplement face-to-face planning meetings. The necessary processes involved in the formation of collaborative relationships and the conduct of research have included both successes and challenges. Successes were found in the number of matches in research interests that were shared between faculties at the two universities. Successful proposals and a strengthened interest in research among faculty were other positive outcomes.

## Matches in Research Interests

Matches in research interests were influenced by faculty interests as well as the focus of the P20 grant to develop researchers who would be able to study minority health issues and disparities. Although much was accomplished among the Pilot Core directors using e-mail and telephone correspondence, the on-site visits of Pilot Core personnel were effective in generating interest and enthusiasm from faculty and PhD students through these face-to-face meetings. Potential for collaboration among Hampton University and University of Pennsylvania faculty was explored through informal meetings and discussion between Pilot Core personnel and faculty and students. Equally important was the preparation for the on-site visits. Students and faculty were polled to assess their research interests related to minority health and health disparities issues. Lists of those interests were generated and used to identify potential collaborations in relation to topics, experience, and willingness to partner. Timely announcements, requests for proposals, and follow-up by Pilot Core members facilitated the formation of successful partnerships.

## Successful Proposals

Successful funding of pilot proposals was another outcome of the partnership within the Pilot Core group. Pilot Core personnel committed themselves to effectively soliciting, reviewing, and giving constructive feedback to applicants on their proposals. Specifically, prospective investigators were encouraged to submit drafts of proposals to the Pilot Core members in advance of the posted deadline in order to receive helpful feedback. Face-to-face meetings were also helpful in assisting prospective investigators in clarifying their aims and design of their proposed pilot studies. This resulted in strengthening the proposals and enhancing their feasibility and funding potential. This activity also provided valuable experience in reviewing proposals for those Pilot Core members who were less experienced in the review process. A sense of shared purpose and open communication within the group developed and was sustained. Sharing of expertise in terms of research knowledge and some culture brokering were other positive aspects of the Pilot Core collaboration between the two institutions.

## Renewed Interest in Research

Another successful outcome of the Pilot Core activity was the enhancement of faculty research interest and competence. The Pilot Core activity has positively influenced how research activity is viewed, particularly among faculty at Hampton University, a school that has not been research intensive in the past. Because faculty expectations have changed with respect to research, their ability to effectively function as thesis and dissertation committee members and advisors is enhanced. Through the Pilot Core activities, faculty members are motivated to evaluate and expand their understanding of nursing theory and research methods. It is also gratifying to faculty to know that they are able to contribute to the cultural sensitivity and competence of researchers at Penn and other majority and non-majority institutions, whose experiences differ from their own.

The primary challenge has been time constraints and the competing demands faced by faculty at minority serving institutions who are seeking to initiate research projects on health disparities among vulnerable populations. Many minority serving institutions, including Hampton University, are teaching-intensive universities, their faculty often carry larger teaching loads than faculty at research-intensive universities. Nursing faculty are often particularly challenged by the need to balance classroom teaching and clinical teaching and practice with the time required to plan and prepare research proposals and conduct studies.

## Federally Funded Research and Scholarship by HPC Members

HPC members are conducting extramurally funded research on health disparities. Three examples of federally funded HPC studies in which multiple-level influences of health behaviors are addressed include Jemmott, Jemmott, Hutchinson, Icard, and Gadsden's (2003) "Church-Based Parent-Child HIV Prevention Project" (R01 MH63070), Hutchinson's (2001) "Dyadic Ecological Analysis of Adolescent HIV Risk" (R03 MH63659), and Gennaro, Macones, and Douglas's (2003) "Physiologic Mechanisms in Preterm Labor in African American Women" (R03 NR008548). The first is a randomized controlled trial intervention study, in which abstinence-based HIV risk reduction interventions are tested with both young adolescents and their parents through the Black Baptist churches in Philadelphia, PA. After participating in either a parent-child abstinence program, a faith-based parent-child abstinence program, or a parent-child health promotion control condition, young adolescents and their parents are followed for 18 months to examine adolescents' HIV-risk-related attitudes, intentions and behaviors (adolescents') and parents' attitudes, and intentions and behaviors related to communicating and helping their children avoid HIV-risk-related behaviors. Although data collection for this study is ongoing, qualitative reports from participants have been very positive.

The second study is a secondary analysis of data from adolescent females, their mothers, their male dating partners, and their male dating partners' mothers undertaken to examine the relative influence of parents and partners on sexual decision-making within an adolescent dyad. In this study, baseline data from over 1,000 adolescent dating couples and their parents from the National Longitudinal Survey of Adolescent Health are linked and used to model reports of sexual activity and condom use 1 year later (Hutchinson, 2001).

Another federally funded study examines the physiologic basis of causes for within-group variations and health disparities in birth outcomes. Dr. Susan Gennaro's study, "Physiologic Mechanisms in Preterm Labor in African American Women" (R03 NR008548) compares African American pregnant women who experience preterm labor and birth with African American pregnant women who experience preterm labor but deliver at term and African American women who have normal term deliveries not preceded by preterm labor. Stress, nutrition, infections, and serum, cervical, and vaginal cytokines are being examined to determine their influence in increasing the heightened risk of African American women for preterm birth (Gennaro et al., 2003). In addition, Dr. Gennaro has served as a consultant to NINR's Workgroup on Health Disparities and Pregnancy Outcomes, convened in 2003, to identify future directions for research in improving pregnancy outcomes in minority populations. The recommendations of this group were recently published in the *American Journal of Obstetrics and Gynecology* (Gennaro, 2005).

Several related publications have also been generated by HPC members during the past few years. These include a report on the family influences of adolescent sexual risk behaviors among inner-city African American and Latino females (Hutchinson, Jemmott, Jemmott, Braverman, & Fong, 2003). The state of the science in pregnancy outcomes research among minority populations was reviewed by Gennaro (2005). Another study reported work conducted by Dr. Amar (HPC center member and former predoctoral fellow in the center) in collaboration with Susan Gennaro (Amar & Gennaro, 2005). Additional manuscripts are in progress or under review. For example, a manuscript is in development which describes the culture-specific factors contributing to HIV risk among Jamaica adolescent females (Hutchinson et al., under review). A manuscript under review highlights the use of ecological models to promote our understanding of adolescent sexual risk among vulnerable populations (Hutchinson & Vasas, under review).

## Summary and Recommendations

The HPC experience illustrates the importance of comprehensively addressing health disparities among vulnerable populations by studying the multi-system level factors contributing to health disparities, enhancing the cultural competence of health disparities researcher, and promoting the recruitment and training of health researchers who are themselves members of vulnerable, marginalized, and underserved populations. The HPC experience, and the experiences of the other P20-funded partnership centers for health disparities, demonstrate that partnerships between research-intensive majority institutions and minority-serving institutions can be mutually beneficial and productive in meeting these three aims.

Efforts such as those initiated by the HPC to increase the recruitment, training, and promote the career trajectories of nurse researchers who are themselves members of racial and ethnic minority groups are critically important (Wallen et al., 2005) and consistent with Powell and Gilliss's (2005, p. 34) assertion that ethnic minority researchers are "ideally suited to lead research teams in an effort to reduce health disparities and eliminate unequal treatment among these individuals" because of their similar life experiences. Initiatives to increase the number of minority health disparities researchers should continue and be expanded in order to attract, recruit, retain, and promote minority health professionals across the undergraduate, graduate, predoctoral, and postdoctoral levels. The fruitful efforts of the nursing partnership centers for health disparities should be encouraged and funding for centers such as the HPC should be continued and expanded. Even though these centers are only midway through their initial funding cycles, a number of publications, presentations, workshops, and conferences have resulted. These outcomes further our understanding of the unique health needs and experiences with health disparities among vulnerable populations, and enhance our ability to develop culturally appropriate responses to ameliorate these needs.

Based on the HPC experience, our recommendations are to: (a) extend funding for the existing P20 Nursing Partnership Centers on Health Disparities; (b) expand the program to include additional national and international partnerships to promote research training in health disparities among vulnerable populations, particularly for researchers who are themselves members of minority and vulnerable populations (one such initiative is a new request for proposal jointly issued by NINR and the Fogarty International Center); and (c) address the realities of both the strengths and limitations that exist in majority serving institutions and minority serving institutions that promote or inhibit the faculty's ability to develop a culturally competent research program in health disparities research. These issues include faculty diversity, expertise in transcultural nursing, time constraints, organizational culture, research infrastructure, teaching loads, and policies toward research release time. By collaborating and sharing their expertise, majority serving institutions and minority serving institutions can build on their own strengths, supplement their areas of need, share their expertise and resources, further their own programs of research, and collaboratively build the science needed to alleviate health disparities among vulnerable populations.

## ACKNOWLEDGMENT

The authors of this manuscript and the members of the HPC gratefully acknowledge the NINR and its support. Grant support for the development of this manuscript was provided through P20 NR008361 (L. S. Jemmott and S. Gennaro, Co-PIs) and P20 NR008389 (B. Davis, PI).

## REFERENCES

Aday, L. (2001). At risk in America. San Francisco: Jossey-Bass.

Amar, A., & Gennaro, S. (2005). Dating violence in college women: Associated physical injury, healthcare usage, and mental health symptoms. Nursing Research, 54, 235–242.

American Diabetes Association. (2004). Retrieved September 9, 2005, from http://www.diabetes.org/ diabetes-statistics/african-americans.jsp

Bauman, L., Dramin, B., Levine, C., Hudis, J. (2000). Who will care for me?: Planning the future care and custody of children orphaned by HIV/AIDS. In W. Pequegnat & J. Szapocznik (Eds.), Working with families in the era of HIV/AIDS. pp. 155–188. Thousand Oaks, CA: Sage Publications.

Braithwaite, R. (2001). The health status of Black men. In R. Braithwaite & S. Taylor (Eds.), Health issues in the Black community (pp. 62–80). San Francisco: Jossey-Bass.

Bronfenbrenner, U. (1979). *Ecology of human development: Experiments by nature and design*. Cambridge, MA: Harvard University Press.

Bronfenbrenner, U. (1989). Ecological systems theory. *Annals of Child Development, 6,* 556–581.

Centers for Disease Control. (2004). *HIV/AIDS Surveillance Report, 2003, 15.* Atlanta: U.S. Department of Health and Human Services, Center for Disease Control and Prevention.

Commonwealth Fund. (2002). *Diverse Communities, Common Concerns: Assessing Health Care Quality for Minority Americans.*

Cooper-Patrick, L., Gallo, J., Gonzales, J., Vu, H. T., Powe, N. R., Nelson, C., et al. (1999). Race, gender, partnership in the physician-patient relationship. *Journal of the American Medical Association, 282,* 583–589.

Cornelius, J., and Jemmott, L. S. (2005, July). *Identifying African-American grand families' HIV risk reduction behaviors.* Paper presented at the Sigma Theta Tau International Preconference, Kona, Hawaii.

de Chesnay, M. (2005). Vulnerable populations: Vulnerable people. In M. de Chesnay (Ed.), *Caring for the vulnerable.* pp. 3–12. Boston: Jones and Bartlett Publishers.

Department of Health and Human Services. (2001). *Healthy People 2010.* Retrieved June 20, 2005 from http://www.healthypeople.gov/Document/html/uih/uih_bw/uih_2.htm

DiClemente, R., & Wingood, G. (2000). Expanding the scope of HIV prevention for adolescents: Beyond individual-level interventions. *Journal of Adolescent Health, 26,* 377–378.

DiIorio, C. (2000). Keeping it R.E.A.L. A mother adolescent HIV prevention program. In W. Pequegnat & J. Szapocznik (Eds.), *Working with families in the era of HIV/AIDS* (pp. 113–132). Thousand Oaks, CA: Sage Publications.

Dixon, E. L., Strehlow, A., Davis, C., Copeland, D., Jones, T., Robinson, L. et al. (in press). Generating science by training future scholars in nursing research. *Annual review of nursing research, 25.*

Fawcett, J., & McCorkle, R. (1995). Cultural considerations in postdoctoral nursing research training. In *Successful postdoctoral research training for African American nurses* (pp. 5–9). Washington, DC: American Nursing Association Pamphlet G–191.

Flaskerud, J. H., (2000). Developing leadership and excellence with VPs in research, education, and practice. *Nursing Leadership Forum, 4*(3), 76–84.

Flaskerud, J. H., & Winslow, B. J. (1998). Conceptualizing vulnerable populations health-related research. *Nursing Research, 47,* 69–78.

Gennaro, S. (2005). Overview of current state of research in pregnancy outcomes in minority populations. *American Journal of Obstetrics and Gynecology, 192,* S3–10.

Gennaro, S., Macones, G., & Douglas, S. (2003). *Mechanisms underlying preterm birth in African American women.* R03 NR008548. Bethesda, MD: National Institute of Health/National Institute of Nursing Research.

Grady, P. (2001). *Research partnership program to address health disparities.* Retrieved June 20, 2005, from http://ninr.nih.gov/ninr/news-info/pubs/outlooksept01.html

Grady, P. (2003). *A NINR initiative to address health disparities.* Retrieved June 21, 2005, from http://ninr.nih.gov/ninr/news-info/pubs/NOJan03.pdf

Hampton University, (2003). *25th Annual Conference on the Black Family.* Retrieved July 28, 2005, from http://www.hamptonu.edu/interests/calendar/BFC/index.html

Horowitz, C., Davis, M., Palermo, A., & Vladeck, B. (2000). Approaches to eliminating sociocultural disparities in health. *Health Care Financing Review, 21*(4), 57–71.

Hutchinson, M. K. (2000, January). *Ecological modeling in sexual risk research.* Paper presented at the Proseminar in Health Outcomes Research, University of Pennsylvania School of Nursing, Philadelphia, PA.

Hutchinson, M. K. (2001). *Dyadic ecological analysis of adolescent sexual HIV risk.* (R03 MH63659). Bethesda, MD: National Institute of Health/National Institute of Nursing Research.

Hutchinson, M. K., Jemmott, J. B., 3rd, Jemmott, L. S., Braverman, P., & Fong, G. T. (2003). The role of mother-daughter sexual risk communication in reducing sexual risk behaviors among urban adolescent females: A prospective study. *Journal of Adolescent Health, 33*(2), 98–107.

Hutchinson, M. K., Jemmott, L. S., Vasas, E., Hewitt, H., Kahwa, E., Waldron, N., & Bonaparte, B. (in press). Identifying culture-specific factors contributing to HIV sexual risk among Jamaican adolescents. *Journal of American Nurses in AIDS Care.*

Hutchinson, M. K., & Montgomery, A. (2005, July). *Family influences of sexual risk behavior among African American college students.* Poster presented at Sigma Theta Tau Preconference in Kona, Hawaii.

Hutchinson, M. K., & Vasas, E. (in press). Family-based expansion of the Theory of Planned Behavior: Framework for HIV risk-reduction with adolescents. *Journal of Nursing Scholarship.*

Jemmott, L., Gennaro, S., Davis, B., Hutchinson, M. K., Tulman, L., Medoff-Cooper, B., & Deatrick, J. (2002). *Hampton-Penn Center to reduce health disparities* (P20 NR008361). Bethesda, MD: National Institutes of Health/National Institute of Nursing Research.

Jemmott, L., Jemmott J., Hutchinson, M. K., Icard, L., & Gadsden, V. (2003). *Church-Based Parent-Child HIV Prevention Project* (R01 MH63070). Bethesda, MD: National Institutes of Health/National Institute of Nursing Research.

Meleis, A. I. (1996). Culturally competent scholarship: Substance and rigor. *Advances in Nursing Science, 19*(2), 1–16.

National Center for Health Statistics. (2002). *Health U.S., 2002,* Table 2. Retrieved May 3, 2005, from http://www.cdc.gov/nchs/data/hus/hus02.pdf

National Institutes of Health. (2002). *NIH news release: New initiative to reduce health disparities announced by the National Institute of Nursing Research.* Retrieved April 7, 2005, from http://ninr.nih.gov/ninr/news-info/healthdisp.pdf

National Institute of Nursing Research. (n.d.). *Types of research and research training mechanisms.* Retrieved June 20, 2005, from http://ninr.nih.gov/ninr/research/dea/restype.html

National Institute of Nursing Research. (2001). *RFA-NR-02–004 Nursing Partnership Centers on Health Disparities.* Retrieved June 18, 2005, from http://grants.nih.gov/grants/guide/rfa-files/RFA-NR-02–004.html.

Office of Minority Health. (2000). Retrieved June 28, 2005, from http://www.omhrc.gov/OMH/sidebar/datastats1.htm

Pequegnat, W., & Szapocznik, J. (2000). The role of families in preventing and adapting to HIV/AIDS. In W. Pequegnat and J. Szapocznik (Eds.), *Working with families in the era of HIV/AIDS* (pp. 3–26). Thousand Oaks, CA: Sage.

Powell, D., & Gilliss, C. (2005). Partnering in the cultivation of the next generation of ethnic minority nurse scientists: Responding to a compelling national agenda. *Journal of the National Black Nurses Association, 14*(2), 34–43.

Rockeymoore, M. (2005, June 9). Health discrimination: A 21st century civil rights issue. *The Black Commentator, 141.* Retrieved on August 17, 2005, from http://www. blackcommentator.com/141/141_cover_rockeymoore.html

Shapiro, M. F. (1999). Variations in the care of HIV infected adults in the United States: Results from the HIV cost and service utilization study. *Journal of the American Medical Association, 281,* 2305–2315.

Smedley, B., Stith, A., & Nelson, A. (2002). *Unequal treatment: Confronting racial and ethnic disparities in health care.* Institute of Medicine. Washington, DC: National Sciences Press.

Spruill, I., & Riegel, B. (October, 2005). *It takes a whole village to raise a healthy child.* Paper presented at the annual conference of the Society of Nurses in Genetics (ISONG), Salt Lake City, Utah.

Wallen, G. R., Rivera-Goba, M. V., Hastings, C., Peragallo, N., & De Leon Siantz, M. (2005). Developing the research pipeline: Increasing minority nursing research opportunities. *NLN: Nursing Education Perspectives, 26,* 29–33.

Wenneker, M., & Epstein, A. (1989). Racial inequalities in the use of procedures for patients with ischemic heart disease in Massachusetts. *Journal of the American Medical Association, 261*(2), 253–257.

Wingood, G., & DiClemente, R. (2000). The Willow program: Mobilizing social networks of women living with HIV to enhance coping and reduce sexual risk behaviors. In W. Pequegnat & J. Szapocznik (Eds.), *Working with families in the era of HIV/AIDS* (pp. 281–298). Thousand Oaks, CA: Sage Publications.

# Chapter 6

## Generating Science by Training Future Scholars in Nursing Research Addressing the Needs of Vulnerable Populations

Elizabeth L. Dixon, Aaron J. Strehlow, Claudia M. Davis,
Darcy Copeland, Tonia Jones, Linda A. Robinson,
Jan Shoultz, and Jacquelyn H. Flaskerud

ABSTRACT

*This chapter focuses on the National Institutes of Health (NIH) T32 National Research Service Award (NRSA) funding mechanism, designed to enhance the development of nurse scientists. The general history and principles underlying NIH funding for T32s as well as the National Institute of Nursing Research's (NINR) involvement in the NRSA program is described, highlighting the University of California Los Angeles School of Nursing's T32 training program in vulnerable populations research and the program and career trajectory data from close to two-thirds of NINR-funded T32s directors. Recommendations for the improvement of NINR-funded T32*

*training programs are identified. Findings include the need for increased collaboration
between institutions receiving T32 funding from the NINR.*

Keywords: nurse scientist training; pre- and postdoctoral support; financial
support; T32; NINR; vulnerable populations; research fellowships; national
research service award

# INTRODUCTION

The National Institutes of Health (NIH) initiated sponsorship of the National
Research Service Award (NRSA) training program in 1975. Since its inception,
the NRSA program has been used by the NIH as the primary mechanism of support for predoctoral and postdoctoral research training in the health sciences.
The NRSA program provides both institutional training grants (known as T32s)
and individual fellowships (known as F31s and F32s). The aim of the NRSA program is to ensure an adequate and continuing supply of diverse scientists trained
to conduct innovative health-related research in areas considered important to
the Nation's health (NIH, 2002a; Pion, 2001).

This chapter focuses on the T32 NRSA funding mechanism and, specifically,
how the T32 has influenced the development of a cadre of nurse scientists trained
to conduct vulnerable populations research. Vulnerable populations are defined as
social groups who experience differential patterns of morbidity, mortality, and life
expectancy because of fewer resources and increased exposure to risks (Flaskerud
& Winslow, 1998). Vulnerable groups include individuals living in poverty, ethnic
and racial minorities, and socially marginalized populations. The general history
and principles underlying NIH funding for T32s as well as the National Institute
of Nursing Research's (NINR) involvement in the NRSA program is described.
Through support from the NINR, 28 universities had T32s in place in 2003 (NINR,
n.d.). A case study of the University of California Los Angeles (UCLA) School of
Nursing's experience with a T32 as well as data from a sample of all 28 T32 training programs is presented. This information illustrates the operational functioning
of NINR-funded T32s and types of training in vulnerable populations research.
Moreover, it provides an indication of the career paths of T32 funding recipients,
and identifies suggested areas for enhancement of T32 training programs in nursing. Although the NINR and its National Advisory Council for Nursing Research
(NACNR) are involved in an ongoing evaluation of nurse scientist training programs and have provided initial findings of this evaluation (NINR, 2003), relatively little is known about how T32 participation influences the development of
nursing scholars trained to conduct vulnerable populations research.

Before proceeding, the authors would like to note that the Internet sites cited in the following discussion were valid on the date indicated in the reference list. The NINR Web site, in particular, has been redesigned and Web addresses have changed. For NINR references, readers are referred to http://www.ninr.nih.gov/.

## HISTORY OF T32 MECHANISM AND NURSE SCIENTIST TRAINING

### NIH Funding for T32s

An overview of the history of the NIH's NRSA training program is described by Pion (2001) as part of a study detailing the early achievement of former NRSA predoctoral award recipients on various career outcome measures. Although the NIH had been providing support for research training since 1930, the legislation creating the NRSA program specifically targeted the training of a broader group of scientists (as opposed to health professionals) and redirected funds to fields in which there was an identified need for a larger pool of biomedical and behavioral researchers.

Since their initiation in 1975, the overriding goal of the NRSA program has been to identify and support the pre- and postdoctoral education of talented individuals who desire to pursue careers in biomedical and behavioral research. This goal is accomplished by awarding two types of training support: (a) T32 institutional training grants (institutions choose award recipients and mentor them through their research training); and (b) fellowships to individuals for supervised study with senior scientists. At the current time, approximately 80% of NIH's NRSA training funds are directed toward the funding of T32s (Pion, 2001).

According to the National Research Council (1980), the fundamental purpose of the NRSA programs is to: (a) influence the career decisions of individuals by providing an opportunity to become involved in scientific study in a targeted area, while making this training more affordable through the provision of financial support; and (b) provide award recipients with training experiences that lay the foundation for success as independent investigators.

The aforementioned study by Pion (2001) is significant to this discussion as this author compared the early career outcomes of NRSA predoctoral trainees with doctorally prepared individuals who were graduate students in the same discipline and at the same time as the NRSA predoctoral trainees. This study's findings found that NRSA predoctoral trainees in the biomedical and behavioral sciences: (a) completed their degrees in less time; (b) were more likely to pursue postdoctoral training; (c) were more likely to secure tenure-track faculty positions;

and (d) were more likely submit a grant to the NIH or National Science Foundation. These findings provide evidence that the NRSA training programs are achieving their goal of facilitating the development of active and productive research scientists.

## NINR and T32 funding

The predecessor to the NINR, the National Center for Nursing Research, funded its first seven T32 training programs in 1987. Since that time, the number of NINR T32 awards steadily increased to 28 in 2003 (NINR, n.d.). In accordance with the aim of the NIH's NRSA training program, the expectation is that the funding of T32s within nursing would result in the development of future nursing scholars. Given the nature of the nursing shortage in the United States, the need for the development of nursing scholars and a productive nursing workforce is magnified.

With respect to the NINR budget for T32s, the NINR devoted 5% of its overall budget to the funding of T32s in 2004 and projected estimates indicate that this amount will increase to 6% in 2006. Comparing the amount of money directed toward individual NRSA fellowships as opposed to T32 grants, the NINR spent 71% of its training budget on institutional training (T32) in 2004 as opposed to 29% for individual fellowships. The NINR proposes to increase the institutional training amount to 80% in 2006 (NINR, 2005a). According to Dr. Patricia Grady, Director of the NINR, the percent of the NINR budget allocated for training is approximately twice the NIH average and the NINR is consistently among the top three NIH institutes or centers with the highest percent of budget dedicated to training (NINR, 2005b).

As previously indicated, the NINR and NACNR are currently involved in an evaluation of nurse scientist training programs (NINR, 2003). This evaluation, which will cover a 10-year period from 1992–2001, will provide data addressing multiple facets of the NINR training programs including the career outcomes and trajectories for recipients of T32 funding. Pertaining to T32s, the initial findings of this evaluation include the following: (1) The majority of postdoctoral fellowships are supported by T32s; (2) Approximately one-half of T32 predoctoral fellows were supported for about 2 years; and (3) Since 1996, institutions without T32 funding have received more predoctoral individual NRSAs than institutions with T32s. Further preliminary data indicate that fewer T32-supported fellows received subsequent NIH research grants (R series) or NIH career development awards (K series) as compared to recipients of individual NRSA awards.

In response to this evaluation, the NACNR recommended that the NINR collect additional data from T32 applications; such data included past trainees' receipt of all types of funding and awards, types of employment secured following training, age at time of award, and qualitative measures such as the factors that might make the T32 awardees of some institutions more productive than those of other institutions. Another suggestion was that the identification of mechanisms of support for mentorship so that mentors might enhance training outcomes. The analyses of these outcomes of T32 training are currently underway (NINR, 2003).

## Principles Underlying NINR Support for T32s Focused on Vulnerable Populations Research

Various principles underlie NINR's support for the training of nurse scientists in vulnerable populations research. The following section identifies and discusses two of these principles: (a) NINR's commitment to the elimination of health disparities, and (b) the value of mentorship in the sponsorship of vulnerable populations research training.

## NINR Commitment to the Elimination of Health Disparities

The first principle underlying NINR support for T32s focused on vulnerable populations research is its commitment to the elimination of health disparities. In 1999, the NIH developed a strategic plan to address disparities in health care access and health outcomes. This group provided the NIH with its first definition of health disparities, "differences in the incidence, prevalence, mortality, and burden of diseases and other adverse health conditions that exist among specific population groups in the United States" (NIH, n.d.). Vulnerable populations suffer disproportionately from health disparities and the existence of health disparities is a characteristic generally associated with vulnerable populations.

In 2001, $20 million of the NIH budget was allocated to establish a trans-NIH Coordinating Center for Research on Health Disparities within the Office of the Director (NIH, n.d.). This group developed a strategic plan including goals, timetables, and methods of tracking accomplishments. The NIH now requires each individual institute to create a strategic plan for addressing health disparities.

The NINR began addressing health disparities and targeting the health needs of vulnerable populations prior to this mandate. In 1999, 20% of the NINR's budget was devoted to minority health issues; $11.29 million of which was set aside for research on health disparities (NINR, 2000a). Since that time, NINR funding opportunities continue to emphasize the importance of increasing the number of studies which both include minority participants and are conducted by minority researchers, as well as disseminating research findings to underserved groups. The NINR mission statement explicitly states that it supports health disparities research, and eliminating health disparities is an area of research emphasis in the NINR Strategic Plan for 2006–2010.

The NINR's Strategic Plan on Reducing Health Disparities is derived from its overall Strategic Plan for the 21st Century and is comprised of three domains, each with specific goals (NINR, 2000b). The first domain is *Areas of Focus*. This refers to an overall leadership emphasis on incorporating cultural and ethnic dimensions into scientific inquiry occurring under the purview of the NINR. The two goals under this domain are "to solicit research applications in targeted areas that will address significant questions related to health disparities, and to support the investigator-initiated research proposals that address significant questions related to health disparities and offer the best prospects for new knowledge and better health" (NINR, 2000b). In accordance with the first goal, program announcements and requests for applications have targeted various vulnerable populations and topics including low birth weight in minority populations, centers for research to reduce oral health disparities, diabetes self-management in minority populations, and cancer prevention among minority populations. Individual research funding has been provided to investigate chronic disease management in Spanish-speaking individuals, care of frail elderly African American nursing home residents, cultural variations in end of life care, and reducing sexual risk behaviors among economically challenged adolescents of color.

The second domain of the Strategic Plan is *Infrastructure*, which focuses on the development and expansion of research capabilities within schools of nursing including training and career development opportunities. The two goals of this domain are "to enhance research infrastructure allowing for an increased emphasis on projects relating to health disparities, and to enhance mentorship, training, and research opportunities for minority students and researchers" (NINR, 2000b). The provision of T32 training grants focused on health disparities or vulnerable populations falls in this domain, as do research supplements for underrepresented minorities and mentored research scientist development awards for minority investigators. There are currently 28 institutions receiving support from NINR T32 grants. Of these, 13 specifically emphasize research training that targets one or more vulnerable populations.

The final domain of the strategic plan on reducing health disparities is *Public Information Outreach*, focusing on promoting research training programs and enhancing dissemination of findings. Goals of this domain are to maintain involvement with minority nursing organizations to support identification and dissemination of minority health priorities and strategies and to help minority students and researchers advance their scientific careers, to enhance communication and dissemination of research activities and findings, and to continue sponsorship of annual training programs and involvement with other NINR and NIH initiatives (NINR, 2000b).

In an effort to meet these goals, the NINR has collaborated with the National Coalition of Ethnic Nursing Associations in conducting workshops addressing minority health nursing research, summarizing research results from NINR-funded studies on health disparities, and participating in activities with minority nursing organizations as well as the Hispanic Youth Initiative and the Society for the Advancement of Chicanos and Native Americans (NINR, 2000b).

In addition to the commitment to eradicate health disparities among vulnerable populations outlined by the NINR Strategic Plan, in 2001, the NINR in collaboration with the National Center on Minority Health and Health Disparities (NCMHD), established a program creating partnerships between schools of nursing with established research programs and schools of nursing with a significant number of minority students that are attempting to develop more intensive research programs (Grady, 2001). Between the NINR and the NCMHD, roughly $15 million was earmarked to create 17 centers and 8 partnerships to specifically address research in health disparities (NIH, 2002b). These partnerships aim to increase both the number of research studies involving minority participants, address health disparities, as well as increase the number of ethnic minority scholars conducting research. Each partnership has a specific focus and includes: health needs of Asian and Pacific Islanders; health promotion and restoration in the Hispanic population; access to care, process of care, and health outcomes; minority groups living with HIV disease; culturally competent nursing research; the influence of culture, race, and ethnicity on health promotion and disease prevention; health needs of rural, low-income Mexican American and American Indian populations; and self-management and self-assessment strategies to promote positive health and lifestyle changes in minority populations (Grady, 2003).

One of the Department of Health and Human Services' (DHHS) two overarching goals for Healthy People 2010 is the elimination of health disparities (DHHS, 2001). This goal cannot be attained without research funding. By providing significant financial support to individuals, institutions, and research centers, the NINR is playing an active role in helping to eliminate health disparities among vulnerable populations. Funding experienced researchers as well as training future researchers to address the wide range of issues involved in creating and perpetuating health disparities among vulnerable populations are crucial steps in this process.

## MENTORSHIP

A second principle underlying NIH and NINR support for T32s focused on vulnerable populations research is the recognition of the value of mentorship.

A number of documents within the NINR Web site refer to mentoring, or pairing new investigators with more experienced nurse researchers, as a valuable aspect of nursing training. At a meeting of T32 directors in 2003, the directors noted that T32 participants benefited from having multiple mentors. The mentors themselves considered the experience rewarding and also stated they benefited by the additional exposure to new research topics and methods (NINR, 2004). In addition, the NACNR has suggested to the NINR that it might consider identifying mechanisms of support for mentors involved with the training of nurse researchers (NINR, 2003). In both words and action, the NINR demonstrates acknowledgment of the value of mentorship.

Given the importance of mentorship to the development of nursing scholars in vulnerable populations research and other areas, this section addresses the concept of mentorship. There has been considerable attention of the development of nursing science over the past several years, yet less attention has been devoted to the development of the nurse scientist (Williams, 1988). With increasing enrollments in doctoral nursing programs (American Association of Colleges of Nursing, 2004), the concept of mentorship is essential to the development and productivity of nursing scholars in academia and in other nursing research positions.

The relationships between mentors and their protégés has been well described in the nursing, medicine, psychology, and business literature (Andrews & Wallis, 1999; Ford, 2004; Johnson, 2002; Marks & Goldstein, 2005; Staveley-O'Carroll et al., 2004; Tobin, 2004). Mentors may be identified as role models, counselors, and teachers (Johnson, Koch, Fallow, & Huwe, 2000). Generally, mentors are individuals who have accomplished significant career milestones and are able to pass on to others the wisdom they have attained through their experiences. Berk, Berg, Mortimer, Moss-Walton, and Yeo (2005) identified various attributes of mentors, such as commitment to the concept of mentoring, ability to challenge the protégé to explore his or her potential, and respectful of the protégé's potential for unique contributions.

To facilitate identification of the training needs of T32 fellows and to promote communication between fellows and their mentors, the NIH advocates the creation of an Individual Development Plan (IDP) (J. H. Flaskerud, personal communication, June 26, 2005). The IDP, developed by the Federation of American Societies for Experimental Biology and described in a series of articles that appeared in *The Scientist* (Clifford, 2002; Preston, 2002; Rieff, 2002), provides a formal plan to identify trainees' short-term performance needs and long-term career goals. The NIH recommendation that IDPs be incorporated into a broader mentoring program for T32 fellows again points to the recognition that mentors play an important role in the development of future research scientists.

In relating the value of mentorship and the training of nurse scientists prepared to conduct research with vulnerable populations, one wonders whether the mentors are guided by different or additional set of principles and skills that will ensure that their trainees continue a research career working with vulnerable populations. Relevant guiding principles could conceivably include commitments to social and distributive justice. Distributive justice, for instance, implies that society has a duty and responsibility to individuals with health needs such that all people are entitled to equal access and equitable health care (Putsch & Pololi, 2004). A mentor's skills and knowledge in the research applications of the concepts of cultural and linguistic competence or health literacy could be additional factors important for the development of trainees in vulnerable populations research. The specific qualities that enhance a mentor's ability to translate their knowledge and skills to their trainees pursuing vulnerable populations research careers is unknown and would be an important topic for future research.

Overall, mentoring is an extremely powerful process that can promote the intellectual, personal, and professional development of nursing scholars. Effective mentors are an absolute necessity for advancement of nursing science relating to the health of vulnerable populations.

## CASE STUDY AND DATA FROM INSTITUTIONS WITH NINR-FUNDED T32S

### Case Study of the UCLA T32 in Nursing Research With Vulnerable Populations History

The UCLA School of Nursing initially received an NINR T32 training grant in vulnerable populations research in 1994. As Flaskerud (2000) identified, building excellence and scholarship in nursing science requires a synergy among practice, education, research, and community involvement. The origins of this scholarship began in practice with UCLA's academic nursing center that has been providing direct patient care to the homeless and indigent population in Los Angeles since 1983. The majority of the clientele served by this health center are ethnic and racial minorities living at, or well below, national poverty levels. The health center provides a site for clinical training for nursing students, faculty practice, and a setting for community-based research.

With the clinic's development, education at the school expanded to incorporate knowledge and skills relevant to the care of underserved populations. Early faculty research led to the identification of concepts relevant to the health problems among vulnerable populations. These early identified research concepts ultimately led to the development of the underlying constructs in the

Vulnerable Populations Conceptual Model (VPCM) by Flaskerud and Winslow (1998), namely, resource availability, relative risk, and health status. The VPCM was further substantiated by a large body of research relating socioeconomic status, social status, and social and human capital with morbidity, mortality, knowledge, and power (Flaskerud & Winslow, 1998). Over the years, nursing faculty have developed research training careers based on health disparities and vulnerable populations. These vulnerable populations have included, but are not limited to, homeless populations, adolescents, ethnic minorities, women of color infected with HIV, adolescents in detention, and adolescents experiencing unplanned pregnancies.

The UCLA School of Nursing's experience in working with vulnerable populations provided the strong foundation for receipt of its first vulnerable populations T32 award. With this grant, a graduate level course in the health-related problems of vulnerable populations was developed, and an affiliated interdisciplinary scientific team, the Vulnerable Populations Research Interest Group, was formed.

## Description of the UCLA Vulnerable Populations T32 Training Program

The purpose of UCLA's vulnerable populations T32 training program was to prepare nursing scholars to conduct and disseminate nursing research in the area of the health-related problems of vulnerable populations. The program was designed to build the body of nursing science and knowledge relating to vulnerable populations. UCLA's T32 training program was unique in that it had a specific conceptual framework, the VPCM, which influenced the research of all the fellows. Vulnerable groups investigated in the training program were those living below the poverty level, ethnic and racial minorities, and socially marginalized populations.

Trainees in the T32 program were expected to meet the following objectives:

1. Plan, conduct, evaluate, and disseminate culturally competent research in the health-related problems of vulnerable populations;
2. Generate and test theory concerned with health disparities among vulnerable populations;
3. Contribute to the development of science in this area, both the knowledge base and methods, as a foundation for education and practice;
4. Collaborate with research participants, clinicians, and other researchers in the design and conduct of research and the development of science in the health-related problems of vulnerable populations;

5.  Contribute to health and social policy and ethical decision making as it affects vulnerable populations;

6.  Develop skills to contribute as educators, mentors, and leaders in nursing and health care; and

7.  Complete an extramural grant application to study health disparities in vulnerable populations (applies to postdoctoral fellows only).

The training program sponsored three predoctoral and two postdoctoral fellows each year. Predoctoral fellows were asked to submit a curriculum vitae, copies of transcripts, results of their scores on the graduate record examination, examples of scholarly papers or creative works, letters of recommendation, and a statement of purpose clarifying research, career, and program goals. Postdoctoral fellows were required to hold an earned doctorate, with either a masters degree or doctorate in nursing. Fellows were all assigned a faculty advisor that worked closely with them in program planning and career development.

Predoctoral fellows were expected to progress through their doctoral program by completing the required courses and oral and written examinations in a timely fashion. Postdoctoral fellows enrolled in courses that covered health-related problems of vulnerable populations, research on the family, community and health systems, nursing research ethics seminars and courses on accountability in biomedical research. All fellows were required to complete training in participatory research methods, community-based research, grant writing, and writing for publication. Fellows were required to participate in the Vulnerable Populations Research Interest Group monthly meetings and attend colloquia and workshops sponsored by the affiliated Center for Vulnerable Populations Research. It was in these meetings where they discussed their research, manuscripts, and participated in group identified projects that included research conference presentations and the development of publications. This publication is an example of one of the projects in which the T32 fellows participated.

Since its inception, UCLA enrolled 13 predoctoral and 7 postdoctoral fellows. Over the last 10 years, these fellows authored over 153 publications, conducted 155 conference and symposia presentations, and obtained over $2,036,997 in extramural grants for research. Graduates of the fellowship training have gone on to work in academic, research, and clinical practice settings.

## Examples of Scientific Contributions to Vulnerable Populations Research

Fellows associated with the UCLA School of Nursing's T32 in vulnerable populations research have expanded the body of knowledge and science relating to vulnerable populations in many domains. These domains include knowledge about the health and risk exposures of vulnerable populations as well as community-based participatory research methods.

To illustrate the innovative research on the health of vulnerable populations conducted by UCLA's T32 fellows, selected examples of published research results are provided. African American men are not generally considered an at-risk population for osteoporosis. In a study of the bone marrow density in African American men receiving hormonal therapy for prostate cancer, however, Conde et al. (2004) found significant bone loss in the lumbar spine, hip, and Ward's triangle in men over 70 years of age. In another study, Strehlow (2002) found that rhinitis and rhinorrhea were commonly associated with crack cocaine smoking among homeless individuals, a symptom that had never been previously reported. Tullmann (2002) observed that low-income older adults often experienced atypical symptoms of acute myocardial infarction, but did not seek treatment because they were only aware of the more commonly reported symptoms of heart attacks derived from studies of more affluent populations. These findings provide critical information for health care providers.

Daroszewski (2004) examined the dietary risks for cardiovascular disease among a sample of African American women. This fellow found that 77% of the women were consuming diets with more than 30% of their calories from fat. Carter (2003) discovered that even though depression is a normal response to a family member's diagnosis of cancer, caregiver's sleep quality and depression change over time and the use of self-report measures to document these symptoms greatly underestimates their incidence. Dixon (2004) conducted a multilevel epidemiologic analysis of the relationships between neighborhood characteristics and population health. Dixon demonstrated that neighborhood characteristics, including the area's socioeconomic and safety level, significantly predicted the individual health status of people living in the neighborhood (despite the individual's own socioeconomic status). Moreover, this study provided further evidence of the linkage between resource availability and health status as identified in the vulnerable population model developed by Flaskerud and Winslow (1998).

Further, advancing community-based participatory research methods, Cohen (2003) demonstrated the use of a cultural and linguistic adaptation of guided imagery and relaxation methods that were developed with low income, pregnant Latinas in a study on stress and anxiety. Utilizing lay health advisors in an intervention study promoting cardiovascular health, Kim, Koniak-Griffin, Flaskerud, and Guarnero (2004) found that lay health advisors experienced a sense of responsibility for the health of the community in which they lived and worked and concluded that the incorporation of lay health advisors in health promotion programs may enhance the overall success of such programs.

Current T32 fellows are exploring such topics as biologic and psychological factors that may influence hepatitis B vaccination response rates among homeless individuals, factors that affect the relationships between breast cancer survivors and their partners, the experience of violence and help-seeking behaviors among mothers of mentally ill individuals, intimate partner violence among members of multiple Hawaiian ethnic groups, and the complexities home health nurses experience in the provision of medication symptom management to persons with HIV/AIDS. Thus, UCLA T32 fellows have effectively contributed to the body of knowledge in nursing science in the area of the health-related problems of vulnerable populations.

## The Experiences of Other Universities With NINR-Funded T32s

In order to elucidate the experiences of, and activities associated with, other T32 training programs, institutions receiving T32 funds were identified via the NINR Web site (NINR (n.d.). This section includes data gathered from the Principal Investigators (PIs) of these T32 grants. A survey was developed to elicit responses from the PIs pertaining to: (a) their T32 programs; (b) the fellows associated with the program; and (c) the scholarly and career outcomes of former train-ees. To determine their willingness to participate in the survey, e-mail contacts were made with the PIs of the 28 NINR-funded T32 training programs between March and May 2005. Seventeen of the 28 PIs responded within the designated time-frame. From the completed surveys, data were abstracted and the findings are shown in Table 6.1.

In addition to identifying T32 program names, PIs, and affiliated universi-ties, Table 6.1 provides data on the number of years the T32 has been funded, the number of fellows supported by the T32 (to date and per year), and required activities associated with the T32. As indicated by the range of the numbers of years funded (2–18 years), this sample represents a broad range of experience in the operation and administration of T32 awards. The types and frequency of required program activities varies as well. Apart from individualized course-work required for the PhD, the vast majority of T32s (16 out 17 programs or 94%) require specific coursework or participation in educational offerings (seminars, colloquia) for predoctoral fellows. With respect to the frequency of T32-related activities, the University of Washington's T32 in Women's Health, also the longest-running T32 program, conducts the most frequent gatherings of pre- and postdoctoral fellows with weekly nursing research seminars. Participa-tion in mentored or individualized research was identified by nearly all of the T32 program directors.

In terms of the relationship of the information presented in Table 6.1 to vul-nerable populations research, it should be noted that although the T32 program names may not necessarily indicate a connection to vulnerable populations, all

**TABLE 6.1** Characteristics and Activities Associated with NINR-funded T32s

| University | T32 Program Name and PI(s) | Years Funded | Fellows (to date or per year) | Required Program Activities |
|---|---|---|---|---|
| Case Western Reserve University | Childbearing, Child-rearing and Caregiving PIs: Dr. May Wykle & Dr. Carol Musil | 4 | Predoctoral 7 2/yr | Predoc – Topical seminar in childbearing, child-rearing, and caregiving research; course on ethics and research; research practicum. |
| Indiana University School of Nursing | Training in Behavioral Nursing PI: Dr. Joan K. Austin | Predoctoral 15 Postdoctoral 10 | Predoctoral 3/yr Postdoctoral 3/yr | Predoc – Health Behavior Research Seminar, Research in Progress (RIP) meetings, and health behavior workshops. Postdoc – Individualized study, interdisciplinary comentors, Health Behavior Research Seminar, and external consultation. |
| Johns Hopkins University | Training in Health Disparities of Underserved Populations PI: Dr. Jerilyn Allen | 3 | Predoctoral 8 Postdoctoral 1 | Predoc/Postdoc – 4 quarters of (1) credit seminars on health disparities research. Postdoc – up to 15 hours/week of research residency. |

| Oregon Health Science University | Research Training: Nursing Care for Older People PI: Dr. Patricia G. Archbold | Predoctoral 15 Postdoctoral 13 | Predoctoral 3/yr Postdoctoral 5/yr | Predoc/Postdoc – Course to present their research ideas; identification of an NRSA research sponsor; submission of a written report; be a research assistant/conduct research under faculty direction; pilot work for dissertation. Postdoc – Responsible conduct of research, prepare proposals; review/critique research proposals with NIH format; review manuscripts; work with faculty to carry out research; pilot work with supervision; dissemination of work; may also participate in augmented program. |
| University of Arizona | Injury Mechanisms and Related Responses PI: Dr. Ki Moore | 3 | Predoctoral 3 Postdoctoral 2 | Predoc – Write individual NRSA; attend monthly seminar series. Postdoc – Write individual post-doc: K07 or K08 and/or R21; attend monthly seminar series. |

*(Continued)*

**TABLE 6.1** Characteristics and Activities Associated with NINR-funded T32s (*Continued*)

| University | T32 Program Name and PI(s) | Years Funded | Fellows (to date or per year) | Required Program Activities |
|---|---|---|---|---|
| University of California, Los Angeles | Nursing Research with Vulnerable Populations PI: Dr. Jacquelyn Flaskerud | 10 | Predoctoral 13 Postdoctoral 7 | Predoc – Monthly T32 group meetings; complete required courses; monthly colloquia; joint development of symposia and publications; mentored research activities. Postdoc – Monthly T32 group meetings; proposal development for extramural funding; monthly colloquia; joint development of symposia and publications; individualized study and mentored research activities. |
| University of California, San Francisco | Nursing Research Training in Symptom Management PI: Dr. Kathryn A. Lee | 9 | Predoctoral 24 Postdoctoral 19 | Predoc/Postdoc – Three quarters of symptom management seminars. |

| University of Illinois at Chicago | Primary Health Care (PHC) Research Training PI: Dr. Beverly J. McElmurry | 10 | Predoctoral 13 Postdoctoral 7 | Three courses in PHC—theory, ethics, & research/evaluation; Also, mentored research field experience; ongoing PHC brown bag series for trainees and others; individualized outcome goals such as presentations, publications, applications for funding, and global mentored activity. |
| University of Illinois at Chicago | Biobehavioral Nursing Research PI: Dr. Janet L. Larson | 11 | Predoctoral – 1 new position each year, total n=17 Postdoctoral - 1 new position each year, total n=9 | All fellows are required to participate in the Biobehavioral Nursing Research Seminar which is offered for credit each semester. Predoc – Required to take a graduate level physiology and biochemistry course; Biobehavioral research for dissertation. Postdoc – Mentored research activities. |

(Continued)

**TABLE 6.1** Characteristics and Activities Associated with NINR-funded T32s (*Continued*)

| University | T32 Program Name and PI(s) | Years Funded | Fellows (to date or per year) | Required Program Activities |
|---|---|---|---|---|
| University of Iowa | Clinical Genetic Nursing Research PI: Dr. Janet Williams | 5 | Postdoctoral 5 | Postdoc – Individual study with mentor; genetics classes if needed; weekly/monthly research seminars. |
| University of Michigan | Health Promotion/Risk Reduction (HPRR) Interventions PI: Dr. Carol Loveland-Cherry | 13 | Predoctoral 4/yr Postdoctoral 4/yr | Predoc – Three T32 meetings per month with faculty and postdoc fellows; 3 required HPRR specialty courses. Postdoc – Four T32 meetings per month with faculty and predocs (One is only postdocs); individual mentoring and study. |
| University of Michigan | Neurobehavior PIs: Dr. Bonnie Metzer & Dr. Barbara Therrien | 12 | Predoctoral 4/yr Postdoctoral 2/yr | Predoc – Finish coursework, work with mentor to develop research proposal and complete dissertation. Postdoc – Extend their research training via coursework and development of individual research program with mentor(s). |

| University of North Carolina at Chapel Hill | Interventions for Preventing and Managing Chronic Illness PI: Dr. Merle Mishel | 9 | Predoctoral 37 Postdoctoral 16 | Predoc/Postdoc – Bimonthly seminars in writing for publication. Two courses: From Theory to Intervention and Advanced Design; proposal generation for NRSA and other funding; involvement in mentor's research. Postdoc – Mentored research activity at one Center at UNC-CH; submission of proposal for extramural funding. |
| University of Rochester School of Nursing | Interventions with High Risk Children and Youth PI: Dr. Harriet Kitzman | 4 | Predoctoral 6/yr Postdoctoral 2/yr | Predoc/Postdoc – Two semesters of required specialty courses and participation in research forum. Postdoc – mentored research with sponsor and individual study. |
| University of Washington | Women's Health Nursing Research Training PI: Dr. Marcia Killien | 18 | Predoctoral 6/yr: to date = 31 Postdoctoral 4/yr: to date = 30 | Predoc/Postdoc – Weekly women's health nursing research seminars; Summer: participate in scientific integrity groups. Postdoc – Mentored research activity with sponsor. |

*(Continued)*

179

**TABLE 6.1** Characteristics and Activities Associated with NINR-funded T32s (*Continued*)

| University | T32 Program Name and PI(s) | Years Funded | Fellows (to date or per year) | Required Program Activities |
|---|---|---|---|---|
| University of Washington | Biobehavioral Nursing Research Training PI: Dr. Pam Mitchell | 6 | Predoctoral 6/yr Postdoctoral 4/yr | Predoc/Postdoc – Biobehavioral nursing research seminar and a research residency each quarter; summer: participate in scientific integrity groups. Postdoc – Mentored research activity with sponsor. |
| University of Wisconsin–Madison | Patient-Centered Informational Interventions PI: Dr. Sandra Ward | 4 | Predoctoral 10 Postdoctoral 5 | Predoc – Bimonthly informal T32 group discussions; complete required courses; monthly colloquia; guidance in development of F31 applications; joint development of symposia; work as an assistant with funded investigators. |

| | | | |
|---|---|---|---|
| Yale University School of Nursing | Research Training: Self- and Family Management PI: Dr. Margaret Grey | 2 | Predoctoral 4 Postdoctoral 4 | Postdoc – Individualized study; Biweekly T32 research forums; Proposal development for R03 or R21 type mechanisms; monthly colloquia; joint development of symposia. Predoc – Monthly seminars; Two courses on self and family management of chronic illnesses. Postdoc – Individual study with mentor; monthly seminars; two courses on self and family management of chronic illnesses. |

of the programs either focus on groups that would be considered vulnerable (i.e., women, older adults, children) or involve research areas that can be applied to vulnerable groups (i.e., symptom management, targeted biobehavioral interventions, genetics, and risk reduction strategies). As a result, the T32 fellows have many opportunities to incorporate research addressing the needs of vulnerable populations and this research can then be translated into practice.

In addition to the information displayed in Table 6.1, PIs were asked questions related to the career outcomes of former T32 fellows. They were also asked to provide suggestions for improvement of NINR funded T32 training programs. When asked about the estimated percentage of former T32 trainees that go on to pursue research careers, two PIs from one school estimated that 100% of both pre- and postdoctoral fellows engaged in nursing research activities following the training program. However, the PIs added that a limited number of these former trainees have attained federal funding for their research. At five schools, the PIs estimated that 100% of their postdoctoral fellows pursued research careers. In one school, 83% of their predoctoral fellows have gone on to careers in academia. At the other schools, the PIs estimated that most pre- and postdoctoral fellows go on to become nurse researchers as a part of the multiple responsibilities of an academic career.

Of the two more recently funded T32 programs, long-term outcomes were less clear; however, it was noted that one of the PIs indicated that all of the predoctoral fellows are currently participating in the program and one postdoctoral fellow has integrated research into his or her faculty role. At a second program, the predoctoral participants are currently enrolled in coursework and two postdoctoral fellows are completing their training; one of whom has been hired at a research-intensive institution and another is currently interviewing for a nursing research position.

In summary, the funding for training of pre- and postdoctoral fellows through the T32 mechanism is producing nursing scholars who integrate research within their multifaceted roles. This federally funded program is supporting the mission and strategic plans of the NIH and NINR by increasing the pool of scholars who can build the science of nursing and participate in interdisciplinary scientific teams.

## Recommendations and Conclusions

The NINR is the only institute at the NIH that supports research training for a target discipline. The shortage of nurse scientists persists, especially among Hispanic and African American nurses (Fawcett & McCorkle, 1995; Wallen, Rivera-Goba, Hastings, Peragallo, & DeLeon Siantz, 2005). While the NINR is committed to a small increase in its budget allocated to NRSAs, allocating an even greater percentage of its budget to development of nurse researchers through funding T32s and other research training mechanisms (i.e., K awards or individual NRSAs) is an important strategy to increase the numbers of nurse scientists prepared to conduct nursing research in the future. It is also recommended that the NINR continue to engage in its evaluation of the activities and posttraining scientific productivity of T32 fellows, and more publicly, disseminate this information to both institutions with current T32 funding as well as to institutions interested in applying for T32 funding. Though a major undertaking, a compilation and publication of this data may help identify best practices to maximize the benefits of T32 research training.

Training nurse scientists is different from the training of other health scientists. The pool of applicants is older and often geographically immobile. The T32 stipend, which has recently increased, remains a barrier for many nurses, especially at the postdoctoral level. The limited support for research expenses can hamper the postdoctoral fellow's ability to conduct pilot work necessary to submit a competitive research proposal or for a predoctoral fellow to complete a dissertation with an adequate sample size. These federally set financial limits are frequently not practical considering the usual career trajectory among nurse scientists. McGivern (2003) calls for accelerated research tracks that link baccalaureate preparation with doctoral preparation. This model could potentially yield a pool of predoctoral and postdoctoral fellows that are younger, more geographically mobile, and less dependent on a full-time salary.

On an institutional level, several of the NINR-funded T32 directors surveyed recommended increased collaboration and communication between T32 directors, particularly in terms of recruiting fellows. A recent conference bringing together T32 directors was viewed positively as a way to share innovative and effective practices. Other suggestions included joint sponsorship of annual or biannual conferences and summer institutes involving T32 fellows, their mentors, and T32 directors, as it is difficult to sponsor these events individually and secure adequate attendance. Additional recommendations for the enhancement of T32 training come from a report to the NACNR (NINR, 2004). These suggestions include promotion of the establishment of interdisciplinary research teams of students, training faculty in mentorship, and the consideration of funding non-nurse postdoctoral fellows.

The following recommendations for enhancing T32 nurse training programs come from the fellows associated with the UCLA T32 in vulnerable populations research. Fellows identified perceived facilitators of an effective T32 learning experience and challenges experienced as a participant. Apart from individualized mentoring, fellows considered required group-initiated research activities as critical to their growth as nurse scientists. These activities included participation in symposia development and presentation at professional meetings as well as manuscript preparation and publication. In addition to helping them build their resumes, these activities provided fellows with real-world skills and experiences in disseminating research. Requiring that T32 fellows engage in collectively supported projects is strongly recommended.

UCLA T32 fellows in vulnerable populations research further identified the opportunity to engage in an informal social network of pre- and postdoctoral fellows as a facilitator of an effective T32 learning experience. As a group of peers, the fellows exchanged resources and ideas that were both instructive and mutually beneficial. Consequently, the nurturance of collegial relationships and social cohesion between T32 fellows may be a valuable strategy for creating an effective T32 training environment.

Time constraints and commuting distances created a challenge to fostering opportunities for social networking between the UCLA T32 fellows. This challenge can be addressed in a variety of ways. For instance, fellows in their second year of T32 training could be paired with new fellows for the informal mentoring that is necessary to learn about the institution's resources and for creating a culture to groom nurse scientists into the role. In addition, greater utilization of electronic communications could be established between fellows, faculty, and T32 affiliates when personal meetings cannot take place because of time or geographic constraints. Establishing a cyber café to facilitate electronic communications would be one method to expand the opportunities for networking and improve communication about opportunities to present, publish, and fund nursing research. Since each funded T32 has a limited number of fellows at any given time, cyber connections could link fellows with similar interests to accelerate the learning process. Cyber connections could also be used to maintain communication among fellows after their training has been completed.

In summary, the incorporation of suggested enrichments to NINR-funded T32s combined with continued analytic evaluation of the program will result in the identification of a best practice model. NINR-funded T32s have afforded many developing nurse scholars the opportunity to learn from, and be mentored by, knowledgeable and experienced leaders in nursing research. T32s represent an investment in the future of nursing and the generation of nursing science.

## ACKNOWLEDGMENTS

Authors of this manuscript, all current or former fellows of the NINR-funded Nursing Research on Vulnerable Populations T32 training program at the UCLA School of Nursing gratefully acknowledge the NINR and the UCLA faculty for the training they have received as nurse scientists. We are also grateful for the candid responses from Directors of NINR-funded T32s from across the nation who have shared their thoughts on how T32 research training is currently operating and could be improved upon. Grant support for the development of this manuscript comes from NINR 5 T32 NR 07077 and NINR 2P30NR005041.

## REFERENCES

Andrews, M., & Wallis, M. (1999). Mentorship in nursing: A literature review. *Journal of Advanced Nursing, 29*(1), 201–207.

American Association of Colleges of Nursing. (2004). AACN *Annual state of the schools*. Retrieved March 20, 2005, from http://www.aacn.nche.edu/media/pdf/annualreport04pdf

Berk, R., Berg, J., Mortimer, R., Moss-Walton, B., & Yeo, T. (2005). Measuring the effectiveness of faculty mentoring relationships. *Academic Medicine, 80*(1), 66–71.

Carter, P. A. (2003). Family caregivers' sleep loss and depression over time. *Cancer Nursing, 26*(4), 253–259.

Clifford, P. S. (2002). Quality time with your mentor. *The Scientist, 16*(19), 59.

Cohen, J. (2003). Effects of an intervention program to decrease distress in pregnant Latina women at risk for preterm birth. *Dissertation Abstracts International, 63*(07), 3227 (UMI No. AAT 3059571).

Conde, F. A., Sarna, L., Oka, R. K., Vredevoe, D. L., Retting, M. B., & Aronson, W. J. (2004). Age, body mass index, and serum prostate-specific antigen correlate with bone loss in men with prostate cancer not receiving androgen deprivation therapy. *Urology, 64*, 335–340.

Daroszewski, E. B. (2004). Dietary fat consumption, readiness to change, and ethnocultural association in midlife African American women. *Journal of Community Health Nursing, 21*(2), 63–75.

Dixon, E. L. (2004). Neighborhoods and adult health status: A multi-level analysis of social determinants of health disparities in Los Angeles County. *Dissertation Abstracts International, 65*(05), 2341 (UMI No. AAT3132998).

Fawcett, J., & McCorkle, R. (1995). Cultural considerations in postdoctoral nursing research training. In *Successful postdoctoral research training for African American nurses* (pp. 5–9). American Academy of Nursing: Washington, DC.

Flaskerud, J. H. (2000). Developing leadership and excellence with vulnerable populations in research, education, and practice. *Nursing Leadership Forum, 4*(3), 76–84.

Flaskerud, J. H., & Winslow, B. J. (1998). Conceptualizing vulnerable populations health-related research. *Nursing Research, 47*, 69–78.

Ford, H. (2004). Mentoring, diversity, and academic surgeon. *Journal of Surgical Research, 118*, 1–8.

Grady, P. (2001). *Research partnership program to address health disparities*. Retrieved April 8, 2005, from http://ninr.nih.gov/ninr/news-info/pubs/outlooksept01.html

Grady, P. (2003). *An NINR initiative to address health disparities*. Retrieved April 7, 2005, from http://ninr.nih.gov/ninr/news-info/pubs/NOJan03.pdf

Johnson, B. (2002). The intentional mentor: Strategies and guidelines for the practice of mentoring. *Professional Psychology: Research and Practice, 33*(1), 88–96.

Johnson, B., Koch, C., Fallow, G., & Huwe, J. (2000). Prevalence of mentoring in clinical versus experimental doctoral programs: Survey findings, implications, and recommendations. *Psychotherapy, 37*(4), 325–334.

Kim, S., Koniak-Griffin, D., Flaskerud, J. H., & Guarnero, P. A. (2004). The impact of lay health advisors on cardiovascular health promotion: Using a community-based participatory approach. *Journal of Cardiovascular Nursing, 19*(3), 192–199.

Marks, M., & Goldstein, R. (2005). The mentoring triad: Mentee, mentor, and environment. *The Journal of Rheumatology, 32*(2), 216–218.

McGivern, D. O. (2003). The scholar's nursery. *Nursing Outlook, 51,* 59–64.

National Institutes of Health. (n.d.). *Addressing health disparities: The NIH program of action.* Retrieved April 8, 2005, from http://healthdisparities.nih.gov/whatare.html

National Institutes of Health. (2002a). *NIH National Research Service Award institutional research training grants.* Retrieved April 5, 2005, from http://grants.nih.gov/grants/guide/pa-files/PA-02-109.html

National Institutes of Health. (2002b). *NIH news release: New initiative to reduce health disparities announced by the National Institute of Nursing Research.* Retrieved April 7, 2005, from http://ninr.nih.gov/ninr/news-info/healthdisp.pdf

National Institute of Nursing Research. (n.d.). *Current NINR National Research Training Award institutional research training grants.* Retrieved June 10, 2005, from http://ninr.nih.gov/ninr/research/dea/2002T32.html

National Institute of Nursing Research. (2000a). *News from NINR: Health disparities.* Retrieved April 8, 2005, from http://ninr.nih.gov/ninr/news-info/pubs/outlookjuly00.htm

National Institute of Nursing Research. (2000b). *Strategic plan on reducing health disparities.* Retrieved April 5, 2005, from http://ninr.nih.gov/ninr/research/diversity/mission.html

National Institute of Nursing Research. (2003). *Minutes of the National Advisory Council for Nursing Research—January 28–29, 2003.* Retrieved June 5, 2005, from http://ninr.nih.gov/ninr/about/adv-council/meetings/minutes0103.pdf

National Institute of Nursing Research. (2004). *Minutes of the National Advisory Council for Nursing Research—January 27–28, 2004.* Retrieved June 5, 2005, from http://ninr.nih.gov/assets/Documents/NACNRminutesjan2004.doc

National Institute of Nursing Research. (2005a). *Congressional justification, 2006.* Retrieved June 5, 2005, from http://ninr.nih.gov/assets/Documents/NINRCJFY2006.pdf

National Institute of Nursing Research. (2005b). *Minutes of the National Advisory Council for Nursing Research—January 25–26, 2005.* Retrieved June 5, 2005, from http://ninr.nih.gov/assets/Documents/Jan2005CouncilMinutes-final.pdf

National Research Council. (1980). *Personnel needs and training for biomedical and behavioral research.* Washington, DC: National Academy Press.

Pion, G. M. (2001). *The early career progress of NRSA predoctoral trainees and fellows.* NIH Publication Number 00–4900. Retrieved June 11, 2005, from http://grants.nih.gov/training/career_progress/

Preston, J. R. (2002). Mentors are made, not born. *The Scientist, 16*(17), 54–55.

Putsch, R., & Pololi, L. (2004). Distributive justice in American health care: Institutions, power, and the equitable care of patients. *The American Journal of Managed Care, 10*(10), SP45–SP53.

Rieff, H. I. (2002). A mentor maintenance program. *The Scientist, 16*(20), 65.

Staveley-O'Carroll, K., Pan, M., Meier, A., Han D., McFadden, D., & Souba, W. (2004). Developing the young academic surgeon. *Journal of Surgical Residence, 118,* 109–113.

Strehlow, A. J. (2002). The presence of rhinitis and rhinorrhea and body system problems in homeless crack-cocaine smokers. *Dissertation Abstracts International, 62*(08), 3558 (UMI No. AAT3024023).

Tobin, M. (2004). Mentoring: Seven roles and some specifics. *American Journal of Respiratory and Critical Care Medicine, 170*, 114–117.

Tullmann, D. (2002). The effects of an intervention to reduce delay on the knowledge, attitudes, beliefs, perceived control and anxiety in older adults at risk for acute myocardial infarction. *Dissertation Abstracts International, 63*(07), 3236 (UMI No. AAT3059604).

U.S. Department of Health and Human Services. (2001). *Healthy People 2010*. Retrieved April 8, 2005, from http://www.healthypeople.gov/Document/html/uih/uih_bw/uih_2.htm#goals

Wallen, G. R., Rivera-Goba, M. V., Hastings, C., Peragallo, N., & De Leon Siantz, M. (2005). Developing the research pipeline: Increasing minority nursing research opportunities. *NLN: Nursing Education Perspectives, 26*, 29–33.

Williams, C. A. (1988). Career development of the nurse-scientist: The new doctorate faces a postdoctoral. *Journal of Professional Nursing, 4*, 73.

# PART III

## Integrating Biologic Methods in Vulnerable Populations Research

# Chapter 7

## Genomics and Proteomics Methodologies for Vulnerable Populations Research

Christine E. Kasper

### ABSTRACT

*This chapter describes common genomic and proteomic methods and their application to the study of vulnerable population groups. The International HapMap project is discussed in relation to unique Haplotype single nucleotide polymorphisms (htSNPs) in population groups. In addition, studies, which have used these methods to investigate aging, ethnic, and racial specific conditions, as well as psychiatric diseases, are reviewed. Advantages and limitations of various genomic and proteomic approaches are discussed in relation to population admixture and sample selection.*

Keywords: genomics; proteomics; vulnerable population methods

## GENOMIC AND PROTEOMIC METHODS

The recent popularity of genomic and proteomic methods is enticing to those who seek a way to ease the pain and disparities to which vulnerable populations are subject. While the precision of techniques provides a means to uncover mechanistic causes, such as poverty, abuse, and their sequelae, genomics and proteomics are fundamentally no more than tools capable of revealing information about a biologic system. How we use that information and understand its meaning will illumine how we better the lives of those we serve.

Genomics seeks to study the molecular organization and physical mapping of the nucleotides on a genome (Khoury, 2003). There are two major subfields of study, structural and functional genomics. Borrowing heavily from other disciplines such as biophysics and bioinformatics, structural genomics studies the three-dimensional shape, macromolecular folding classifying the molecules into functional families. Functional genomics studies the function of the entire genome, integration of the structure of DNA, the molecular function, and interaction of genes and gene products (Wu et al., 2002).

Examining genomic information in terms of regulation and function is proteomics. The study of proteomics was born from the completion of the Human Genome Project as was the study of genomics. It consists of all the proteins encoded by cellular DNA and reveals the detailed function of a cell (Cavalli-Sforza, 2005). Proteomic function varies with developmental age, nutrition, environmental stressors, metabolic rate, organ system, and general health of the organism (Rédei & Rédei, 2003). All of these factors are known to be important variables in the study of vulnerable population groups. Recently, there has been an exponential expansion of this field as proteins are the functional molecules of the cell and targets of drug interventions. Pharmacogenomic drugs are under development targeting complex diseases and related conditions, such as hypertension, obesity, and type II diabetes, known to be disproportionately higher in vulnerable populations than in the general population (Ioannidis, Ntzani, Trikalinos, 2004; Kahn, 2005).

Proteomic methods seek to resolve and identify groups of interacting proteins (Gromov et al., 2002). Cellular proteins interact to form molecular machines, regulatory pathways, and biologic systems. When proteins are altered due to genetic defects or modification by nutritional or environmental factors, the interaction of that protein with others is also changed, becoming causal factors in disease, and potent sites of drug intervention. Proteomic studies seek to understand the behavior of biologic systems and map the relationships between proteins (Uetz & Finley, 2005). These maps provide data for the construction of predictive models of metabolic behavior and signal transduction through the defined system (Apic, Ignjatovic, Boyer, & Russell,

2005; Vidal, 2005). Protein information in the form of two-dimensional poly-acrylamide gel electrophoresis (2DPE) databases form the basis of exploratory investigations. International 2DPE databases, such as SwissProt, serve as repositories for protein data and contain protein sequences along with descriptions of the function of the protein, its domain structure, post-translational modifications, their known variants, and diseases associated with deficiencies in proteins (Bairoch et al., 2005; Boeckmann et al., 2003; Yip et al., 2004) (see Figure 7.1).

Proteins are produced in highly complex interacting systems requiring a high level of precision and variable control. When the genome produces RNA, the products can be processed in multiple ways and translated into multiple polypeptides. The translated products can be modified by a host of various epigenetic mechanisms. The multiple alternative ways of transcription result in numerically more proteins than genes. Further, these proteins then undergo substantial additional post-translational modifications to adapt them to the developmental state, and other needs of the organism. While the genome is stable and remains essentially the same throughout the life cycle, proteomic functions and the proteins produced over time will vary greatly in response to external factors as well as interactions with other proteins (Demirel & Keskin, 2005; Hao, Zhu, Huang, & Li, 2005; Liu, Liu, & Zhao, 2005). Estimates of the total number of proteins produced by the human genome vary widely in the range of 23,000 to 40,000 genes (Harrison & Gerstein, 2002; Harrison, Kumar, Lang, Snyder, & Gerstein, 2002).

Epidemiologic research has clearly demonstrated that persons belonging to vulnerable populations by virtue of ethnicity, race, or socioeconomic status are often disadvantaged in relation to health care and response to conventional treatment (Burchard et al., 2003; Foster & Sharp, 2002; Marshall, 1998). Stressors, such as nutrition, toxic chemical exposure, and psychological stressors alter protein manufacture and may result in disease (Dierick, Eliaers, et al., 2002; Hayes et al., 2005; Kim et al., 2004; Waters & Fostel, 2004; Young, 2003). It is thought by many that application of genomic and proteomic technologies to complex diseases in vulnerable populations may reveal unique genetic markers and responses to external factors which will be used to create customized pharmacologic agents and other targeted therapies (Halapi, Stefansson, Hakonarson, 2004; Lewin & Weiner, 2004).

## PURPOSE

This chapter reviews and summarizes selected research papers which use genomic and proteomic approaches to determine fundamental structural and functional changes in proteins arising from altered transcription and translation

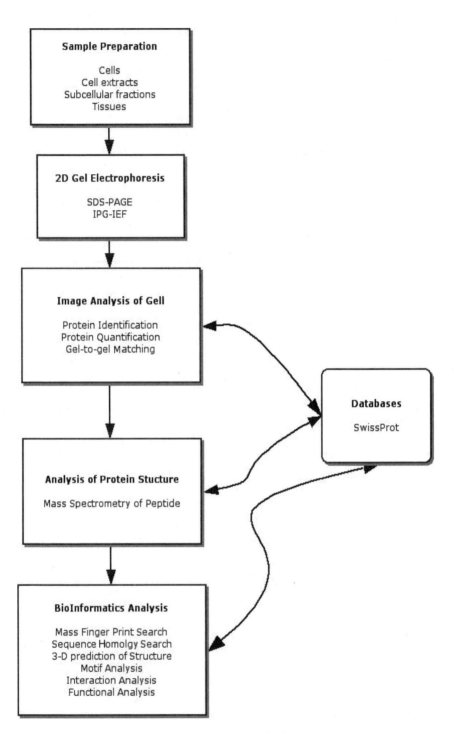

FIGURE 7.1    International 2DPE database, SwissProt.

of the genome underlying health disparities in vulnerable populations, such as ethnic and racial minority groups, gender differences, geriatric populations, and those with psychiatric illness (Bonham, Warshauer-Baker, & Collins, 2005). The study of health disparities has been monitored by the long-standing use of social and political constructs especially with regard to ethnicity and race (Atkin, 2003).

In the context of health services research, the use of these categories allows the monitoring and measurement of racial and ethnic disparities in health status, access, quality of care, and outcomes, which are the result of systematic disadvantages, such as chronic nutritional deficits, environmental exposure to toxins, or exposure to chronic stress (Shields et al., 2005). If these population characteristics are used for the purposes of basic genetic biomedical research, it may falsely appear that certain groups or races possess an inherent vulnerability to a disease.

The critical difference is that the use of ethnic or racial characterization variations, appropriate for monitoring the health impact of racial, ethnic, or socioeconomic disparities, are not necessarily the same as those required for biologic studies structured to find the underlying causal pathways of disease (Duster, 2005; Lee, Mountain & Koenig, 2001; Ossorio & Duster, 2005; Parra, Kittles, & Shriver, 2004; Shields et al., 2005; Whitfield & McClearn, 2005). The genetic composition of an individual is the sum of all of their ancestors. In six generations, an individual has 126 ancestors. Each genetic contribution contains multiple genetic variants, and assuming that categorical population identities, such as Asian or European, can imply single origins or genetic similarity, the concept is biologically inaccurate.

Categorization of people by race and ethnicity fundamentally reflect the viewpoint, values, norms, and traditions of a country's belief system and the majority groups (Wilkinson & King, 1987). These factors are logically studied within the context of the social sciences; however, biology is universal, devoid of social constructs, governed by fundamental laws of physics, mathematics, and chemistry. Biology can adapt or be influenced by the environment, nutrition, toxins, and chronic stressors. The interface of human biology and society is where the study of vulnerable populations is of value. However, to understand these effects fully, one needs to determine the factors imbedded within the concepts of race and ethnicity, such as stress or nutrition, which have geologic effects. These so-called health behaviors are the variables of interest, which can alter genetic expression.

## SCOPE OF REVIEW

Genomics and proteomics, inherently transdisciplinary in nature, are reported in a wide variety of scientific research journals. Computerized searches for research reports were made using PubMed, Medline, and Cumulative Index of Nursing and Allied Health Literature. The key words race, ethnicity, aging, psychiatry, vulnerable populations, nursing, proteomics, and genomics were used. In addition, specific ethnic and racial populations were used with the key words (i.e., African American, Chinese, Native American, etc.). Other sources of information included the NIH Center for Scientific Review's CRISP database, and the Internet based search tool Google Scholar. Papers that only used genetic methods or examined the function of a single gene were excluded (Rédei & Rédei, 2003). Studies reporting the use of genomic techniques first appeared in the early 1990s and did not fully emerge until an accurate high quality sequence of the Human Genome was available in 2003 (Collins et al., 1998). To date, there have been 5,236 papers on genomics since 1988 and 2,428 using proteomic methods since 1998. Papers reporting studies on human genomics and proteomics reduce the numbers to 1,259 and 432, respectively. Papers citing the use of these methods with various racial or ethnic population groups or other vulnerable populations have only been reported in the past 5 years and number less than 50. It is interesting to note that when searches crossed authors names with faculty of schools of nursing, 12 of these papers had at least one author who was also a member of a nursing faculty.

The innovative programs of the National Institute of Nursing Research such as the summer Genetics Institute and the funding of investigator training grants (Grady & Collins, 2003) have fostered nursing research in these areas. Many laboratories in Schools of Nursing are beginning programs of research in genomics and proteomics; however, few have yet to publish papers.

## Overview of Contextual Issues

Both genomic and proteomic methodologies ideally require a stringent level of control of the organism of interest. The precision of the methods is only as precise as the initial controls imposed on the sample; and, the genetic consistency of the sample. Application of sophisticated genomic or proteomic techniques to determine a change in diet or toxic effects of a chemical on a specific strain, for example Fisher 344 rats, usually leads to fairly precise findings, as the precision and limited variance is derived from a known genetic pedigree reared under highly controlled environmental conditions. Research subjects, on the other hand, do not present themselves to our studies similarly well documented. Therefore, the investigator needs to consider their sample populations in biologic terms and not groups commonly associated with epidemiologic or population health studies.

## Vulnerability

The concept of vulnerability has been widely studied within nursing, public health, and social science disciplines. Depending on the scientific question, various population factors, such as ethnicity, race, socioeconomic status, and age, have been used to define population membership (Duster, 2005; Ioannidis et al., 2004; Ossorio & Duster, 2005; Shields et al., 2005; Wang & Sue, 2005; Whitfield & McClearn, 2005). These social constructs serve to define characteristics that are useful within the context of social and behavioral research. However, neither ethnicity nor race is sufficiently stringent to serve as proxies for inter-individual biologic differences. Largely, these variables are assigned by self-identification or appearance. Both methods have been demonstrated to be notoriously inaccurate especially within highly admixed North American population groups (Duster, 2005; Ossorio & Duster, 2005; Shields et al., 2005; Wang & Sue, 2005; Whitfield & McClearn, 2005).

However, the underlying uncritical reliance on such population character-istics as ethnicity, language, religion, culture, nationality, proves to be insufficient when examining vulnerable populations from the viewpoint of genomics or pro-teomics. One of the most important findings of the Human Genome Project was that there is 99.9% sequence similarity shared by all humankind (Bonham et al., 2005; Collins, 2004). This is an important paradigm shift for the researcher from vague socially based variables of race and ethnicity to a more subtle and nuanced consideration of the distribution and structure of genetic differences among humans (Foster & Sharp, 2002, 2004). What might be the origins of the various diseases, syndromes and other health related problems, which arise for the < 0.1% genetic variation?

Inter individual differences begin with a single mutation, which is then amplified and reproduced over time with each generation and over space and distance with the migration and inter mating of that generation. Sampling of the mutation at a fixed point in time would reveal the inheritance of the mutation at different rates and frequencies in different groups and individuals in those groups over time. While these may appear in ethnic or racial popu-lation groups, the actual overall variation of the genome would reflect the accumulated genomic history, which contains exponentially more variance. Therefore, substitution of race or ethnicity for historical genetic variation could lead to confusion regarding the attribution of biologic significance to the marker (Foster & Sharp, 2002, 2004). These distinctions become more important as disease and drug related genes common to vulnerable popula-tions are sought.

There are currently 48 genes, which have pharmacogenetic variants (Goldstein & Hirschhorn, 2004), reported to influence drug response between African Americans and European Americans (Serre & Paabo, 2004). However, of all genetic variation that exists in humans, only a very small number are explained to be due to between group variations. The vast majority of genetic variations are due to inter individual differences in a group. Part of the reason for this phenomenon is that all humans are believed to have genetically origi-nated in Africa. Therefore, we all carry so-called African genes, which, from a genomic-proteomic view, gives a different concept to what it means to be African American.

## Design and Methodological Limitations

Scientifically, the study of proteomics has altered some of the traditional means of structuring experiments. Most scientific experimentation is driven by first posing hypotheses. However, hypotheses are not always used for proteomic research; more direct methods, using the simultaneous expression patterns of interacting genetic networks, are employed (Wagner, Miliotis, Marko-Varga, Bischoff, & Unger, 2002). The general aim of these experiments is to compare the expression level of as many proteins as possible at a given point in time, under specific experimental conditions in a chosen organism. The unknown proteins expressed in the experimental system are then compared to a known control in the hope of finding new proteins or altered protein expression. Strictly speaking, this is a classic experimental design.

## Linkage Analysis and Association Studies

In general, there are two major approaches to determine susceptible genes for complex disorders, linkage analysis, and association studies. Linkage analysis is hypothesis neutral and searches for markers that statistically segregate with a disease. Most of these studies seek to construct detailed maps of the chromosome segment to identify the actual gene or genes causal to the disease. Association studies ask if certain genetic variants are more likely to occur in patients with a specific disease than by statistical chance. This method has the increased chance for false positives or the identification of effects that are too small to be found in linkage studies. Often association studies are also limited by smaller sample sizes and self-identification of race or ethnic characteristics. Of the selected studies, the most robust are those using admixture analysis rather than self-classification (Arya et al., 2002; Fernandez et al., 2003; Ioannidis et al., 2004; Thompson et al., 2004; Zhu et al., 2005).

## Proteomic Methods

The "Current Protocols in Human Genetics" (Dracopoli et al., 2005) series provides the authoritative repository of current methods in genomics and proteomics. The online e-Book format changes continuously with updated releases every week. Every methodology included has been tested and peer reviewed and represents the cutting edge techniques for these fields. Unique to these invaluable guides are the inclusion of historical background information and evolution of the methods along with key citations.

A standard array of methods has been developed to study the genome such as polymerase chain reaction, sequencing after cloning, and microarrays. However, there are no established procedures applicable to all proteins. Two-dimensional gel electrophoresis (2DGE) is widely used to separate most proteins and monoclonal antibody techniques are used to tag and identify the location of proteins alone or together (colocalized) with other proteins.

Proteome analysis is usually a two-part process. The sample is collected and analyzed using 2DGE. Proteins expressed by the genome and located in the sample at the time of collection are separated as so-called spots in the gel, visualized with a stain or label and quantified (Lauber et al., 2001). Current instrumentation permits the separation of 1,000–2,000 proteins on a single 2D gel (Dierick, Dieu et al., 2002; Toda, 2001). The proteins, which have been separated on the 2D gels, are then stained or labeled in order to see or visualize the protein. Stains and labels differ in their sensitivity, cost, toxicity, and must be compatible with mass spectroscopy analysis. Following visualization of the proteins, the 2D gel pattern is digitally imaged and analyzed for proteins of interest. Image analysis of 2DGE is the most time consuming, labor intensive, and crucial part of proteomic comparisons. The gels are compared to databases such as SwissProt and the proteins of interest are identified or further studied using mass spectrometry (Gorg et al., 2000; Lauber et al., 2001). Recent software programs have assisted in this process but have not significantly reduced the time these comparisons entail.

The proteins present in the sample are the limiting factor in 2DGE. Often, sampled proteins are lost during transfer from the sample to the initial 1-dimensional immobilized pH gradient gel or cannot be solubilized by the selected buffer solution. If large numbers of proteins are present (e.g., >100–2,000), it may be necessary to subdivide the sample into isolated subcellular components prior to running the 2DGE (Jung, Heller, Sanchez, & Hochstrasser, 2000). Subdividing the sample into cellular locations limits the number or proteins separated on each gel, permitting better visual spacing between each, and easier isolation of the proteins (Dracopoli et al., 2005). Newer methods have been developed to examine isoforms, structure, and modulational changes during development; post-transcriptional and post-translational modifications; and interactions with other proteins or substances, such as drugs or toxins (Table 7.1). Proteomics has emerged as a key discipline in the post-genomic tool chest over the last few years; and, proteomic technology has become extraordinarily powerful. Mass spectrometry, array-based protein methods, and single cell imaging methods have combined to give us rich data of all the expressed proteins of the cell, its so-called proteome. While the technology is still developing rapidly, data collection efforts are coalescing. Sophisticated bioinformatics programming

**TABLE 7.1**    Genomic and Proteomic Methods

| Genomic: Sequence methods | Proteomic methods |
| --- | --- |
| • Chromatogram | • Domain functions |
| • PCR | • Yeast 2 hybrid |
| • Cycle sequencing | • Arabidopsis |
| • Automated megabase sequencing | • ICAT (silent version) |
| • Capillary electrophoresis | • Transposons |
| • Whole genome sequencing | • Cre/lox P recombination |
| • RT-PCR | • Epitope Tags |
| • Nested PCR | • Barcode knockout yeast |
| • Northern blot | • Biotin and Avidin binding |
| • Southern blot | • Affinity chromatography |
| • Western blot | • Kinase and enzyme assays |
| • SDS and Coomassie stain of protein gel | • Relative sizes |
| • Knockout mouse | • RNAi (RNA interference) |
| • FACS: fluorescence activated cell sorting | • Mass Spectroscopy |
| • Elisa | • Visualization of data |
| • Dendrograms | • 2DGE |

and databanks are needed to keep track of the wealth of data and beginning efforts are underway to integrate disparate large-scale data sets.

## Vulnerable Populations and the HapMap

In the case of vulnerable population research, it is assumed that nutrition, stress, environmental toxins, or so-called racial and ethnic factors create or influence differences in protein expression. Experiments will be limited by differences between subjects in their exposure to these factors or differences in their genetic mixture of historic ancestral groups. To minimize these limitations, subjects need to be as similar as possible in their history and genetic background. In studies where race or ethnicity is a factor, ideally subjects are screened and compared to the HapMap database for known genetic markers of ancestral continental origin (International HapMap Consortium, 2003; Liu, Johnson, Casella, & Wu, 2004). Microsatellite or single nucleotide polymorphism (SNP) markers are used to look for genes that contribute to disease risk in whole-genome association studies. In these studies, DNA from people with a disease of interest is compared to others without respect for ancestry or population groups (Foster & Sharp, 2002, 2004). Unlike studies that rely on disease associations, the HapMap provides a data source to look for similarities or patterns of genetic variation between persons with a disease, known as an association study.

Haplotypes are linear sequences between 100 to 100,000 bases long, located on a single chromosome, and can be identified by an altered chromosomal segment. It is known that alleles close to the altered segment are frequently inherited together as a group known as linkage disequilibrium (LD). Using the LD groups to search rather than a single genetic change, increases processing speed. When complete, the HapMap will allow the identification of a few SNPs or haplotype SNPs (htSNPs) to locate longer segments for study. In addition, haplotypes are conserved within populations over time. The HapMap will record common genetic variants from subjects in genetic studies. However, there are no genomic equivalents to so-called race or ethnic groupings, nor can SNPs or haplotypes be grouped in this manner. The complex diseases, which may result in certain ancestral groupings, appear as clusters of similar patterns of different magnitudes across a large geographical space. Historically, newer SNPs, haplotypes, and alleles are more likely to be found within some population groups who share common localities and social groups. This assumes that there has been less time for these factors to be dispersed into the larger gene pool. It is not yet known how databases of common genetic variations across populations, such as HapMap will contribute to the elucidation of such limited genetic variants (Tishkoff & Kidd, 2004).

Differences in genetic background of either the experimental or control groups can yield false positive or false negative findings. It is crucial to match race, ethnicity, and verify genetic admixture of the subjects (Halder & Shriver, 2003; Parra, Kittles, & Shriver, 2004; Patterson et al., 2004; Smith et al., 2004a). This factor alone is a major source of error in genomic and proteomic studies. For example, classifying subjects as European in origin rather than Southern European or Northern European may be sufficient to increase the risk of error in the study. Another potential source of error involves the sampled tissues. One cannot always use peripheral blood or serum samples as a proxy for a specific tissue due to marker dilution in the peripheral blood supply (Taback & Hoon, 2004). This phenomenon is especially important when conducting studies of the central nervous system and behavioral factors (Zhang et al., 2005). In certain conditions, the environment is a very important variable to attempt to control. Similar duration and magnitude of exposure to the environmental factor is optimal. Consideration of the consistency of the environmental factor in different locations is also an important factor.

## Reviewed Study Groupings

While many studies have been published using genomic and proteomic methods and approaches, very few have specifically targeted groups that could be designated as vulnerable populations. At this time, studies of this nature have been limited by gaps in data resident in the key databases such as the HapMap. Study of vulnerable populations will be facilitated as more SNPs and htSNPs data from various population groups is entered into the HapMap. The reviewed studies are grouped into characteristics of vulnerable populations, such as ethnicity or race, aging, cancer, and psychiatric illness; these characteristics are derived from the keywords designated by the studies themselves. While these studies often use sociologic constructs, genomic or proteomic studies seek genetic mechanisms of disease. Studies that used genomic or proteomic methods to determine the success of clinical interventions will not be discussed here (Table 7.2). In addition, redundant studies or those reporting negative results were also eliminated.

## Aging

Experimental gerontology or experimental aging research has focused on progressively accumulating errors in genetic structures with aging and is generally known as error catastrophe theory or generalized error theory of aging (Orgel, 1963, 1973). These theories propose that aging is due to accumulating DNA sequence errors, which then produce inaccurate protein synthesis and degraded proteins. Altered forms of proteins are known as isoforms and form the basis of much of the scientific work using various methods of gel electrophoresis. Based on these methods, experimental gerontology uses methods of differential patterns displayed by these aging altered protein structures on 2DGE gels. Differential display visually and physically separates the altered protein from those of controls.

To date, there are three significant studies conducted on human populations with respect to aging. The first, and most significant, by Ioannidis et al. (2004) is a large-scale (N = 297,911) study of disease associations across various ages and so-called racial groups: European, East Asian, Hawaiian, African, Arabic, Turkish, and Native Indian (Table 7.2). The important question addressed by this study was whether ancestry influences the impact of each gene variant on the disease risk. It was convincingly demonstrated for 43 validated gene-disease associations across 697 study populations of various descents that genetic markers for gene-disease associations vary greatly in frequency across populations, but their biological impact on the risk for common diseases appears to be consistent across traditional racial boundaries. In general, common diseases occur across racial and continental boundaries. It would then appear that environmental and life-style factors may indeed negatively impact this control genomic baseline giving credence to the study of vulnerable population groups.

Two smaller, but substantial, studies used linkage analysis to search for genomic changes specifically due to aging. Weeks et al. (2000) searched and located candidate genes for age-related maculopathy. Age-related maculopathy

**TABLE 7.2** Selected Research Papers

| Citation | Sample | Populations | Design | Purpose | Results |
|---|---|---|---|---|---|
| **Aging** | | | | | |
| (Ioannidis et al., 2004) | N = 697 studies, total N = 297,411 | Human, aging, European East Asian African Hawaiian Turkish Arabic Native Indian | Meta analysis, gene-disease association | To determine if ancestry influences the impact of each gene variant on the disease risk | Frequency of markers in control population showed large statistical variability between races. Large heterogeneity in genetic effects (odds ratios) between races in only 14% of cases. Markers for proposed gene disease associations vary in frequency across populations, biological impact on risk for common diseases consistent across traditional so-called racial boundaries. |
| (Weeks et al., 2000) | N = 2129, N = 364 families | Human, aging, origins not specified | Genome wide screen, linkage analysis | To test the hypothesis that the genes responsible for monogenic macular dystrophies and other retinal degenerations may play a role in the etiology of ARM (age-related maculopathy) | Excluded up to nine candidate regions, identified other regions of potential linkage. Chr. 5 near D5S1480, where a reasonable candidate gene, glutathione peroxidase 3, resides. |
| (Zhang et al., 2005) | Ages 25–31: N = 10 female & 12 male, ages 66-85: N = 6 female & 10 male | Human, aging, origins not specified | Genomic linkage analysis | Identification of cerebrospinal fluid (CSF) biomarkers of the common age-related neurodegenerative | Identified more than 300 proteins in CSF and found that there were 30 proteins with >20% change in concentrations between older and younger individuals. |

*(Continued)*

**TABLE 7.2**   Selected Research Papers (*Continued*)

| Citation | Sample | Populations | Design | Purpose | Results |
|---|---|---|---|---|---|
| **Asthma** | | | | | |
| (Choudhry et al., 2005b) | N = 684 | Human, Puerto Rican, MexAm | Genetic association | To determine if genetic predisposition to asthma or to greater asthma severity differs among subgroups within the Latino population. | Ethnic specific pharmacogenetic differences between Arg16Gly genotypes, asthma severity, bronchodilator response. |
| (Choudhry et al., 2005a) | N = 659 families | Human, MexAm, Puerto Rican, AfAm | Genome wide screen | To determine the genetic and environmental factors that contribute to asthma morbidity and mortality being fourfold higher in Puerto Ricans than they are in Mexicans. | Gene-environment interaction between 5q31 region and asthma with those exposed to environmental tobacco smoke. CD14+1437 genotypes associated with asthma severity. |
| **Cancer** | | | | | |
| (Baysal et al., 2004) | N = 726 | Human, AfAm, Hispanic, Caucasian Other | HPLC sequence analysis, and single nucleotide polymorphism (SNP) genotyping by pyrosequencing of CHEK2 gene. | To determine whether the gene CHEK2 contributes to the occurrence of OvCa in various racial / ethnic groups in the US. | Frequencies of del1100C and AA252G variants NSD. Suggesting variations in CHEK2 do not make a significant contribution to the pathogenesis of OvCa in U.S. population. |

**Cardiovascular/Hypertension/Obesity**

| | | | | | |
|---|---|---|---|---|---|
| (Arya et al., 2002) | N = 415 in 27 families | Human, MexAm | Multipoint variance components linkage approach | To determine whether high density lipoprotein levels and diabetes in MexAm could be attributed to markers on Chr. 9p. | Found evidence of linkage of a qualitative trait locus (QTL) for HDL-C level to a genetic location between markers D9S925 and D9S741 on Chr. 9p. Replicated study. |
| (Beery et al., 2003) | N = 15 family members / Long QT syndrome | Human, origins not specified | Candidate locus approach | To determine the potassium channel mutation causing LQT syndrome in multiple generations of one family. | During survey of the KCNQ1 coding region, a G-to-A transition (G502A) identified. Uncovered potassium channel mutation causing LQTS in this family. |
| (Fernandez et al., 2003) | N = 145 | Human, AfAm women | Genotyping | | Significant association of obesity in Chr. 1, 11, 12. Women had known quantitative admixture data. |
| (Giger et al., 2005) | N = 290. | Human, Pre-menopausal AfAm women | Candidate locus | To determine risk markers in premenopausal AfAm women for their association with known coronary heart disease (CHD) risk factors. | Frequency of D6589 allele 185, D6S89 allele 191, TNFα allele 97, and TNFα allele 103 allele in the high-risk > low-risk group; and D6S89 195 allele higher in the low-risk group. Elevated systolic blood pressure associated with HLA-DRB1*09 and TNFα 117 alleles. |

*(Continued)*

205

**TABLE 7.2** Selected Research Papers (*Continued*)

| Citation | Sample | Populations | Purpose | Design | Results |
|---|---|---|---|---|---|
| (T. Liu et al., 2004) | N = 270 yielding N = 4,196,970 SNPs. Proof of model on N = 155. | Human, Han Chinese, Japanese, Yoruba in Nigeria, and northern and western Europe | HapMap analyses of linkage disequilibrium (LD) for SNPs | To develop a statistical model for directly characterizing specific sequence variants that are responsible for disease risk based on the haplotype structure provided by HapMap. | Patients carrying a haplotype constituted by allele Gly16 at codon 16 and allele Gln27 at codon 27 genotyped within the beta2AR candidate gene had significantly lower body mass index than patients carrying the other haplotypes. |
| (Reiner et al., 2005) | N = 810 | Human, AfAm | Association study | To characterize the genetic background heterogeneity among self-identified African American subjects sampled as part of a multi site cohort study of cardiovascular disease in older adults | Using 24 ancestry-informative biallelic SNP markers, there was evidence of substantial population substructure and admixture to four genetically distinct subpopulations. Blood glucose level correlated with individual Afr. ancestry, BMI was associated more strongly with genetic similarity. BP, HDL cholesterol level, C-reactive protein level, and carotid wall thickness were not associated with genetic background. BP and HDL cholesterol level varied by geographic site, and CRP level differed by occupation. |

| Citation | N | Sample | Study Type | Objective | Findings |
|---|---|---|---|---|---|
| (Thompson et al., 2004) | N = >1,000 | Human, 52 worldwide samples. European, AfAm, Han Chinese, unrelated | Comparative genomics | To determine if genetic variants that influence salt homeostasis are linked to differences in response to blood pressure medication. | CYP3A5*1/*3 polymorphism, influences salt and water retention and risk for salt-sensitive hypertension, CYP3A5*3 extreme frequency variation across populations, correlated with distance from the equator. Large differences between AfAm and non-African populations. |
| (Zhu et al., 2005) | N = 1,310 | Human, 82% African ancestry | Genome wide admixture mapping | To identify genetic variants contributing to the risk of hypertension. | Results suggest that Chr. 6q24 and 21q21 may contain genes influencing risk of hypertension. |
| **Psychiatric** | | | | | |
| (Abkevich et al., 2003) | N = 1,890 | Human, major depressive disorder, sex linked; origins unspecified | Genome wide scan | To identify chromosomal loci contributing to genetic predisposition to major depression. | Identified significant linkage to MDD in males at marker D12501366 and 1 or more genes at Chr. 12q with sex specific predisposition on 12q22-q23.2. |
| (Elvidge et al., 2001) | N = 454 | Human, Bipolar; origins unspecified | Family-based association study | To determine if the Ball RFLP is a possible susceptibility factor for both schizophrenia and bipolar disorder. | Excluded Ball RFLP (restriction fragment length polymorphism) in the dopamine D3 receptor gene as a possible susceptibility factor for schizophrenia and bipolar disorder. |

(Continued)

**TABLE 7.2** Selected Research Papers (*Continued*)

| Citation | Sample | Populations | Design | Purpose | Results |
|---|---|---|---|---|---|
| (Jones et al., 2000) | N = 219 unrelated bipolar probands, N = 219 controls | Human, Bipolar disorder; origins unspecified | Case control association study | To exclude known polymorphisms associated with to bipolar disorder and puerperal psychosis. | Excluded polymorphisms within the estrogen receptor alpha gene (ESR 1) from an important contribution to susceptibility to bipolar disorder and puerperal psychosis. |
| (Kirov et al., 1999) | N = 131 mothers and their children | Human, Bipolar disorder; origins unspecified | Family-based association design | To search for polymorphisms in three genes involved in the metabolism of dopamine. | Found a non-significant trend for ultra-rapid cycling patients, to have higher frequency of low-activity alleles compared with 92 bipolar non-rapid patients. |
| (Licinio et al., 2004) | N = 80 | Human, Mexican Americans | Haplotype association | To determine if the response to antidepressant treatment is heterogeneous and if the CRHR1 gene and other genes in stress-inflammatory pathways are involved in response to antidepressant treatment. | Variations in the Corticotrophin-releasing hormone receptor 1 (CRHR1) gene and 8-week response to daily antidepressant treatment. |
| (McCandless et al., 1998) | Father-daughter pair | Human, Bipolar disorder; origins unspecified | Genomic, case study, positional cloning | To determine the chromosomal changes associated with bipolar disorder. | Found pericentric inversion of Chr. 9. |

(ARM) is a leading cause of visual impairment in geriatric population and is a complex genetic disorder. These authors have identified multiple pathways in the etiology of ARM, including pathways involved with fatty acid biosynthesis and the complement system. This study is the most recent in an extensive list of maculopathy studies by this group. It should be noted that Yvette P. Conley, PhD, of the University of Pittsburgh School of Nursing, is one of the group's prolific principal investigators.

In another study of the aging genome, Zhang et al. (2005) used cerebral spinal fluid (CSF) to search for age-related protein changes. They quantified more than 300 CSF proteins of which there were 30 demonstrating >20% changes in conformation due to aging. This study demonstrated the efficacy of using CSF as an uncontaminated source to study aging proteins.

## Asthma

There are only two publications, which examine asthma in the context of vulnerable populations. Choudhry et al. (2005a) segregated Latino subjects by geography, Puerto Ricans versus Mexican Americans, and also considered the different qualities of exposure to environmental tobacco smoke in different geographical locations. The Latino groups in this study were split as it was recognized that the two groups represented significantly different admixtures of African, Native American, Spanish, and other groups. These authors reported that these groups responded differently to albuterol and asthmatic therapy (Choudhry et al., 2005b). In this case, reliance alone on self-identification of ethnic or racial group is ultimately insufficient for the study of disease and drug response. It should be noted that although differences have been found between Latino groups, studies have not yet looked for these markers in European or Asian populations.

## Cancer

There is a scarcity of published studies using genomic or proteomic methods to investigate specific forms of cancer in vulnerable populations. Baysal et al. (2004) reported findings from a large (N = 726) study of ovarian cancer in African-Americans, Hispanics, and Whites. Currently the etiology of ovarian cancer is unknown, but a number of endocrine, environmental, and genetic factors have been associated with ovarian cancer risk: advancing age, Whites race, residence in North America and Northern Europe, low parity, infertility, and family history. In this study, they examined the potential role of CHEK2 gene in ovarian cancer susceptibility using cases obtained in the United States through Gynecologic Oncology Group protocols 144, 172, 182; the University of Hawaii Cancer Research Center; and Creighton University. Controls were identified from Pittsburgh and Hawaii. While the researchers did not find statistically significant evidence that mutations and the two common variants in the CHEK2 gene play an important role in the etiology of ovarian cancer in the United States, they concluded that functional variations in linkage disequilibrium do not play an important role in ovarian cancer susceptibility.

## Cardiovascular/Hypertension/Obesity

Genomic and proteomic studies of cardiovascular disease, hypertension, or obesity form the largest group of studies involving vulnerable populations. Most of these studies in this group have focused on environmental and dietary influences on African Americans' health, whereas another group has directly studied these same variables in various African populations. As previously discussed, one of the difficulties of studying African Americans is the highly varied genetic admixture of each subject. A limitation of many of these studies is their small sample size (e.g., approximately 250), along with a failure to quantify the genetic admixture of each subject. Many individuals may have some of the characteristics of their African ancestors but also carry a larger contribution from Native American, European, or Asian ancestors. Without further clarification, significant findings may erroneously be attributed solely to African ancestry rather than other ancestral origins.

Of the studies in this grouping (Table 7.2), two of the most intriguing used comparative genomics and genome-wide admixture mapping to identify factors from African populations which might contribute to cardiovascular disease and hypertension (Thompson et al., 2004; Zhu et al., 2005). The Thompson group found some genes that may contribute to the altered handling of salt and water retention in salt-sensitive hypertension between African American and African, populations. Zhu et al. (2005) located two chromosomes that were likely to contain genes influencing hypertension in persons with African ancestry.

## Psychiatric Illness

To understand genetic variations in disease, data are needed on family history and behavior manifestations of the disease. Psychiatric illnesses represent a large percent of the genomic and proteomic studies conducted to date. This is likely due to the availability of subjects and their families along with extensive histories of disease clustering in a family. Families are studied rather than large population groups and provide sufficient power for analysis. However, inherent problems exist in diagnosis of psychiatric diseases. Psychiatric disorders such as depression may manifest different clusters of symptoms with varying intensities among patients. Often patients are misdiagnosed as they present with ambiguous symptoms. Another difficulty is phenotypic heterogeneity. In this situation, a similar set of symptoms may be caused by a number of distinct genetic variations (Hamet & Tremblay, 2005).

Most genomic and proteomic studies in psychiatric illness have focused on depression and bipolar disorders, which have been long known to have a strong genetic component. Samples are often selected from families with known diagnoses or small case studies to control for admixture variation. Only one study was found that examined depression in an ethnic/racial group (Mexican Americans; Licinio et al., 2004). This study demonstrated that there were certain variations in corticotrophin-releasing hormone receptor 1 (CRHR1) that contributed to altered responses among patients to treatment with antidepressant drugs.

## Translating Findings Into Practice

The ultimate goal of the studies reviewed in this chapter is to determine mechanistic origins of complex diseases in order to develop therapies that directly address genetic errors or genetic responses to the environment. This aim is very different than research to inform practice or to build a body of evidence-based clinical interventions. At this time, their direct application to practice is limited. Nonetheless, some of the findings with regard to susceptibility to conditions such as hypertension or obesity have potential implications for development of early intervention strategies for vulnerable populations of African American and Latino populations. It should be cautioned that these genetic predispositions might also be found in other populations. Until demonstrated otherwise, patients should be encouraged to construct medical pedigrees of their families. To this end, the U.S. Surgeon General's Family History Initiative was launched last year to encourage families to record and communicate those conditions, which run in their family (Dept. of Health and Human Services, 2004). Given that few individuals have recorded their family medical history, it is important for nurses to encourage patients and special populations to do so. Recorded family medical histories will also provide for early recognition of conditions known to occur in their families. It is hoped that targeted therapeutics and less expensive methods of testing for genetic errors in the population at large will soon be available (Carmona & Wattendorf, 2005; Guttmacher, Collins, & Carmona, 2004).

## Implications for Future Research and Policy

Genomic and proteomic technologies hold promise to change the ways in which disease is prevented, diagnosed, and treated in the near future. Because the application of these methods will be expensive, only developed countries are likely to have the finances and infrastructure needed to apply these advances in their health care systems. The World Health Organization has identified the development of potential disparities in genomic care between the third world and industrialized nations (Smith, Thorsteinsdottir, Daar, Gold, & Singers, 2004b).

Over time, genomics technologies should aide in the control of complex diseases such as asthma, diabetes, and cardiovascular pathologies. While genetic causes may be found, the interacting environmental causes will also need to be linked to genetic predisposition. As these factors will vary by geographical location and specific toxic element, extensive research will be needed. At all times, cost benefit analyses should be conducted to determine whether these new methods are truly better ways to deliver health care (Wilkinson & Targonski, 2003).

The views expressed are those of the author and do not reflect the official policy or position of the Uniformed Services University of the Health Sciences, the Department of Defense, the Department of Veterans Affairs, or the United States Government.

## REFERENCES

Abkevich, V., Camp, N. J., Hensel, C. H., Neff, C. D., Russell, D. L., Hughes, D. C., et al. (2003). Predisposition locus for major depression at chromosome 12q22–12q23.2. *American Journal of Human Genetics, 73*(6), 1271–1281.

Apic, G., Ignjatovic, T., Boyer, S., & Russell, R. B. (2005). Illuminating drug discovery with biological pathways. *FEBS Letters, 579*(8), 1872–1877.

Arya, R., Duggirala, R., Almasy, L., Rainwater, D. L., Mahaney, M. C., Cole, S., et al. (2002). Linkage of high-density lipoprotein-cholesterol concentrations to a locus on chromosome 9p in Mexican-Americans. *Nature Genetics, 30*(1), 102–105.

Atkin, K. (2003). Ethnicity and the politics of the new genetics: Principles and engagement. *Ethnicity and Health, 8*(2), 91–109.

Bairoch, A., Apweiler, R., Wu, C. H., Barker, W. C., Boeckmann, B., Ferro, S., et al. (2005). The universal protein resource (UniProt). *Nucleic Acids Research, 33*(Database issue), D154–159.

Baysal, B. E., DeLoia, J. A., Willett-Brozick, J. E., Goodman, M. T., Brady, M. F., Modugno, F., et al. (2004). Analysis of chek2 gene for ovarian cancer susceptibility. *Gynecologic Oncology, 95*(1), 62–69.

Beery, T. A., Dyment, M., Shooner, K., Knilans, T. K., & Benson, D. W. (2003). A candidate locus approach identifies a long QT syndrome gene mutation. *Biologic Research for Nursing, 5*(2), 97–104.

Boeckmann, B., Bairoch, A., Apweiler, R., Blatter, M. C., Estreicher, A., Gasteiger, E., et al. (2003). The Swiss-Prot protein knowledgebase and its supplement TrEMBL in 2003. *Nucleic Acids Research, 31*(1), 365–370.

Bonham, V. L., Warshauer-Baker, E., & Collins, F. S. (2005). Race and ethnicity in the genome era: The complexity of the constructs. *American Psychology, 60*(1), 9–15.

Burchard, E. G., Ziv, E., Coyle, N., Gomez, S. L., Tang, H., Karter, A. J., et al. (2003). The importance of race and ethnic background in biomedical research and clinical practice. *New England Journal of Medicine, 348*(12), 1170–1175.

Carmona, R. H., & Wattendorf, D. J. (2005). Personalizing prevention: The U.S. Surgeon General's family history initiative. *American Family Physician, 71*(1), 36, 39.

Cavalli-Sforza, L. L. (2005). The human genome diversity project: Past, present and future. *Nature Reviews Genetics, 6*(4), 333–340.

Choudhry, S., Avila, P. C., Nazario, S., Ung, N., Kho, J., Rodriguez-Santana, J. R., et al. (2005a). CD14-tobacco gene-environment interaction modifies asthma severity and IGE levels in Latino asthmatics. *American Journal of Respiratory Critical Care Medicine, 172*(2), 173–182.

Choudhry, S., Ung, N., Avila, P. C., Ziv, E., Nazario, S., Casal, J., et al. (2005b). Pharmacogenetic differences in response to albuterol between Puerto Ricans and Mexicans with asthma. *American Journal of Respiratory Critical Care Medicine, 171*(6), 563–570.

Collins, F. S. (2004). What we do and don't know about 'race', 'ethnicity', genetics and health at the dawn of the genome era. *Nature Genetics, 36*(11 Suppl), S1315.

Collins, F. S., Patrinos, A., Jordan, E., Chakravarti, A., Gesteland, R., & Walters, L. (1998). New goals for the U.S. Human Genome Project: 1998–2003. *Science, 282*(5389), 682–689.

Demirel, M. C., & Keskin, O. (2005). Protein interactions and fluctuations in a proteomic network using an elastic network model. *Journal of Biomolecular Structure and Dynamics, 22*(4), 381–386.

Department of Health and Human Services. (2004). *The U.S. Surgeon General's family history initiative.* Retrieved April 15, 2005, from http://www.hhs.gov/familyhistory/

Dierick, J. F., Dieu, M., Remacle, J., Raes, M., Roepstorff, P., & Toussaint, O. (2002). Proteomics in experimental gerontology. *Experimental Gerontology, 37*(5), 721–734.

Dierick, J. F., Eliaers, F., Remacle, J., Raes, M., Fey, S. J., Larsen, P. M., et al. (2002). Stress-induced premature senescence and replicative senescence are different phenotypes, proteomic evidence. *Biochemical Pharmacology, 64*(5–6), 1011–1017.

Dracopoli, N., Haines, J., Korf, B., Moir, D., Morton, C., Seidman, C., et al. (Eds.). (2005). *Current protocols in human genetics.* New York: John Wiley Current Protocols.

Duster, T. (2005). Medicine: Race and reification in science. *Science, 307*(5712), 1050–1051.

Elvidge, G., Jones, I., McCandless, F., Asherson, P., Owen, M. J., & Craddock, N. (2001). Allelic variation of a Bali polymorphism in the DRD3 gene does not influence susceptibility to bipolar disorder: Results of analysis and meta-analysis. *American Journal of Medical Genetics, 105*(4), 307–311.

Fernandez, J. R., Shriver, M. D., Beasley, T. M., Rafla-Demetrious, N., Parra, E., Albu, J., et al. (2003). Association of African genetic admixture with resting metabolic rate and obesity among women. *Obesity Research, 11*(7), 904–911.

Foster, M. W., & Sharp, R. R. (2002). Race, ethnicity, and genomics: Social classifications as proxies of biological heterogeneity. *Genome Research, 12*(6), 844–850.

Foster, M. W., & Sharp, R. R. (2004). Beyond race: Towards a whole-genome perspective on human populations and genetic variation. *Nature Reviews Genetics, 5*(10), 790–796.

Giger, J. N., Strickland, O. L., Weaver, M., Taylor, H., & Acton, R. T. (2005). Genetic predictors of coronary heart disease risk factors in pre-menopausal African-American women. *Ethnicity and Disease, 15*(2), 221–232.

Goldstein, D. B., & Hirschhorn, J. N. (2004). In genetic control of disease, does 'race' matter? *Nature Genetics, 36*(12), 1243–1244.

Gorg, A., Obermaier, C., Boguth, G., Harder, A., Scheibe, B., Wildgruber, R., et al. (2000). The current state of two-dimensional electrophoresis with immobilized pH gradients. *Electrophoresis, 21*(6), 1037–1053.

Grady, P. A., & Collins, F. S. (2003). Genetics and nursing science: Realizing the potential. *Nursing Research, 52*(2), 69.

Gromov, P. S., Ostergaard, M., Gromova, I., & Celis, J. E. (2002). Human proteomic databases: A powerful resource for functional genomics in health and disease. *Progress in Biophysics and Molecular Biology, 80*(1–2), 3–22.

Guttmacher, A. E., Collins, F. S., & Carmona, R. H. (2004). The family history—more important than ever. *New England Journal of Medicine, 351*(22), 2333–2336.

Halapi, E., Stefansson, K., & Hakonarson, H. (2004). Population genomics of drug response. *American Journal of Pharmacogenomics, 4*(2), 73–82.

Halder, I., & Shriver, M. D. (2003). Measuring and using admixture to study the genetics of complex diseases. *Human Genomics, 1*(1), 52–62.

Hamet, P., & Tremblay, J. (2005). Genetics and genomics of depression. *Metabolism, 54*(5 Suppl 1), 10–15.

Hao, Y., Zhu, X., Huang, M., & Li, M. (2005). Discovering patterns to extract protein-protein interactions from the literature: Part II. *Bioinformatics, 21*(15), 3294–3300.

Harrison, P. M., & Gerstein, M. (2002). Studying genomes through the aeons: Protein families, pseudogenes and proteome evolution. *Journal of Molecular Biology, 318*(5), 1155–1174.

Harrison, P. M., Kumar, A., Lang, N., Snyder, M., & Gerstein, M. (2002). A question of size: The eukaryotic proteome and the problems in defining it. *Nucleic Acids Research, 30*(5), 1083–1090.

Hayes, K. R., Vollrath, A. L., Zastrow, G. M., McMillan, B. J., Craven, M., Jovanovich, S., et al. (2005). Edge: A centralized resource for the comparison, analysis, and distribution of toxicogenomic information. *Molecular Pharmacology, 67*(4), 1360–1368.

International HapMap Consortium. (2003). The International HapMap Project. *Nature, 426*(6968), 789–796.

Ioannidis, J. P., Ntzani, E. E., & Trikalinos, T. A. (2004). 'Racial' differences in genetic effects for complex diseases. *Nature Genetics, 36*(12), 1312–1318.

Jones, I., Middle, F., McCandless, F., Coyle, N., Robertson, E., Brockington, I., et al. (2000). Molecular genetic studies of bipolar disorder and puerperal psychosis at two polymorphisms in the estrogen receptor alpha gene (ESR 1). *American Journal of Medical Genetics, 96*(6), 850–853.

Jung, E., Heller, M., Sanchez, J. C., & Hochstrasser, D. F. (2000). Proteomics meets cell biology: The establishment of subcellular proteomes. *Electrophoresis, 21*(16), 3369–3377.

Kahn, J. (2005). Ethnic drugs. *Hastings Center Report, 35*(1), 1.

Khoury, M. J. (2003). Genetics and genomics in practice: The continuum from genetic disease to genetic information in health and disease. *Genetics Medicine, 5*(4), 261–268.

Kim, S. I., Voshol, H., van Oostrum, J., Hastings, T. G., Cascio, M., & Glucksman, M. J. (2004). Neuroproteomics: Expression profiling of the brain's proteomes in health and disease. *Neurochemical Research, 29*(6), 1317–1331.

Kirov, G., Jones, I., McCandless, F., Craddock, N., & Owen, M. J. (1999). Family-based association studies of bipolar disorder with candidate genes involved in dopamine neurotransmission: DBH, DAT1, COMT, DRD2, DRD3 and DRD5. *Molecular Psychiatry, 4*(6), 558–565.

Lauber, W. M., Carroll, J. A., Dufield, D. R., Kiesel, J. R., Radabaugh, M. R., & Malone, J. P. (2001). Mass spectrometry compatibility of two-dimensional gel protein stains. *Electrophoresis, 22*(5), 906–918.

Lee, S. S., Mountain, J., & Koenig, B. A. (2001). The meanings of "race" in the new genomics: Implications for health disparities research. *Yale Journal of Health Policy Law Ethics, 1*, 33–75.

Lewin, D. A., & Weiner, M. P. (2004). Molecular biomarkers in drug development. *Drug Discovery Today, 9*(22), 976–983.

Licinio, J., O'Kirwan, F., Irizarry, K., Merriman, B., Thakur, S., Jepson, R., et al. (2004). Association of a corticotropin-releasing hormone receptor 1 haplotype and antidepressant treatment response in Mexican-Americans. *Molecular Psychiatry, 9*(12), 1075–1082.

Liu, T., Johnson, J. A., Casella, G., & Wu, R. (2004). Sequencing complex diseases with HapMap. *Genetics, 168*(1), 503–511.

Liu, Y., Liu, N., & Zhao, H. (2005). Inferring protein-protein interactions through high-throughput interaction data from diverse organisms. *Bioinformatics, 21*, 3279–3285.

Marshall, E. (1998). DNA studies challenge the meaning of race. *Science, 282*(5389), 654–655.

McCandless, F., Jones, I., Harper, K., & Craddock, N. (1998). Intrafamilial association of pericentric inversion of chromosome 9, inv (9)(p11-q21), and rapid cycling bipolar disorder. *Psychiatric Genetics, 8*(4), 259–262.

Orgel, L. E. (1963). The maintenance of accuracy of protein synthesis and its relevance to aging. *Proceeding of the National Academy of Science USA, 67*, 517–521.

Orgel, L. E. (1973). Ageing of clones of mammalian cells. *Nature, 243*, 441–445.

Ossorio, P., & Duster, T. (2005). Race and genetics: Controversies in biomedical, behavioral, and forensic sciences. *American Psychologist, 60*(1), 115–128.

Parra, E. J., Kittles, R. A., & Shriver, M. D. (2004). Implications of correlations between skin color and genetic ancestry for biomedical research. *Nature Genetics, 36*(11 Suppl), S54–60.

Patterson, N., Hattangadi, N., Lane, B., Lohmueller, K. E., Hafler, D. A., Oksenberg, J. R., et al. (2004). Methods for high-density admixture mapping of disease genes. *American Journal of Human Genetics, 74*(5), 979–1000.

Rédei, G. P., & Rédei, G. P. (2003). *Encyclopedic dictionary of genetics, genomics, and proteomics* (2nd ed.). Hoboken, NJ: Wiley-Liss.

Reiner, A. P., Ziv, E., Lind, D. L., Nievergelt, C. M., Schork, N. J., Cummings, S. R., et al. (2005). Population structure, admixture, and aging-related phenotypes in African-American adults: The cardiovascular health study. *American Journal of Human Genetics, 76*(3), 463–477.

Serre, D., & Paabo, S. (2004). Evidence for gradients of human genetic diversity within and among continents. *Genome Research, 14*(9), 1679–1685.

Shields, A. E., Fortun, M., Hammonds, E. M., King, P. A., Lerman, C., Rapp, R., et al. (2005). The use of race variables in genetic studies of complex traits and the goal of reducing health disparities: A transdisciplinary perspective. *American Psychologist, 60*(1), 77–103.

Smith, M. W., Patterson, N., Lautenberger, J. A., Truelove, A. L., McDonald, G. J., Waliszewska, A., et al. (2004a). A high-density admixture map for disease gene discovery in African-Americans. *American Journal of Human Genetics, 74*(5), 1001–1013.

Smith, R. D., Thorsteinsdottir, H., Daar, A. S., Gold, E. R., & Singers, P. A. (2004b). Genomics knowledge and equity: A global public goods perspective of the patent system. *Bulletin of the World Health Organization, 82*(5), 385–389.

Taback, B., & Hoon, D. S. (2004). Circulating nucleic acids and proteomics of plasma/serum: Clinical utility. *Annals of the New York Academy of Science, 1022*, 1–8.

Thompson, E. E., Kuttab-Boulos, H., Witonsky, D., Yang, L., Roe, B. A., & Di Rienzo, A. (2004). CYP3a variation and the evolution of salt-sensitivity variants. *American Journal of Human Genetics, 75*(6), 1059–1069.

Tishkoff, S. A., & Kidd, K. K. (2004). Implications of biogeography of human populations for 'race' and medicine. *Nature Genetics, 36*(11 Suppl), S21–27.

Toda, T. (2001). Proteome and proteomics for the research on protein alterations in aging. *Annals of the New York Academy of Science, 928*, 71–78.

Uetz, P., & Finley, R. L., Jr. (2005). From protein networks to biological systems. *FEBS Letters, 579*(8), 1821–1827.

Vidal, M. (2005). Interactome modeling. *FEBS Letters, 579*(8), 1834–1838.

Wagner, K., Miliotis, T., Marko-Varga, G., Bischoff, R., & Unger, K. K. (2002). An automated on-line multidimensional HPLC system for protein and peptide mapping with integrated sample preparation. *Anal Chemistry, 74*(4), 809–820.

Wang, V. O., & Sue, S. (2005). In the eye of the storm: Race and genomics in research and practice. *American Psychologist, 60*(1), 37–45.

Waters, M. D., & Fostel, J. M. (2004). Toxicogenomics and systems toxicology: Aims and prospects. *Nature Review Genetics, 5*(12), 936–948.

Weeks, D. E., Conley, Y. P., Mah, T. S., Paul, T. O., Morse, L., Ngo-Chang, J., et al. (2000). A full genome scan for age-related maculopathy. *Human Molecular Genetics, 9* (9), 1329–1349.

Whitfield, K. E., & McClearn, G. (2005). Genes, environment, and race: Quantitative genetic approaches. *American Psychologist, 60*(1), 104–114.

Wilkinson, D. Y., & King, G. (1987). Conceptual and methodological issues in the use of race as a variable: Policy implications. *Milbank Quarterly, 65*(Suppl 1), 56–71.

Wilkinson, J. M., & Targonski, P. V. (2003). Health promotion in a changing world: Preparing for the genomics revolution. *American Journal of Health Promotion, 18*(2), 157–161.

Wu, L. F., Hughes, T. R., Davierwala, A. P., Robinson, M. D., Stoughton, R., & Altschuler, S. J. (2002). Large-scale prediction of saccharomyces cerevisiae gene function using overlapping transcriptional clusters. *Nature Genetics, 31*(3), 255–265.

Yip, Y. L., Scheib, H., Diemand, A. V., Gattiker, A., Famiglietti, L. M., Gasteiger, E., et al. (2004). The Swiss-Prot variant page and the modsnp database: A resource for sequence and structure information on human protein variants. *Human Mutation, 23*(5), 464–470.

Young, V. R. (2003). Trace element biology: The knowledge base and its application for the nutrition of individuals and populations. *Journal of Nutrition, 133*(5 Suppl 1), 1581S-1587S.

Zhang, J., Goodlett, D. R., Peskind, E. R., Quinn, J. F., Zhou, Y., Wang, Q., et al. (2005). Quantitative proteomic analysis of age-related changes in human cerebrospinal fluid. *Neurobiology of Aging, 26*(2), 207–227.

Zhu, X., Luke, A., Cooper, R. S., Quertermous, T., Hanis, C., Mosley, T., et al. (2005). Admixture mapping for hypertension loci with genome-scan markers. *Nature Genetics, 37*(2), 177–181.

# Chapter 8

## Psychoneuroimmunology and Related Mechanisms in Understanding Health Disparities in Vulnerable Populations

Teresita L. Briones

### ABSTRACT

*The nervous system as well as the endocrine system maintain extensive communication with the immune system through the influence of hormones and neurotransmitters and also by way of the hardwiring of sympathetic and parasympathetic nerves to the lymphoid organs. There is now convincing evidence that the communication between these three body systems is bidirectional. This chapter will provide a succinct review of how neuroendocrine and immune functions are affected in factors that impact vulnerability, such as aging, acute infection, and central nervous system injury. Given that the relevant literature on these topics is vast, the presentation in this chapter will serve to highlight primary references that reflect state of the science in these systems of focus.*

Keywords: psychoneuroimmunology; health disparities; vulnerable populations

## INTRODUCTION

The nervous, endocrine, and immune systems are complex entities that interact with each other to mount a variety of essential and coordinated responses important in maintaining homeostasis and survival. These three systems communicate through intricate chemical messengers; the broad interdisciplinary field involved in the study of the interactions among the central nervous system (CNS), endocrine, and immune systems is called psychoneuroimmunology (PNI). Researchers in the field of PNI have developed a body of knowledge that demonstrates the bidirectional communication between the neuroendocrine and immune systems.

The purpose of this review is to succinctly summarize the existing evidence concerning interactions between these systems in populations experiencing vulnerable conditions, and to demonstrate how data generated in the field of PNI are relevant to the practice of nursing. In doing this review, a PubMed search using keywords such as *nervous, neuroendocrine,* and *immune* limited to the last 5 years was performed and returned more than 5,000 results; less than 1% were published in nursing journals. The search was limited to the last 5 years because of the rapidly evolving technological advances in the field of PNI research. More focused searches using keywords *aging, infection,* and *CNS injury* returned less than 2,000 results; the majority of which were review articles. The greater part of research studies obtained from the PubMed search was conducted using animal models; some studies involved human subjects. Inclusion criteria in this review comprised studies that: (a) were original databased papers, (b) used established animal models, or (c) used both objective and subjective measures of outcome variables in research conducted using human subjects, and (d) addressed factors that made populations vulnerable, such as injury, acute infection, and being elderly. None of the articles included in the review were from nursing journals, as PNI papers published in nursing journals are mostly review articles with the exception of two databased papers that did not meet the criteria set out for inclusion in this review.

## PNI: A BRIEF REVIEW

The basic foundation of PNI research rests within the communication between the hypothalamic-pituitary-adrenal (HPA) axis and the autonomic nervous system, with the immune system as key pathways for regulating health and disease. Although the factors initiating physical and psychological stress are fundamentally different, the ways they impact the neuroendocrine and immune systems have many similarities. The HPA axis and the sympathetic-adrenal-medullary (SAM) axis are the central sensors of stress; both of these systems can influence the immune system (Steinman, 2004). The hypothalamus integrates information from physical and psychological stimuli and, in response to stress, releases corticotropin-releasing hormone (CRH) from the paraventricular nucleus. CRH acts upon the pituitary gland to induce release of adenocorticotropic hormone (ACTH), which stimulates the adrenal gland to produce glucocorticoids (cortisol) and the androgenic hormone dehyroepiandrosterone (DHEA) from the adrenal cortex (Butcher & Lord, 2004). The adrenal gland is also regulated by the sympathetic nervous system, secreting catecholamines in response to acetylcholine release from preganglionic sympathetic fibers innervating the adrenal medulla (Glaser & Kiecolt-Glaser, 2005). For example, the catecholamines (epinephrine and norepinephrine), ACTH, and cortisol are all influenced by stress, and each of these hormones can induce quantitative and qualitative suppression of immune function. In contrast, DHEA is primarily immune enhancing, producing some degree of counterbalance to the potentially detrimental effects of long-term stimulation of the HPA-SAM axis (Butcher & Lord, 2004).

Almost all immune cells have receptors for one or more of the hormones that are released during activation of the HPA and SAM axes (Steinman, 2004). Immune modulation by the adrenal hormones may be accomplished through two pathways: directly, through binding of the hormone to its cognate receptor at the surface of the cells, or indirectly, by increasing the production of cytokines, such as interferon-γ (IFN-γ), interleukin-1 (IL-1), IL-2, IL-6, tumor necrosis factor (TNF), and chemokines (Maier, 2003). Cytokines are intercellular signaling peptides released by most nucleated cells and are involved in cellular growth and differentiation as well as immune modulation, frequently classified as pro-inflammatory and anti-inflammatory (Dantzer, 2001). Pro-inflammatory cytokines are those involved in the inflammatory response, are pyrogenic, and are involved in the acute phase response seen in infection. Anti-inflammatory cytokines are those that exert their influence in a negative feedback manner to reduce the inflammatory response. Chemokines, on the other hand, are small cytokines that are multifunctional and initially believed to modulate leukocyte trafficking. Recently, chemokines have been found to be involved in cell adhesion, phagocytosis, cell proliferation, and angiogenesis (Cartier, Hartley, Dubois-Dauphin, & Krause, 2005).

Interactions between the CNS and the immune system can occur in several ways: (a) the CNS can act reciprocally with the immune system, (b) the CNS can drive immunity, and (c) the immune system can regulate CNS function. For instance, IL-1 influences the production of CRH by the hypothalamus (Glaser & Kiecolt-Glaser, 2005; Steinman, 2004). CRH in turn, can affect the HPA axis, and thereby trigger increases in cortisol secretion and influence immune function. Furthermore, lymphocytes can be activated by hormones such as ACTH and prolactin because almost all immune cells have receptors for one or more of HPA-SAM hormones (Table 8.1) (Elenkov & Chrousos, 2002). The role of lymphocyte-derived hormones in immune responses is not fully understood at this time, however, they may play a part in modulating cell function within the microenvironment of lymphoid organs (Glaser & Kiecolt-Glaser, 2005). Moreover, studies that show nerve fibers in the spleen and thymus that connect to the autonomic nervous system suggest that hard-wiring exists between the sympathetic nervous system and lymphoid organs (Steinman, 2004). Hence, it is not surprising that neurotransmitters such as acetylcholine, norepinephrine, vasoactive intestinal peptide, substance P, and histamine can modulate immune activity. Figure 8.1 provides an illustration of the neural pathways involved in immune regulation and some of the bidirectional signals between the neuroendocrine and immune systems that modulate the immune response.

## CONTEXTUAL ISSUES

In this section, the different contextual changes that occur within an individual that activates the bidirectional communication between the neuroendocrine and immune systems are highlighted. The contextual changes that will be reviewed include: physiological changes that occur with aging, during an episode of acute infection, and with a CNS injury. Given the tremendous physiological impact of the aforementioned conditions which produce detrimental effects, individuals experiencing these contextual changes are considered vulnerable; thus, this underscores the need for better understanding of the complexity of the neuroendocrine system and immune system communication in this population.

## AGE-RELATED IMMUNE RESPONSE

The alteration in secretion of adrenocortical hormones seen during aging may potentially impact the immune response in the elderly. Although production of cortisol remains reasonably constant with age, levels of DHEA decrease gradually from the third decade and reaching levels that are only 10–20% of their maximum by the eighth decade (Ferrari, Arcaini et al., 2000; Ferrari et al., 2001). As a result, a status of relative glucocorticoid excess is commonly seen in the elderly, which may have a negative impact on baseline immune function, leading to an exaggerated response to stressors. This decline in immune function is termed immune senescence, and is defined as the state of dysregulated immune function that contributes to the increased susceptibility of the elderly to infection and possibly to autoimmune disease and cancer

**TABLE 8.1**    HPA-SAM Axes Hormones and Immune Cell Receptors

| Hormone | Location of receptors in immune cells |
|---|---|
| Glucocorticoids | T and B cells<br>Neutrophils<br>Macrophages |
| Corticotropin-releasing hormone | T cells<br>Macrophages |
| Prolactin | T and B cells<br>NK cells<br>Macrophages<br>Granulocytes |
| Growth hormone | T and B cells<br>NK cells<br>Macrophages |
| Catecholamines | T and B cells<br>NK cells<br>Macrophages |
| Substance P | T and B cells<br>Eosinophils<br>Mast cells<br>Macrophages |
| Neuropeptide Y | T and B cells<br>Macrophages |
| Serotonin | T and B cells<br>NK cells<br>Macrophages |

(Grubeck-Loebenstein & Wick, 2002). Research in immune senescence has addressed both the innate and adaptive arms of the immune system, though most of the cellular components of the innate immune system are less well studied than adaptive responses. B cells, key players in the adaptive immune response, are known to increase with age and may be the source of the increased levels of autoantibodies in the elderly (Johnson, Rozzo, & Cambier, 2002; Linton, Habertson, & Bradley, 2000). While some researchers have reported that levels of natural killer (NK) cells are not affected by aging (Di Lorenzo et al., 2000), others have shown increased numbers of NK cells with age, with reduced cyto-toxic activity on a per cell basis (Miyaji et al., 2000; Solana & Mariani, 2000; Tarazona et al., 2000). These latter data may explain why some investigators

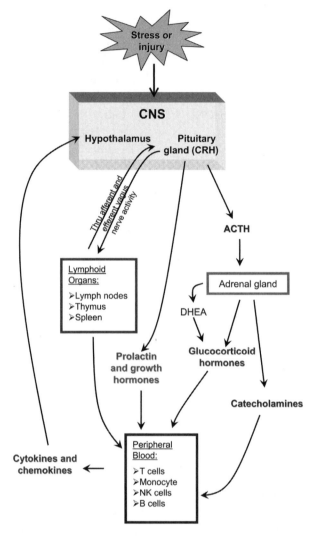

**FIGURE 8.1** Physiological and psychological stress or injury can stimulate the HPA and SAM axes. This stimulation will lead to the production of ACTH by the pituitary gland and then release it to activate the adrenal gland to secrete glucorticoid hormones, catecholamines and DHEA. DHEA has a modulating influence on glucocorticoids. In addition to the hormonal influence, the SAM axis is also activated through innervation of the lymphoid organs. Lymphoid organs can influence the production of immune cells in the peripheral blood and these cells can then be activated by hormones released through the HPA and SAM axes. The immune cells can produce both pro-inflammatory and anti-inflammatory cytokines which can then modulate the activity of the hypothalamus.

who have only considered total NK activity may have failed to detect the loss of cytotoxic activity in individual cells.

Studies on innate immune senescence primarily focus on changes in macrophage and neutrophil function. Macrophages from aged mice express lower levels of most toll-like receptors (TLRs) and their function is also reduced (Boehmer, Goral, Faunce, & Kovacs, 2004; Renshaw et al., 2002). Since TLRs are the key receptors by which the macrophage responds to pathogens, and ultimately initiates both adaptive and innate immune responses, such a decline has significant implications for immune function in the elderly. Reduced TLR function in aged mice is demonstrated by the decreased ability of macrophages to support T-cell activation; resulting in induced inhibition of T-cell responses to mitogens (substances that can cause lymphocytes to undergo cell division) (Renshaw et al., 2002). It is believed that the reduced TLR function associated with age is caused by the actions of cortisol (Boehmer et al., 2004). Additionally, the secretion of cytokines and chemokines by aged macrophages is also altered, with a skewing toward an inflammatory response indicated by enhanced production of the pro-inflammatory cytokine IL-6 (Kiecolt-Glaser et al., 2003; Leng, Yang, & Walston, 2004).

There is also evidence that aging is accompanied by a change in how HPA axis activation communicates with the immune system, which will likely have an impact on the neuroendocrine response to stress (Ferrari, Fioravanti, Magri, & Solerte, 2000). In a study using animal models wherein old and young mice were compared following burn injury, it was found that elderly mice had lower survival rates and were more immunosuppressed compared to young burn injury mice (Kovacs, Plackett, & Witte, 2004). The age-related immune suppression seen in these studies was associated with increased expression of the pro-inflammatory cytokine IL-6 in the plasma. Similar findings have been reported in healthy subjects (Butcher et al., 2001; Butcher, Killampalli, Chahal, Alpar, & Lord, 2003) and in patients who suffered from mild traumatic injury (young patients with a single limb fracture compared to elderly patients with a fractured neck of the femur). While almost 50% of the elderly cohort succumbed to bacterial infection within 5 weeks of trauma, no infections were seen in the young trauma group (Butcher et al., 2003). In all studies, a modest increase in neutrophil phagocytic capacity was seen in the elderly group at the time of injury followed by suppression in phagocytic function that persisted for 5 weeks. Interestingly, when phagocytic function returned in the elderly group, it was at a level significantly lower than that in the young cohort. The separate contribution of age and trauma to immune functional decline and susceptibility to infection in the clinical study was effectively partialed out because both patient groups had no significant comorbidity. These results suggest that the combination of stress and aging can influence clinical outcome in elderly trauma victims.

Studies have suggested that the combination of decreased serum DHEA and elevated cortisol seen with increasing age and in trauma combine to reduce immunity in the elderly to below critical threshold, resulting in increased susceptibility to infection (Butcher et al., 2001; Marsland, Bachen, Cohen, Rabin, & Manuck, 2002). In another clinical study of young and elderly trauma patients, it was reported that cortisol was elevated approximately twofold in the young cohort, but seven fold in the elderly (Jarrar, Kuebler, Wang, Bland, & Chaudry, 2001). The dramatic increase in cortisol in the elderly may be attributed to: (a) higher baseline cortisol/DHEA ratio associated with aging, and (b) a failure to trigger an increase in serum DHEA in response to trauma, resulting in increased ratio of cortisol to DHEA production (Grubeck-Loebenstein & Wick, 2002). It is not clear whether supplementation with DHEA or its downstream products might be beneficial to elderly trauma patients. There is a dearth of information in human studies that could support or refute the hypothesis that DHEA supplementation would improve immune function or prognosis for elderly trauma victims.

In another study using a small double-blind trial, 25 elderly patients with hip-fracture were supplemented with either 50 mg per day DHEA or placebo for 5 weeks; infection rates and neutrophil function were also assessed in both groups (Butcher & Lord, 2004). No differences in infection rates or neutrophil function were found between the two groups, suggesting that either DHEA treatment is not effective or that, due to the high baseline levels of cortisol in the elderly, modest DHEA supplementation alone may not be effective in influencing immunity.

## ACUTE SICKNESS BEHAVIOR IN INFECTION

During an acute infection, a cluster of non-specific symptoms such as fever, increased need to sleep, hyperalgesia, anorexia, loss of interest in usual activities, decreased social interaction and body care, depression, and impaired concentration are demonstrated by both animals and humans (Dantzer, 2004). This collection of symptoms known as sickness behavior is attributed to the increased production of pro-inflammatory cytokines. Studies have shown that release of pro-inflammatory cytokines in acute illness are a highly organized and evolved strategy employed by the body to combat infection and function to conserve energy (Dantzer, 2004; Vollmer-Conna, 2001). The production of the pro-inflammatory cytokines such as tumor necrosis factor (TNF), interleukin (IL)-1, and IL-6 by activated immune cells (monocyte/macrophages, lymphocytes) play a role in inducing sickness behavior as these cytokines act as signaling molecules in orchestrating the acute phase response (Kelley et al., 2003). The first demonstration of the involvement of cytokines in the induction of acute sickness behavior comes from clinical trials using purified or recombinant cytokines as therapy for cancer wherein the patients developed fever, fatigue, malaise, headaches, anorexia, depression, and, at high doses, delirium (Dantzer, 2001).

Experimental animal models using systemic injection of lipopolysaccharide (LPS), the active fragment of endotoxin from Gram-negative bacteria, have confirmed that most aspects of sickness behavior can be induced by increased production of pro-inflammatory cytokines (Bluthé et al., 2000; Chen, Zhou, Beltran, Malellari, & Chang, 2005; Palin et al., 2001; Sparkman, Kohman, Garcia, & Boehm, 2005; Sparkman, Martin, Calvert, & Boehm, 2005). Conversely, in the presence of pro-inflammatory cytokine antagonists, production of these cytokines are inhibited in the CNS; LPS injection did not result in sickness behavior (Bluthé, Dantzer, & Kelley, 2002; Palin et al., 2001). Yet, the pleiotropism (having more than one biologic function) and redundancy of the cytokine network make it difficult to determine the precise contribution of individual cytokines to sickness behavior. However, there is evidence to suggest that TNF-$\alpha$ and IL-1$\beta$, which are synthesized very early in the immune response, are more potent than the cytokines that are induced later (e.g., IL-6) and act in synergy to induce sickness behavior (Brebner, Hayley, Zacharko, Merali, & Anisman, 2000). Further, the role of IL-6 in sickness behavior is more complex compared to the other cytokines, as evidence suggests that IL-6 has both pro- and anti-inflammatory functions; the latter of which include the induction of natural antagonists to TNF and IL-1 and stimulation of the HPA axis (Bluthé, 2000). Additionally, experimental animal models reveal that aside from inducing acute sickness behavior, a classic stress response is produced following systemic administration of pro-inflammatory cytokines or LPS (Brebner et al., 2000; De Jongh et al., 2003; Grinevich et al., 2001). Activation of the sympathetic nervous system and release of plasma catecholamines, as well as activation of the HPA system leading to the release of ACTH and glucocorticoids, characterize the cytokine- or LPS-induced stress response. IL-6 appears to be a particularly potent stimulator of the HPA axis in humans as well. For example, daily administration of recombinant IL-6 over a week for cancer therapy was found to produce a remarkable activation and enlargement of the adrenal glands, similar to that seen in patients with Cushing's disease (Mastorakos, Chrousos, & Weber, 1993).

To date, very few studies have systematically examined the potential relationships between pro-inflammatory cytokines and mental and behavioral symptoms in sick humans. In a study involving adult patients who have either common cold (rhinovirus) or were receiving interferon-$\alpha$ therapy, cognitive performance was assessed. Both common cold and interferon-$\alpha$ therapy produced impairments in stimulus detection tasks, whereas common colds were associated with impaired hand-eye coordination (Marshall, O'Hara, & Steinberg, 2000, 2002; Scheibel, Valentine, O'Brien, & Meyers, 2004). Interestingly, these cognitive performance deficits were also demonstrated in patients with subclinical infections. Moreover, it has been demonstrated that patients with influenza-like illnesses were impaired on aspects of everyday memory (Capuron, Lamarque, Dantzer, & Goodall, 2000), suggesting the possibility that infections not directly affecting the brain may result in the impairment of cognitive performance and that such impairment appears to be related to the action of cytokines.

In view of the documented involvement of cytokines in cognitive functioning, there is little doubt that cytokines are capable of providing signals to the brain to alter neural activity. The mechanism through which these peripherally produced cytokines might act on the brain is still not fully understood despite much debate on this issue. Cytokines are not thought to cross the blood-brain barrier because of their large molecular weight and hydrophilic (water-attracting) properties. However, a number of specialized mechanisms have been identified that would allow blood-borne cytokines to signal the brain (Banks, Farr, & Morley, 2003). For example, this may occur as a result of cytokine entry at regions of the brain where the blood-brain barrier is weak or absent (e.g., circumventricular organs) to trigger the production of second messengers (e.g., prostaglandins) to target specific neural structures (e.g., hypothalamic regions) to induce local cytokine production. In addition, peripherally secreted cytokines may affect the CNS through the vagus nerve as an alternative route to gain entry into the brain. Most studies provide support to the notion that local production of cytokines by glial cells in the brain plays an important role in the induction of sickness behavior. While the exact mechanism responsible to translate the immune signal into a neural signal is still unclear, it appears that alterations in a variety of neuropeptide (e.g., CRH, substance P, opioids) and neurotransmitter systems (non-adrenaline, serotonin, gamma-aminobutyric acid) are also involved (Dantzer, 2004; Delgado, McManus, & Chambers, 2003).

## IMPACT OF CNS INJURY IN IMMUNE RESPONSE

Previously, the brain was considered to be an immunologically privileged site. Immunological privilege pertains to the inability of immune cells to enter the CNS under both normal physiologic and pathologic conditions to protect the brain from the potential harmful effects of an immune response. Immune privilege was thought to be maintained by the blood-brain barrier because it provides separation between the circulating cells and molecules of the immune system on the one hand and the brain tissues on the other (Schwartz, 2003). The lack of lymphatic vessels and the paucity of constitutive expression of major histocompatibility complex (MHC) class I and II molecules in brain tissues lent further support to the hypothesis of immune privilege (Schwartz, 2003). However, this view has now changed because of the existence of structures in the brain with functions similar to those of lymphatic vessels. Evidence has also emerged on the existence of lymphatic trafficking within brain tissues (Olson & Miller, 2004; Shaked, Porat, Gersner, Kipnis, & Schwartz, 2004).

In addition, brain resident cells, such as microglia and astrocytes, are now considered to play a key role in the immune response of the CNS. The microglia, a class of specialized brain mononuclear phagocytes, distinct from either blood monocytes or peripheral macrophages, are present in the mature brain at a resting state. These resting microglia become activated immediately when the brain micro-environment is disturbed. Activation of these cells involve changes in their shape, enhanced expression of MHC molecules, proliferation, mobilization to the site of injury, and release of pro-inflammatory cytokines (Beschorner, Nguyen et al., 2002; Lau & Yu, 2001; Schwartz, 2003). In addition, activated microglia secrete growth factors that stimulate the activation of astrocytes, which are also among the first cells to respond to CNS injury (Lenzlinger, Morganti-Kossman, Laurer, & McIntosh, 2001).

Further supporting evidence that the brain is a site of immunological activity is the presence of antigen-specific immune response to infection in the brain (Schwartz, 2003; Yoles et al., 2001). In addition, a growing body of evidence points to the development of inflammatory responses in brain tissues in response to primarily so-called non-immune neuronal insult such as brain trauma and cerebral ischemia (commonly seen after stroke and cardiac arrest). Both clinical and animal studies of brain injury show localized increase in the production of cytokines such as IL-1$\beta$, IL-6, TNF, and chemokines (Jander, Schroeter, Peters, Witte, & Stoll, 2001; Jander, Schroeter, & Stoll, 2002; Lau & Yu, 2001; Lenzlinger, Hans, et al., 2001; Perini et al., 2001; Vila et al., 2003). Cytokines and chemokines contribute to the development of inflammation by stimulating endothelial cells to express adhesion molecules allowing influx and accumulation of leukocytes in the damaged brain tissue. Cell adhesion molecules, such as E-selectin and endothelin-1, are increased early after cerebral ischemia and traumatic brain injury (Cherian et al., 2003; Ho et al., 2001). Evidence also exists that neutrophils and T lymphocytes accumulate in the vicinity of the lesion, followed by infiltration of macrophages in the damaged brain tissue in stroke patients (Beschorner, Schluesener, Gözalan, Meyermann, & Schwab, 2002). Yet in brain contusion injury, few neutrophils are evident and the cellular inflammatory reaction consists mostly of activated macrophages, CD4- and CD8-expressing T cells, and NK cells (Barnum et al., 2002; Beschorner, Nguyen, et al., 2002; Shaked et al., 2004). However, commonly seen in both ischemic and traumatic CNS injury are activation of astrocytes and expression of MHC class II molecules within a few days after the injury, suggesting the presence of an immunological response after CNS damage (Shaked et al., 2004). As a result of the influx of inflammatory cells after CNS injury, it is possible that secondary brain damage can occur by (a) plugging of the surrounding capillaries, (b) production of toxic oxygen radicals and enzymes leading to oxidative stress, and eventually, cell death, (c) triggering edema and tissue-destruction, and (d) increasing the tendency to develop thrombosis in the surrounding blood vessels.

Interestingly, some pro-inflammatory cytokines display protective properties in the CNS. For example, IL-6 also acts as a growth factor, being able to induce differentiation of neurites (branches arising from the neuronal cell body such as axons and dendrites) (Winter, Pringle, Clough, & Church, 2004). TNF-α, a powerful cytokine inducing apoptosis (programmed cell death) in peripheral cells, has also been found to protect neurons in the hippocampus, septum, and cortex, and facilitate the regeneration of injured axons (Lenzlinger, Morganti-Kossman et al., 2001). Taken together, these findings argue for an important role for cytokines in the development of inflammation, and possibly, neuroprotection in the injured brain.

Data are also available on the role of complement proteins in injury-induced CNS inflammation (Barnum et al., 2002; Bellander, Singhrao, Ohlsson, Mattsson, & Svensson, 2001; Schafer et al., 2000). The complement system is part of the innate immune system that consists of approximately 30 plasma proteins involved in the recognition and killing of invading pathogens while preserving normal so-called self cells. Complement activation refers to the process of complement cascade initiation resulting in the production of inflammatory mediators, opsonization (coating of microbes to enhance phagocytosis) of cells for phagocytosis by macrophages, and destruction of tissue by formation of membrane attack complexes (Van Beek, El Ward, & Gasque, 2003). Although there is considerable evidence that both glial cells and complement proteins are activated following cerebral ischemia, little is known about the temporal overlap between increased glial expression and complement activation after ischemic injury. We recently studied the time course of glial (microglia and astrocytes) and corresponding complement activation. This included the study of neuronal loss as it relates to the examination of C3 complement proteins and opsonization, C5 and the initiation of phagocytosis, and C9 in the formation of membrane attack complexes for tissue destruction) following cerebral ischemia (Briones, Wadowska, Suh, & Woods, 2003). Our results showed early activation of microglia followed by astrocytes. Complement activation was seen within 24 hours after ischemia with C3 activation, followed by C5 and C9. Peak glial activation was seen 3 days after reperfusion, whereas peak complement activation was seen 7 days after reperfusion. Peak glial activation was significantly correlated with the time that initial neuronal loss was seen whereas peak complement activation was significantly correlated when maximal neuronal loss was evident, suggesting that complement proteins may play a role in secondary damage after cerebral ischemia (see Figures 8.2a and 8.2b).

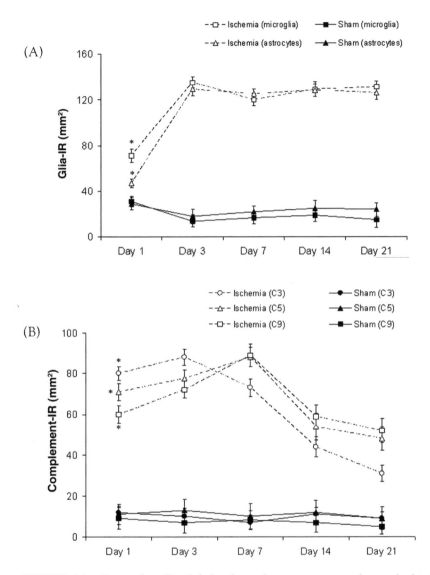

**FIGURE 8.2**    Temporal profile of glial and complement activation after cerebral ischemia. (A) Increased expression of activated glial cells was seen within 24 hrs of ischemia with increased microglial expression seen first followed by astrocytes. Glial expression peaked at day 3 after ischemia and remained elevated until day 21. (B) Increased C3, C5, and C9 expression were seen within 24 hrs of ischemia with C3 activation seen first followed by C5 then C9. Elevations in C3 peaked at day 3 after ischemia while both C5 and C9 expression peaked at day 7. Down regulation of C3 started at day 7 while C5 and C9 expression started to decrease at day 14 after ischemia. *p <0.05—significantly different from shams. Legend: IR-immunoreactivity.

All in all, this review (Table 8.2) demonstrates that extensive communications and interactions exist between the CNS, endocrine system, and immune system. A number of neurotransmitters, hormones, cells, and molecules such as cytokines and other factors participate and regulate this interaction, although among the elderly, this response is blunted (Butcher & Lord, 2004). Additionally, the commonly ignored nonspecific symptoms associated with systemic infection are now beginning to be understood as important for survival (Dantzer, 2004). Knowledge gained about the impact of CNS injuries on immune responses will lead to better insight into the pathophysiological mechanisms leading to brain damage, and thereby, improved treatment strategies.

## DESIGN AND METHODOLOGICAL LIMITATIONS

The complex nature of PNI research requires consideration of multiple methodological issues in the design and interpretation of results. Although most of the studies reviewed were well conceptualized, some design and methodological problems were found. The study limitations that were identified include: (a) gender bias in sampling, (b) variability in the measurement of physiological parameters, and (c) limited clinical implications of the study findings. First, a large number of the research was done using male subjects and this is evident in both animal and human subjects. For instance, gonadal hormones affect cells of the immune system evidenced by variation in NK cell activity across the menstrual cycle; the greatest activity was seen in post menses and least activity seen during menses (Ben-Eliyahu & Shakhar, 2001). Although the gender bias in sampling seen in these studies is reasonable to avoid the confounding effects of gonadal hormones on immune function, generalizations of the study results are limited. In some studies that included female participants, consideration given on the cyclic variation in hormone secretion across the menstrual cycle was not clear. It has been suggested that when women are included in the studies, all participants should be at the same stage of their menstrual cycle when physiological samples are obtained (Kiecolt-Glaser & Glaser, 1988); yet, this is very impractical and often impossible. A reasonable recommendation then to limit the gender bias in sampling is to assess the menstrual cycle and make every effort to randomly distribute participants to minimize variation related to differences in menstrual cycle.

Second, physiological measurement of neuroendocrine activation was not consistent across studies; this is especially true in clinical studies. The commonly measured parameter to detect neuroendocrine activity is the level of cortisol as activation of the HPA and SAM axes results in increased glucocorticoid production. However, this provides a limited view, because both cortisol

**TABLE 8.2** Summary of Articles Reviewed

| Citation | Sample | Purpose/Objective of Study | Variables Measured | Results |
|---|---|---|---|---|
| ***Immune and Aging*** | | | | |
| Boehmer et al. (2004) | Young and old male mice | Investigated whether aging is associated with alterations in cytokine production | • TLR levels in macrophages<br>• TNF-α production<br>• IL-6 production | Macrophages in aged mice showed decreased levels of TLRs and demonstrated suppressed pro-inflammatory cytokine production compared to young mice. |
| Butcher et al. (2001) | Healthy young and elderly male and female volunteers | Examined the effects of aging on neutrophil activity following bacterial infection | • CD16 expression 1<br>• Phagocytic index | CD16 expression in neutrophils correlated with phagocytic index and these measures were reduced in elderly patients with infection compared to the healthy subjects. |
| Butcher et al. (2003) | Patients with fractured neck of femur and healthy volunteers (young and old) | Investigated the effects of age on susceptibility to infection and neutrophil function in elderly patients following mild trauma | • Phagocytic function<br>• Neutrophil levels | No significant difference was seen in neutrophil levels between the two groups but phagocytic function was markedly decreased in the trauma group compared to the healthy group and this decrease persisted for 5 weeks. |
| Di Lorenso et al. (2000) | Young and old male and female volunteers | Examined the effects of age on NK cell activity | • NK cell count<br>• NK cell activity<br>• Apoptosis molecule in NK cells | Decreased NK cell count and NK cell activity was found in the elderly volunteers compared to the young subjects. Furthermore, an age-related increase in the apoptosis molecule was observed. |

*(Continued)*

233

**TABLE 8.2** Summary of Articles Reviewed (*Continued*)

| Citation | Sample | Purpose/Objective of Study | Variables Measured | Results |
|---|---|---|---|---|
| Ferrari et al. (2000) | Elderly patients with either vascular dementia of Alzheimer's disease Healthy elderly volunteers | Examined neuroendocrine changes occurring in physiological and pathological brain aging | • Serum DHEA levels<br>• Serum cortisol during evening and night times | Significant increased in serum cortisol levels were seen in both evening and night times in the elderly subjects, particularly in those with dementia compared to the young subjects. In addition, serum DHEA levels were significantly lower in elderly subjects and even more in patients with dementia compared to the young controls. Consequently, a significant increase in the cortisol/DHEA molar ratio was seen in the elderly. |
| Ferrari et al. (2000) | Healthy young and old subjects Patients with Alzheimer's dementia | Examined NK cell function and cytokine production in physiological and pathological brain aging | • NK cell function<br>• NK cell cytotoxic activity (NKCC)<br>• Morphometric analysis of the brain by magnetic resonance imaging (MRI)<br>• TNF-$\alpha$<br>• Interferon-$\gamma$ (IFN-$\gamma$) | Decreased NK cell function was seen in the elderly especially in those with dementia compared to the young subjects. Increased NKCC and cytokine production was seen in elderly patients with dementia compared to the healthy elderly group. Moreover, this increased NKCC and TNF-$\alpha$ levels were associated with decreased cognitive function. |

| | | | | |
|---|---|---|---|---|
| Jarrar, et al. (2001) | Male trauma patients ages 18 to 44 | Examined the effects of the adrenal steroid dehydroepiandrosterone (DHEA) on immune function following hemorrhagic trauma | • Serum cortisol level<br>• Serum DHEA level | Increased serum cortisol levels were seen in all patients. However, a decrease in serum cortisol levels was seen in patients that received DHEA. |
| Johnson et al. (2002) | Aged wild-type and transgenic (immunoglobulin gene) male mice | Analyzed the effects of aging on B cell production and function | • Total B cell number<br>• Antibody production | No significant difference was seen between the wild-type and transgenic mice in the total number of B cells from the spleen but the transgenic animals produced more autoantibodies that are reactive to DNA products. |
| Kiecolt-Glaser et al. (2003) | Aged volunteers (caregivers of spouse with dementia and noncaregiving spouse) | Determined the effects of chronic stress on IL-6 production and describe its pattern of change | • Serum IL-6 level<br>• Health behaviors | IL-6 levels in caregivers were four-fold greater than the noncaregivers. No differences were seen in health problems, medications, or health-relevant behaviors between the two groups that could account for the caregivers' elevated IL-6 levels. |
| Leng et al. (2004) | Community-dwelling frail and nonfrail older adults | Investigated specific immune system modulation that may contribute to frailty | • Peripheral blood mononuclear cells (PBMC)<br>• IL-6<br>• IL-10<br>• TNF-$\alpha$ | Frail subjects had significantly lower PBMC proliferation compared to non-frail individuals. In addition, frail individuals had higher IL-6 levels compared to the nonfrail subjects but no significant differences were observed in IL-10 and TNF-$\alpha$ production between the two groups. |

(Continued)

**TABLE 8.2** Summary of Articles Reviewed (*Continued*)

| Citation | Sample | Purpose/Objective of Study | Variables Measured | Results |
|---|---|---|---|---|
| Linton et al. (2000) | Aged wild-type and knockout (B cell deficient) male mice | Examined the role of B cells in adaptive immune response in the elderly | • B cell production<br>• Memory B cells<br>• IL-2 | No significant difference was found in IL-2 and B cell production between the two groups. However, development of memory B cells was absent in the knockout mice compared to the wild-type group. |
| Miyaji et al. (2000) | Middle-aged and centenarian volunteers | Examined the immune function in centenarians | • NK cells<br>• NK-T cells<br>• Phagocytic function of granulocytes<br>• IFN-γ | Decreased number of NK cells and NK-T cells were seen in the centenarian group compared to the middle-aged volunteers. Also, the phagocytic function and cytokine production of granulocytes in both healthy and unhealthy centenarians increased compared to the middle-aged group. |
| Renshaw et al. (2002) | Young and aged male mice | Examined whether the decreased immune response in the elderly is a function of TLRs | • IL-6<br>• TNF-α<br>• TLR levels on macrophages | Significantly lower TLRs were observed in the macrophages of aged mice compared to the young group. Furthermore, macrophages from the aged mice secreted significantly lower IL-6 and TNF-α compared to those of young mice. |
| Tarazona et al. (2000) | Young and elderly volunteers | Examined the expression of NK cell markers on T lymphocytes in aging | | Increased expression of NK cell markers were found in a subset of cytotoxic T cells in the elderly group compared to the young volunteers. Additionally, increased proliferation of these T cell subsets was found following stress activation in the aged group compared to the young volunteers. |

## Sickness Behavior

| | | | | |
|---|---|---|---|---|
| Bluthé et al. (2000) | Wild-type and knockout (IL-1β) male mice | Assessed the role of IL-1β in LPS-induced sickness behavior | • Social exploration<br>• Body weight<br>• Mobility<br>• Appetite | Decreased social exploration, appetite, and mobility were observed in wild-type mice that received LPS injection compared to the knockout group. Additionally, increased weight loss was seen in the wild-type mice in comparison to the knockout group. |
| Bluthé et al. (2000) | Wild-type and knockout (IL-6) male mice | Assessed the role of IL-6 in LPS-induced sickness behavior | • Social exploration<br>• Body weight<br>• Mobility<br>• Appetite | Decreased social exploration, appetite, and mobility were observed in the wild-type group compared to the knockout mice after LPS injection. Additionally, increased weight loss was seen in the wild-type mice in comparison to the knockout group. |
| Bluthé et al. (2002) | Adult male rats | Assessed the role of IL-1 in LPS-induced sickness behavior | • Social exploration<br>• Body weight | Decreased social exploration and increased weight loss was seen following LPS injection but these symptoms were reversed following administration of IL-1 antagonist. |
| Brebner et al. (2000) | Adult male rats | Examined the effects of systemic administration of different doses of IL-1β and TNF-α on food consumption | • Appetite<br>• Plasma corticosterone level | Dose-dependent decrease in appetite was seen accompanied by increased plasma corticosterone level. A synergistic effect was seen between IL-1β and TNF-α in increasing plasma corticosterone. |

*(Continued)*

237

**TABLE 8.2** Summary of Articles Reviewed (*Continued*)

| Citation | Sample | Purpose/Objective of Study | Variables Measured | Results |
|---|---|---|---|---|
| Capuron et al. (2000) | Male naval healthy recruits and those with flu-like symptoms, with and without fever | Examined the effects of infectious disease on cognitive functioning and determine the role of fever in the appearance of cognitive impairment | • Short-term memory<br>• Attention | Subjects with flu-like symptoms were impaired in short-term memory and attention task compared to the healthy group. The impairment in short-term memory and attention was not significantly different between those with and without fever. |
| Chen et al. (2005) | Adult male rats | Compared short- and long-term LPS injection on the production of IL-1β, TNF-α, and IL-6 | • IL-1β<br>• TNF-α<br>• IL-6<br>• Plasma corticosterone level | Increased systemic and brain cytokine production was seen after short-term LPS injection. However, with long-term LPS injection only brain cytokine production was increased but systemic levels remained constant. The differential cytokine production was probably mediated by corticosterone. |
| De Jongh et al. (2003) | Adults male rats | Examined the role of IL-6 in HPA axis activation and fever production following laparotomy | • Body temperature<br>• Plasma corticosterone level | Surgical laparotomy induced post-operative hyperthermia but injection of IL-6 antibody accelerated return of body temperature to normal levels. However, injection of IL-6 antibody did not affect the stress-induced plasma corticosterone production. |

| Study | Subjects | Aim | Measures | Findings |
|---|---|---|---|---|
| Grinevich et al. (2001) | Adult male rats | Examined the effect of repeated LPS injection on cytokine production and HPA axis activity | • Plasma ACTH level<br>• Glucocorticoid receptor levels<br>• IL-6 and IL-1β messenger RNA (mRNA)<br>• Plasma corticosterone level<br>• Body weight<br>• Adrenal weight | Glucocorticoid receptor levels, IL-6 and IL-1β mRNA significantly increased after either a single or repeated LPS injection. Plasma corticosterone but not ACTH decreased after repeated LPS injection. Repeated LPS injection decreased body weight while adrenal weight increased compared to the single LPS administration group. |
| Marshall et al. (2000) | Healthy volunteers<br>Volunteers with allergic rhinitis | Examined the effects of symptomatic allergic rhinitis on speed of cognitive processing, attention, and short-term memory | • Short-term memory<br>• Attention<br>• Cognitive processing task | Symptomatic patients with ragweed allergy experience subtle slowed speed of cognitive processing but not deficits in attention and short-term memory. |
| Marshall et al. (2002) | Healthy volunteers<br>Volunteers with allergic rhinitis | Evaluated the effects of symptomatic allergic rhinitis on fatigue level and mood | • Fatigue level (Multi-dimensional Fatigue Inventory)<br>• Mood (Positive Affect-Negative Affect mood-rating scale) | Symptomatic patients with ragweed allergy reported higher levels of mental fatigue but not physical fatigue, as well as reduced motivation. Patients also reported experiencing sadness and reduced feelings of pleasure. |

(*Continued*)

239

**TABLE 8.2** Summary of Articles Reviewed (*Continued*)

| Citation | Sample | Purpose/Objective of Study | Variables Measured | Results |
|---|---|---|---|---|
| Palin et al. (2001) | Adult male rats | Examined the effects of endogenous IL-1 antagonist on LPS-induced sickness behavior | • IL-1β protein level<br>• IL-1β mRNA level<br>• Body weight<br>• Appetite | Increased expression of both mRNA and protein levels of IL-1β antagonist were seen after LPS injection. Correlation was seen between increased IL-β antagonist level and decreased appearance of sickness behavior. |
| Scheibel et al. (2004) | Patients with chronic myelogenous leukemia receiving either IFN-α alone or IFN-α and chemotherapy | Examined the effects of IFN-α on cognitive functioning and the incidence of depression | • Cognitive functioning<br>• Symptoms of depression | Increased depressive symptoms and decreased information processing and cognitive functioning were observed in patients that received interferon therapy alone compared to the group that received interferon in combination with chemotherapy. |
| Sparkman et al. (2005) | Young and old adult female mice | Assessed the effects of age and LPS injection on cognitive functioning | • Water maze performance | Older mice showed significant impairment in the memory task compared to the younger animals. Injection of LPS resulted in a further decrease in cognitive functioning. |
| **CNS Injury** | | | | |
| Barnum (2002) | Adult male rats | Examined the effects of middle cerebral artery occlusion (stroke model) on complement protein activation | • C3 complement protein<br>• C5 complement protein<br>• Leukocyte level | Increased expression of C3 and C5 were seen within 24 hours of occlusion. This activation of the complement system is likely due to massive leukocyte infiltration seen after ischemia. |

| Study | Subjects | Purpose | Measures | Results |
|---|---|---|---|---|
| Bellander (2001) | Male and female traumatic head injury patients who had frontal lobe or temporal lobe resection | Examined the effects of traumatic head injury on complement activation | • C1 complement protein<br>• C3 complement protein<br>• C9 complement protein | Increased expression of all complement proteins examined was seen in the area of injury and also in the penumbral area (surrounding area) of the contusion. No significant difference was seen on complement expression between the frontal and temporal lobes. |
| Beschorner (2002) | Autopsy brains from male and female traumatic closed head injury victims | Examined the effects of traumatic head injury on micrgoglia activation and leukocyte trafficking | • Microglia/macrophages in parenchymal tissues<br>• Microglia/macrophages in perivascular space | Increased number of microglia/macrophages was seen in the perivascular space and parenchyma within 2 days after injury and reached maximum levels within 4–8 days and remained elevated for weeks. The increased microglia/macrophages were seen in the local and surrounding area of the injury. |
| Beschorner (2002) | Autopsy brains from male and female stroke victims | Examined the effects of stroke on micrgoglia activation and leukocyte trafficking | • Microglia/macrophages in parenchymal tissues<br>• Microglia/macrophages in perivascular space | Increased number of microglia/macrophages was seen in the perivascular space and parenchyma within 1–2 days after injury and remained elevated for weeks. The pattern of increased microglia/macrophages was more diffuse than localized. |
| Briones (2003) | Male adult rats | Examined the time course of glial and complement activation following cerebral ischemia and related them to degree of neuronal loss | • C3 complement protein<br>• C5 complement protein<br>• C9 complement protein<br>• Microglia<br>• Astrocytes<br>• Neuron loss | Activation of microglia and astrocytes were seen within 24 hours of injury. Corresponding complement activation was seen with increased in C3 seen first followed by C5 and C9. Peak glial activation was significantly correlated with the time that initial neuronal loss was seen, whereas peak complement activation was significantly correlated with maximal neuronal loss. |

*(Continued)*

241

**TABLE 8.2** Summary of Articles Reviewed (*Continued*)

| Citation | Sample | Purpose/Objective of Study | Variables Measured | Results |
|---|---|---|---|---|
| Cherian (2003) | Hospitalized male and female ischemic stroke patients. Healthy volunteers | Examined concentrations of cell adhesion molecule in stroke patients with different etiologies | • E-selectin in peripheral blood<br>• P-selectin in peripheral blood | Increased E-selectin and P-selectin levels were seen in stroke patients regardless of etiology. The increase was seen within 7 days of stroke onset and is associated with ischemic pathology. |
| Ho (2001) | Wild-type and knockout (endothelin-1) mice | Examined expression of endothelin-1 (ET-1) under normal, hypoxic, and hypoxic/ischemic conditions | • ET-1 mRNA<br>• ET-1 protein | Under normal conditions, no increase in ET-1 mRNA and protein were seen. However, under hypoxic and hypoxic/ischemic conditions, increased ET-1 mRNA and protein were seen in the wild-type mice and this is accompanied by increased morbidity as compared to the knockout group. |
| Jander (2001) | Adults male rats | Examined production of pro-inflammatory cytokines following cotical injury | • IL-1β<br>• TNF-α | A 24-fold increase in both IL-1β and TNF-α was seen in the ipsilateral brain region following cortical injury. |
| Jander (2002) | Adult male rats | Examined production of pro-inflammatory cytokines and apoptosis precursor following middle cerebral artery occlusion | • IL-1β<br>• IL-18<br>• Caspase-1 (precursor for apoptosis) | IL-1β increased within 16 hours after occlusion while IL-18 did not increase until 48 hours after ischemia. The time course of caspase-1 production parallels those of IL-18. Expression of the pro-inflammatory cytokines was seen around the area of infraction and also in the ipsilateral cortex. |

| Lau (2001) | Adult male rats | Assessed the production of pro-inflammatory cytokines after mechanical brain trauma and cerebral ischemia | • IL-1α<br>• TNF-α<br>• IFN-γ<br>• IL-6 | Increased expression of all cytokines measured was seen in both injury models. However, cytokine expression increased within 1 hour after mechanical trauma compared to 4–8 hours following ischemia. |
|---|---|---|---|---|
| Lenzlinger (2001) | Hospitalized male and female traumatic brain injury patients | Examined cell-mediated immune response after severe traumatic brain injury | • β2-microglobulin<br>• IL-2 | Both β2-microglobulin and IL-2 expression increased following traumatic brain injury with concentrations greater in the serum compared to the CSF fluid. The elevation in these cell-mediated immune markers was detected up to 3 weeks. |
| Olson (2004) | Adult mice | Examined TLR expression in microglia after LPS injection in the brain | • TLR level<br>• MHC class II molecules | Elevation in microglia was seen following LPS injection and TLRs in these glial cells were also increased. The activation of TLR was associated with increased MHC class II molecules. |
| Perini (2001) | Male and female stroke patients without signs of infection and healthy volunteers | Examined the immune response to acute stroke and analyzed a possible correlation with clinical outcome | • IL-10<br>• IL-6 | Elevated serum IL-6 level was seen within 24 hours of stroke onset and persisted until day 14 with a maximum increase at day 3. Elevation of serum IL-10 on the other hand did not occur until 7 days after the onset of stroke. Furthermore, increased IL-6 levels correlated with better clinical outcomes while IL-10 elevation did not. |
| Shafer (2000) | Adult male rats | Examined the effects of global cerebral ischemia on C1 complement (initiator of complement activation) activation | • C1 complement protein in neurons<br>• C1 complement protein in astrocytes and microglia | Increased C1 synthesis and activity was seen at 1, 24, and 72 hours after ischemia. This increase in C1 complement proteins was seen only in microglial cells but not in neurons and astrocytes. |

(*Continued*)

**TABLE 8.2** Summary of Articles Reviewed (*Continued*)

| Citation | Sample | Purpose/Objective of Study | Variables Measured | Results |
|---|---|---|---|---|
| Shaked (2004) | Adult female rats | Examined microglial activation and T-cell mediated response following optic nerve injury | • NK cells<br>• Microglia<br>• MHC class II | Increased number of microglia and NK cells were seen immediately following injury that persisted for 3 days. Elevation in MHC class II molecules were seen 3 days after injury with peak expression demonstrated in day 7 and dropped to basla level on day 14. |
| Vila (2003) | Male and female stroke patients | Assessed the effects of pro-inflammatory cytokines on clinical outcomes after ischemic stroke | • IL-4<br>• IL-10<br>• Neurological assessment | Plasma levels of IL-4 and IL-10 increased within 48 hours after onset of stroke. However, concentrations of IL-10 was significantly lower compared to IL-4 and decreased IL-10 levels correlated with worsening of neurological outcome. |
| Winter (2004) | Male and female patients with severe traumatic head injury | Examined the correlation between patient outcome and cytokine expression after traumatic brain injury | • IL-6<br>• IL-1β<br>• Nerve growth factor<br>• Neurological assessment | Increased cytokines levels were seen in the CSF of the head-injured patients within 8–12 hours after insult. Higher levels of IL-6 correlated with improved neurological outcome whereas IL-1β and NGF did not. |
| Yoles (2001) | Adult male rats | Examined T-cell dependent immune response after optic nerve injury | • T-cells<br>• T-cell receptor | Increased number of T cells and T cell receptors were seen following injury. Further, neuronal survival after optic nerve injury was 40% lower in rats with decreased T cell count compared to control animals. |

and DHEA, as well as catecholamines, are released from the adrenal glands during stress activation (Butcher & Lord, 2004). Plasma measurement of cortisol, DHEA, and catecholamines is usually regarded as the more accurate measure of stress-induced neuroendocrine activation (Kiecolt-Glaser & Glaser, 1988); although it is still questionable whether peripheral blood samples could adequately reflect what is transpiring within the CNS and lymphoid tissues or at sites of infection. Some researchers suggest that 24-hour urine sampling is more precise in determining physiological levels of neuroendocrine activation compared to plasma (Dimsdale, Young, Moore, & Strauss, 1987); however, the thoroughness required in performing 24-hour urine collection can result in higher probability of errors. Additionally, it must be considered that secretion of urine metabolites is related to renal function and may be a confounding variable in measuring neuroendocrine activation (Dimsdale et al., 1987). While there are others that suggest using salivary cortisol to measure neuroendocrine activity because it is non-invasive and convenient, the disadvantage of this method of sampling is that it is less accurate (Haus, Nicolau, Lakatua, & Sackett-Lundeen, 1988).

Furthermore, most plasma and salivary sampling in the clinical studies reviewed were done only once. One-time plasma or salivary sampling may not be a true reflection of neuroendocrine activity because hormones secreted during HPA and SAM axes activation is affected by biological rhythms (Sothern & Roitman-Johnson, 2001). When conducting PNI studies, it must be recognized that life is not only structured in space, but also in time. In addition, it should be established that although secretion of biological hormones is synchronized in time, they are not all timed together, as they have their own times of highs and lows. Hormones secreted by the adrenals are good examples as cortisol levels are highest in the morning when a person rises, whereas prolactin and growth hormone levels reach their peak while a person sleeps (Sothern & Roitman-Johnson, 2001). Investigators must be cognizant of the fact that immune parameters are also controlled by circadian variation as illustrated in Table 8.3. Finally, given the complex and probabilistic nature of how immune responses are mounted, significant variation must be expected over time, as a function of situation, and across individuals. Moreover, at any point in time, only a small fraction of the response will be reflected; thus one-time sampling may provide just a fragmentary picture of the bidirectional communication between the neuroendocrine and immune systems, therefore limiting the relevance of the data.

In most of the clinical studies reviewed, either one or two immune parameters were measured. This may be problematic due to the complexity and redundancy in the immune system wherein a change in one parameter can impact the function of other immune players. This is specifically true in cytokine measurement (Glaser & Kiecolt-Glaser, 2005). The most frequently measured immune parameters in the clinical studies, aside from cytokines, were lymphocyte activation and

**TABLE 8.3**  Peak* Values of Endocrine and Immune Parameters in Diurnal Individuals

| Parameter | Time | Reference |
|---|---|---|
| Cortisol (saliva) | 0530 – 0830 | (Sothern & Roitman-Johnson, 2001) |
| Cortisol (plasma) | 0630 – 0830 | (Sothern & Roitman-Johnson, 2001) |
| Cortisol (urine) | 0630 – 0930 | (Sothern & Roitman-Johnson, 2001) |
| Neutrophils, total | 1830 – 2030 | (Haus et al., 1988) |
| Lymphocytes, total | 0000 – 2030 | (Haus et al., 1988) |
| T-helper lymphocytes (CD4) | 0000 | (Levi et al., 1988) |
| T-cytotoxic lymphocytes (CD8) | 1830 | (Levi et al., 1988) |
| NK cells, total | 1700 – 1930 | (Born, Lange, Hansen, Mölle, & Fehm, 1997) |
| NK-cell activity | 1100 – 1300 | (Levi et al., 1988) |
| IL-1$\beta$ | 2130 – 0010 | (Hohagen et al., 1993) |
| IL-2 | 0100 | (Lissoni, Rovelli, Brivio, Brivio, & Fumagalli, 1991) |
| IL-6 | 0200 – 0230 | (Entzian, Linnemann, Schlaak, & Zabel, 1996) |
| IL-10 | 0730 and 1930 | (Young et al., 1995) |
| IL-12 | 2300 | (Petrovsky, McNair, & Harrison, 1998) |
| IFN-$\gamma$ | 0000 – 0130 | (Hohagen et al., 1993) |
| TNF-$\alpha$ | 0730 and 1330 | (Young et al., 1995) |

*peak value or 95% limits from cosinor analysis

NK cell activity. The problem with these measures is that lymphocyte activation is nonspecific as it could reflect either altered lymphocyte distribution or lymphocyte function (Rabin, 1999). Lymphocyte activation could also represent influences of macrophages or of humoral factors, therefore, its clinical relevance is vague (Rabin, 1999). NK cell activity is also nonspecific as its measurement is extremely variable, even in healthy individuals (Daruna, 2004).

Third, clinical implications may be somewhat limited because of the artificial context in which results from some of the human studies were obtained.

That is, stress situations were created specifically for the study and as it is not a random event, it may lack the same significance of real-life challenges. Moreover, the vast majority of the research was done using animal models. Some researchers suggest that rats are not as appropriate as primates for the symptomatic modeling of disease and that human disorders cannot be modeled in animals (Rodgers & Anderko, 2004). Much of the skepticism toward the use of experimental animal models arises from an expectation that disease symptoms should have the same exact physical manifestation in animals as in humans. However, it should be recognized that the modeling of human-like symptoms in animals are made by basic science investigators primarily on the basis of an expectation of functional similarity, rather than one of physical identity. Thus, whereas caution should be taken in translating the implications of research of animal disorders into generalizations about human disorders, the utility of experimental animal models in providing preclinical data is extremely important in providing a better understanding of the mechanisms involved in human disease so that rational therapeutic strategies can be developed.

## CLINICAL IMPLICATIONS

Great strides have been made in the field of PNI toward understanding some of the interactions between the CNS, endocrine, and immune systems, as well as understanding how stress influences the communication between these systems. Although the mechanisms that underlie the interactions between these three systems are not yet fully understood, there are already clear translational implications in the present PNI data. On the basis of present evidence that both aging and stress have a negative impact on immune function, nurses should be very vigilant in caring for elderly patients as they are more prone to infection compared to the younger patients. As seen in recent reports, aging is accompanied by an increase in the incidence of infectious diseases such as influenza and pneumonia (Butcher et al., 2003; Marsland et al., 2002). Although stress is part of our daily lives, the effects of stress are influenced by three variables: magnitude, duration, and the individual's response (Butcher & Lord, 2004). Individual physiological responses to stress in aging may be difficult to control but nurses can have a great impact in modulating the magnitude and duration of stress in their elderly patients. Thus, stress assessment should be incorporated in caring for the elderly. Additionally, the diverse strategies that may be used to modulate the stress response include relaxation techniques, hypnosis, and exercise; all of which have been shown to produce positive endocrine and immune changes (Andersen, 2004; Irwin, Pike, Cole, & Oxman, 2003). Although it is not clear to what extent these positive endocrine and immunological changes have on immunosenescence, results obtained from healthy individuals seem to be promising.

The necessary synchrony between metabolic, physiological, and behavioral components of the systemic response to infection is primarily dependent on cytokines (Dantzer, 2004). Sufficient evidence is now available to accept the concept that immune players such as cytokines are interpreted by the brain as molecular signals of sickness in response to an infectious event. Since it has been demonstrated that the constellation of cytokine-induced symptoms are adaptive in nature (Dantzer, 2001), nurses need to be cognizant that treating so-called sickness behaviors by inhibiting fever formation or by force-feeding may be detrimental to survival. Furthermore, understanding the efficacy of these cytokine-induced symptoms is demonstrated by the fact that both humans and animals have survived infections and injury through evolutionary history; consequently, the nurses' role in this instance should be mainly supportive and ensuring patient comfort. Then again, in the non-acute care setting, nurses should put an emphasis on educating their patients regarding road and work place safety precautions associated with illnesses as innocuous as the common cold. That is, patients who want to continue with their usual daily routine throughout sickness should be warned about accidents in the workplace as there is data demonstrating cognitive impairment even in subclinical symptoms of illness (Vollmer-Conna, 2001).

Lastly, most types of CNS injury lead to a local inflammation in the brain. This inflammatory response is a result of activation of brain resident cells such as astrocytes and microglia (Lau & Yu, 2001; Schwartz, 2003). Evidence that both pro- and anti-inflammatory cytokines as well as growth factors are produced by the resident brain cells suggest that the immune response seen following CNS injury may amplify brain damage on the one hand but, on the other hand, may participate in the healing process and possibly contribute to neuronal regeneration. It is possible that the neuroprotective and neurodegenerative pathways triggered following injury are not two distinct mechanisms but rather they may represent two extremes of a continuum: one may play a role in adaptive responses to injury; the other extreme may mediate neuronal degeneration and cell death when the normal adaptive regulatory mechanisms are overwhelmed. For that reason, it is essential that neuroscience nursing rehabilitation should be aimed at enhancing the protective effects of the immune response following CNS injury. The results of sensory stimulation as a rehabilitation strategy following CNS injury are particularly interesting because it can induce neuronal regeneration and recovery of function that is probably mediated by enhancing the intrinsic regenerative potential of the brain (Briones, Suh, Hattar, & Wadowska, 2005; Briones et al., 2004; Briones, Suh, Jozsa et al., 2005; Briones, Therrien, & Metzger, 2000; Holden, 2005). Studies have also shown that production of growth factors (Mohammed, Winblad, Ebendal, & Lärkfors, 1990), substances necessary for neuronal regeneration by glial cells after CNS injury can be enhanced, increasing the likelihood of early functional recovery (Briones, Woods, Wadowska, Rogozinska, & Nguyen, 2006; Bury, Eichhorn, Kotzer, & Jones, 2000). These studies on sensory stimulation as a rehabilitation tool, suggest that the brain retains a significant residual capacity for mending following insult. Implementing rehabilitation efforts then, especially those undertaken within the window of therapeutic opportunity after CNS injury, may have an effect in enhancing both morphological and behavioral recovery.

## IMPLICATIONS FOR FUTURE RESEARCH

The field of PNI is improving our understanding of the complex physiological changes that take place during neuroendocrine and immune system interaction, providing new insights into various clinical applications. While much progress has been made in the PNI field, several questions still remain unanswered, such as the long-term impact of stressors on the developing CNS, endocrine, and immune systems. The effect of continuous exposure to stressful situations on infants and young children has not been well studied in the PNI field. Indeed, excellent developmental studies of primates indicate that early stressors can reverberate throughout the life of an individual (Coe & Lubach, 2003).

Another question that needs to be answered is the role of genetics in the complex relationship between the CNS, endocrine, and immune systems. This is largely an unknown area at this time and deserves exploration. For example, do individuals who have one or more variants of the polymorphisms associated with increased production of cortisol show greater immunological dysregulation when faced with stressful events? Another question is whether genotype plays a role in an individual's response to stimuli used to enhance the immune response and which immune response is modifiable? Yet another PNI research question relates to the recovery pattern of altered neuroendocrine and immune response induced by stress, and identification of the so-called susceptible period following a stressful episode wherein negative health consequences start to occur.

As shown above, nurses can pose several research questions and make a significant contribution in the PNI field. Through active inter- and intradisciplinary collaborations, utilization of current knowledge in genetics, use of meaningful biomarkers, and a biobehavioral approach, nurse scientists can answer interesting questions that address the remarkable complexities of the interactions between the CNS, endocrine system, and immune system. As new knowledge is generated in the PNI field, we will eventually have an answer to the question of when stress is beneficial or harmful so that strategies can be developed to promote the health of individuals in the future.

## ACKNOWLEDGMENT

Supported by the National Institutes of Health grant # RO1 NR05260.

## REFERENCES

Andersen, B. (2004). Psychological, behavioral, and immune changes after a psychological intervention: A clinical trial. *Journal of Clinical Oncology, 22,* 3570–3580.

Banks, W. A., Farr, S. A., & Morley, J. E. (2003). Entry of blood-borne cytokines into the central nervous system: Effects on cognitive processes. *Neuroimmunomodulation, 10,* 319–327.

Barnum, S. R., Ames, R. S., Maycox, P. R., Hadingham, S. J., Meakin, J., Harrison, D., et al. (2002). Expression of complement C3a and C5a receptors after permanent focal ischemia: An alternative interpretation. *Glia, 38,* 169–173.

Bellander, B. M., Singhrao, S. K., Ohlsson, M., Mattsson, P., & Svensson, M. (2001). Complement activation in the human brain after traumatic head injury. *Journal of Neurotrauma, 18,* 1295–1311.

Ben-Eliyahu, S., & Shakhar, G. (2001). *The impact of stress, catecholamines, and the menstrual cycle on NK activity and tumor development: From in vitro studies to biological significance* (3rd ed.). New York: Academic Press.

Beschorner, R., Nguyen, T., Gözalan, F., Pedal, I., Mattern, R., Schluesener, H., et al. (2002). CD14 expression by activated parenchymal microglia/macrophages and infiltrating monocytes following human traumatic brain injury. *Acta Neuropathologica, 103,* 541–549.

Beschorner, R., Schluesener, H., Gözalan, F., Meyermann, R., & Schwab, J. (2002). Infiltrating CD14+ monocytes and expression of CD14 by the activated parenchymal microglia/macrophages contribute to the pool of CD14+ cells in ischemic brain lesions. *Journal of Neuroimmunology, 126,* 107–115.

Bluthé, R. M. (2000). Role of IL-6 in cytokine-induced sickness behavior: A study with IL-6 deficient mice. *Physiology & Behavior, 70,* 367–373.

Bluthé, R. M., Dantzer, R., & Kelley, K. W. (2002). Effects of interleukin-1 receptor antagonist on the behavioral effects of lipopolysaccharide in rat. *Brain Research, 573,* 318–320.

Bluthé, R. M., Layé, S., Michaud, B., Combe, C., Dantzer, R., & Parnet, P. (2000). Role of interleukin-1 and tumor necrosis factor- in lipopolysaccharide-induced sickness behavior: A study with interleukin-1 type I receptor-deficient mice. *European Journal of Neuroscience, 12,* 4447–4456.

Boehmer, E. D., Goral, J., Faunce, D. E., & Kovacs, E. J. (2004). Age-dependent decrease in Toll-like receptor 4-mediated proinflammatory cytokine production and mitogen-activated protein kinase expression. *Journal of Leukocyte Biology, 75,* 342–349.

Born, J., Lange, T., Hansen, K., Mölle, M., & Fehm, H. L. (1997). Effects of sleep and circadian rhythm on human circulating immune cells. *Journal of Immunology, 158,* 4457–4467.

Brebner, K., Hayley, S., Zacharko, R., Merali, Z., & Anisman, H. (2000). Synergistic effects of interleukin-1beta, interleukin-6, and tumor necrosis factor-alpha: central monoamine, corticosterone, and behavioral variations. *Neuropsychopharmacology, 22,* 566–580.

Briones, T. L., Suh, E., Hattar, H., & Wadowska, M. (2005). Dentate gyrus neurogenesis after cerebral ischemia and behavioral training. *Biological Research for Nursing, 6,* 167–179.

Briones, T. L., Suh, E., Jozsa, L., Hattar, H., Chai, J., & Wadowska, M. (2004). Behaviorally-induced ultrastructural plasticity in the hippocampal region after cerebral ischemia. *Brain Research, 997,* 137–146.

Briones, T. L., Suh, E., Jozsa, L., Rogozinska, M., Woods, J., & Wadowska, M. (2005). Changes in number of synapses and mitochondria in presynaptic terminals in the dentate gyrus following cerebral ischemia and rehabilitation training. *Brain Research, 1033,* 51–57.

Briones, T. L., Therrien, B., & Metzger, B. (2000). Effects of environment on enhancing functional plasticity following cerebral ischemia. *Biological Research for Nursing, 1,* 299–309.

Briones, T. L., Wadowska, M., Suh, E., & Woods, J. (2003). Time course of glial and corresponding complement activation following cerebral ischemia. *Society for Neuroscience Abstract, 29,* 997.

Briones, T. L., Woods, J., Wadowska, M., Rogozinska, M., & Nguyen, M. (2006). Astrocytic changes in the hippocampus and functional recovery after cerebral ischemia are facilitated by rehabilitation training. *Behavioural Brain Research, 171,* 17–25.

Bury, S. D., Eichhorn, A. C., Kotzer, C. M., & Jones, T. A. (2000). Reactive astrocytic responses to denervation in the motor cortex of adult rats are sensitive to manipulation of behavioral experience. *Neuropharmacology, 39,* 743–755.

Butcher, S. K., Chahal, H., Nayak, L., Sinclair, A., Henriquez, N. V., Sapey, E., et al. (2001). Senescence in innate immune responses: Reduced neutrophil phagocytic capacity and CD16 expression in elderly humans. *Journal of Leukocyte Biology, 70,* 881–886.

Butcher, S. K., Killampalli, V., Chahal, H., Alpar, E. K., & Lord, J. M. (2003). Effect of age on susceptibility to post-traumatic infection in the elderly. *Biochemical Society Transactions, 31,* 449–451.

Butcher, S. K., & Lord, J. M. (2004). Stress responses and innate immunity: Aging as a contributory factor. *Aging Cell, 3,* 151–160.

Capuron, L., Lamarque, D., Dantzer, R., & Goodall, G. (2000). Attentional and mnemonic deficits associated with infectious diseases in humans. *Psychological Medicine, 29,* 291–297.

Cartier, L., Hartley, O., Dubois-Dauphin, M., & Krause, K. H. (2005). Chemokine receptors in the central nervous system: Role in brain inflammation and neurodegenerative diseases. *Brain Research Reviews, 48,* 16–42.

Chen, R., Zhou, H., Beltran, J., Malellari, L., & Chang, S. L. (2005). Differential expression of cytokines in the brain and serum during endotoxin tolerance. *Journal of Neuroimmunology, 163,* 53–72.

Cherian, P., Hankey, G. J., Eikelboom, J. W., Thom, J., Baker, R. I., McQuillan, A., et al. (2003). Endothial and platelet activation in acute ischemic stroke and its etiological subtypes. *Stroke, 34,* 2132–2137.

Coe, C. L., & Lubach, G. R. (2003). Critical periods of special health relevance for psychoneuroimmunology. *Brain, Behavior, and Immunity, 17,* 3–12.

Dantzer, R. (2001). Cytokine-induced sickness behavior: Where do we stand? *Brain, Behavior, and Immunity, 15,* 7–24.

Dantzer, R. (2004). Cytokine-induced sickness behaviour: A neuroimmune response to activation of innate immunity. *European Journal of Pharmacology, 500,* 399–411.

Daruna, J. H. (2004). *Introduction to psychoneuroimmunology.* Amsterdam: Elsevier Academic Press.

De Jongh, R. F., Vissers, K. C., Booij, L.H.D.J., De Jongh, K. L., Vincken, P., & Meert, T. F. (2003). Interleukin-6 and perioperative thermoregulation and HPA-axis activation. *Cytokine, 21,* 248–256.

Delgado, A. V., McManus, A. T., & Chambers, J. P. (2003). Production of tumor necrosis factor-alpha, interleukin 1-beta, interleukin 2, and interleukin 6 by rat leukocyte subpopulations after exposure to Substance P. *Neuropeptides, 37,* 355–361.

Di Lorenzo, G., Balistreri, C. R., Candore, G., Cigna, D., Colombo, A., Romano, G. C., et al. (2000). Granulocyte and natural killer cell activity in the elderly. *Mechanisms of Aging and Disease, 108,* 25–38.

Dimsdale, J. E., Young, D., Moore, R., & Strauss, H. W. (1987). Do plasma norepinephrine levels reflect behavioral stress? *Psychosomatic Medicine, 49,* 375–382.

Elenkov, I. J., & Chrousos, G. P. (2002). Stress hormones, proinflammatory and anti-inflammatory cytokines, and autoimmunity. *Annals of the New York Academy of Sciences, 966,* 290–303.

Entzian, P., Linnemann, K., Schlaak, M., & Zabel, P. (1996). Obstructive sleep apnea syndrome and circadian rhythms of hormones and cytokines. *American Journal of Respiratory and Critical Care Medicine, 153,* 1080–1086.

Ferrari, E., Arcaini, A., Gornati, R., Pelanconi, L., Cravello, L., Fioravanti, M., et al. (2000). Pineal and pituitary-adrenocortical function in physiological aging and in senile dementia. *Experimental Gerontology, 35,* 1239–1250.

Ferrari, E., Casarotti, D., Muzzoni, B., Albertelli, N., Cravello, L., Fioravanti, M., et al. (2001). Age-related changes of the adrenal secretory pattern: Possible role in pathological brain aging. *Brain Research Reviews, 37,* 294–300.

Ferrari, E., Fioravanti, M., Magri, F., & Solerte, S. B. (2000). Variability of interactions between neuroendocrine and immunological functions in physiological aging and dementia of the Alzheimer's type. *Annals of the New York Academy of Sciences, 917,* 582–596.

Glaser, R., & Kiecolt-Glaser, J. K. (2005). Stress-induced immune dysfunction: Implications for health. *Nature Reviews Immunology, 5,* 243–251.

Grinevich, V., Ma, X. M., Herman, J. P., Jezova, D., Akmayev, I., & Aguilera, G. (2001). Effect of repeated lipopolysaccharide administration on tissue cytokine expression and hypothalamic-pituitary-adrenal axis activity in rats. *Journal of Neuroendocrinology, 13,* 711–723.

Grubeck-Loebenstein, B., & Wick, G. (2002). The aging of the immune system. *Advances in Immunology, 80,* 243–284.

Haus, E., Nicolau, G. Y., Lakatua, D., & Sackett-Lundeen, L. (1988). *Chronobiology in laboratory medicine*. Baar, The Netherlands: Baker Publishing.

Ho, M. C., Lo, A. C., Kurihara, H., Yu, A. C., Chung, S. S., & Chung, S. K. (2001). Endothelin-1 protects astrocytes from hypoxic/ischemic injury. *Federation of American Societies for Experimental Biology Journal, 15*, 618–626.

Hohagen, F., Timmer, J., Weyerbrock, A., Fritsch-Montero, R., Ganter, U., Krieger, S., et al. (1993). Cytokine production during sleep and wakefulness and its relationship to cortisol in healthy humans. *Neuropsychobiology, 28*, 9–16.

Holden, M. K. (2005). Virtual environment for motor rehabilitation: Review. *Cyber Psychology and Behavior, 8*, 187–211.

Irwin, M. R., Pike, J. L., Cole, J. C., & Oxman, M. N. (2003). Effects of a behavioral intervention, tai chi chih, on varicella-zoster virus specific immunity and health functioning in older adults. *Psychosomatic Medicine, 65*, 824–830.

Jander, S., Schroeter, M., Peters, O., Witte, O. W., & Stoll, G. (2001). Cortical spreading depression induces proinflammatory cytokine gene expression in the rat brain. *Journal of Cerebral Blood Flow and Metabolism, 21*, 218–225.

Jander, S., Schroeter, M., & Stoll, G. (2002). Interleukin-18 expression after focal ischemia of the rat brain: Association with the late stage inflammatory response. *Journal of Cerebral Blood Flow and Metabolism, 22*, 62–70.

Jarrar, D., Kuebler, J. F., Wang, P., Bland, K. I., & Chaudry, I. H. (2001). DHEA: A novel adjunct for the treatment of male trauma patients. *Trends in Molecular Medicine, 7*, 81–85.

Johnson, S. A., Rozzo, S. J., & Cambier, J. C. (2002). Aging-dependent exclusion of antigen-inexperienced cells from the peripheral B cell repertoire. *Journal of Immunology, 168*, 5014–5023.

Kelley, K. W., Bluthe, R.-M., Dantzer, R., Zhou, J. H., Shen, W.-H., Johnson, R. W., et al. (2003). Cytokine-induced sickness behavior. *Brain, Behavior, and Immunity, 17*(1, Suppl. 1), 112–118.

Kiecolt-Glaser, J. K., & Glaser, R. (1988). Methodological issues in behavioral immunology research with humans. *Brain, Behavior, and Immunity, 2*, 67–78.

Kiecolt-Glaser, J. K., Preacher, K. J., MacCallum, R. C., Atkinson, C., Malarkey, W. B., & Glaser, R. (2003). Chronic stress and age-related increases in the pro-inflammatory cytokine IL-6. *Proceedings of the National Academy of Science, 100*, 9090–9095.

Kovacs, E. J., Plackett, T. P., & Witte, P. L. (2004). Estrogen replacement, aging, and cell-mediated immunity after injury. *Journal of Leukocyte Biology, 76*, 36-41.

Lau, L. T., & Yu, C.-H. (2001). Astrocytes produce and release interleukin-1, interleukin-6, tumor necrosis factor alpha and interferon-gamma following traumatic and metabolic injury. *Journal of Neurotrauma, 18*, 351–359.

Leng, S. X., Yang, H., & Walston, J. D. (2004). Decreased cell proliferation and altered cytokine production in frail older adults. *Aging and Clinical Experimental Research, 16*, 249–252.

Lenzlinger, P.M., Hans, V. H., Joller-Jemelka, H. I., Trentz, O., Morganti-Kossmann, M. C., & Kossman, T. (2001). Markers for cell-mediated immune response are elevated in cerebrospinal fluid and serum after severe traumatic brain injury in humans. *Journal of Neurotrauma, 18*, 479–489.

Lenzlinger, P. M., Morganti-Kossman, M. C., Laurer, H. L., & McIntosh, T. K. (2001). The duality of the inflammatory response to traumatic brain injury. *Molecular Neurobiology*, *24*, 169–181.

Levi, F. A., Canon, C., Touitou, Y., Sulon, J., Mechkouri, M., Demey-Ponsard, R., et al. (1988). Circadian rhythms in circulating T lymphocyte subtypes, and plasma testosterone, total and free cortisol in five healthy men. *Clinical and Experimental Immunology*, *71*, 329–335.

Linton, P. J., Habertson, J., & Bradley, L. M. (2000). A critical role for B cells in the development of memory CD4 cells. *Journal of Immunology*, *165*, 5558–5565.

Lissoni, P., Rovelli, F., Brivio, F., Brivio, O., & Fumagalli, L. (1991). Circadian secretions of IL-2, IL-12, IL-6, and IL-10 in relation to the light/dark rhythm of the pineal hormone melatonin in healthy humans. *Natural Immunity*, *16*, 1–5.

Maier, S. F. (2003). Bi-directional immune-brain communication: Implications for understanding stress, pain, and cognition. *Brain, Behavior, and Immunity*, *17*, 69–85.

Marshall, P. S., O'Hara, C., & Steinberg, P. (2000). Effects of seasonal allergic rhinitis on selected cognitive abilities. *Annals of Allergy Asthma and Immunology*, *84*, 403–410.

Marshall, P. S., O'Hara, C., & Steinberg, P. (2002). Effects of seasonal allergic rhinitis on fatigue levels and mood. *Psychosomatic Medicine*, *64*, 684–691.

Marsland, A. L., Bachen, E. A., Cohen, S., Rabin, B., & Manuck, S. B. (2002). Stress, immune reactivity and susceptibility to infectious disease. *Physiology and Behavior*, *77*, 711–716.

Mastorakos, G., Chrousos, G. P., & Weber, J. S. (1993). Recombinant interleukin-6 activates the hypothalamic-pituitary-adrenal axis in humans. *Journal of Clinical Endocrinology and Metabolism*, *77*, 1690–1694.

Miyaji, C.W.H., Toma, H., Akisaka, M., Tomiyama, K., Sato, Y., & Abo, T. (2000). Functional alteration of granulocytes, NK cells, and natural killer T cells in centenarians. *Human Immunology*, *61*, 908–916.

Mohammed, A. K., Winblad, B., Ebendal, T., & Lärkfors, L. (1990). Environmental influence on behavior and nerve growth factor in the brain. *Brain Research*, *528*, 62–72.

Olson, J. K., & Miller, S. D. (2004). Microglia initiate central nervous system innate and adaptive immune responses through multiple TLRs. *Journal of Immunology*, *173*, 13916–13924.

Palin, K., Pousset, F., Verrier, D., Dantzer, R., Kelley, K., Parnet, P., et al. (2001). Characterization of interleukin-1 receptor antagonist isoform expression in the brain of lipopolysaccharide-treated rats. *Neuroscience*, *103*, 161–169.

Perini, F., Morra, M., Alecci, M., Galloni, E., Marchi, M., & Toso, V. (2001). Temporal profile of serum anti-inflammatory and pro-inflammatory interleukins in acute ischemic stroke patients. *Neurological Sciences*, *22*, 289–296.

Petrovsky, N., McNair, P., & Harrison, L. C. (1998). Diurnal rhythms in pro-inflammatory cytokines: Regulation by plasma cortisol and therapeutic implications. *Cytokine*, *10*, 307–312.

Rabin, B. S. (1999). *Stress, immune function, and health: The connection*. New York: Wiley-Liss.

Renshaw, M., Rockwell, J., Engleman, C., Gewirtz, A., Katz, J., & Sambhara, S. (2002). Cutting edge: Impaired toll-like receptor expression and function in aging. *Journal of Immunology, 169,* 4697–4701.

Rodgers, B., & Anderko, L. (2004). Letters to the editor. *Nursing Outlook, 52,* 164.

Schafer, M. K., Schwaeble, W. J., Post, C., Salvati, O., Calabresi, M., Sim, R. B., et al. (2000). Complement C1q is dramatically up-regulated in brain microglia in response to transient global cerebral ischemia. *Journal of Immunology, 164,* 5446–5452.

Scheibel, R. S., Valentine, A.D., O'Brien, S., & Meyers, C. A. (2004). Cognitive dysfunction and depression during treatment with interferon-alpha and chemotherapy. *Journal of Neuropsychiatry and Clinical Neuroscience, 16,* 185–191.

Schwartz, M. (2003). Macrophages and microglia in central nervous system injury: Are they helpful or harmful? *Journal of Cerebral Blood Flow and Metabolism, 23,* 385–394.

Shaked, I., Porat, Z., Gersner, R., Kipnis, J., & Schwartz, M. (2004). Early activation of microglia as antigen-presenting cells correlates with T cell-mediated protection and repair of the injured central nervous system. *Journal of Neuroimmunology, 146,* 84–93.

Solana, R., & Mariani, E. (2000). NK and NK/T cells in human senescence. *Vaccine, 18,* 1613–1620.

Sothern, R. B., & Roitman-Johnson, B. (2001). *Biological rhythms and immune function* (3rd ed., Vol. 2). New York: Academic Press.

Sparkman, N. L., Kohman, R. A., Garcia, A. K., & Boehm, G. W. (2005). Peripheral lipopolysaccharide administration impairs two-way active avoidance conditioning in C57BL/6J mice. *Physiology & Behavior, 85,* 278–288.

Sparkman, N. L., Martin, L. A., Calvert, W. S., & Boehm, G. W. (2005). Effects of intraperitoneal lipopolysaccharide on Morris water maze performance in year-old and two-month old female C57BL/6J mice. *Behavioral Brain Research, 159,* 145–151.

Steinman, L. (2004). Elaborate interactions between the immune and nervous system. *Nature Immunology, 5,* 575–581.

Tarazona, R., DelaRosa, O., Alonso, C., Ostos, B., Espejo, J., Pena, J., et al. (2000). Increased expression of NK cell markers on T lymphocytes in aging and chronic activation of the immune system reflects the accumulation of effector/senescent T cells. *Mechanisms of Aging and Disease, 121,* 77–88.

Van Beek, J., El Ward, C., & Gasque, P. (2003). Activation of complement in the central nervous system: Roles in neurodegeneration and neuroprotection. *Annals of the New York Academy of Sciences, 992,* 56–71.

Vila, N., Castillo, J., Davalos, A., Esteve, A., Planas, A. M., & Chamorro, A. (2003). Levels of anti-inflammatory cytokines and neurological worsening in acute ischemic stroke. *Stroke, 34,* 671–675.

Vollmer-Conna, U. (2001). Acute sickness behaviour: an immune system-to-brain communication? *Psychosomatic Medicine, 31,* 761–767.

Winter, C. D., Pringle, A. K., Clough, G. F., & Church, M. K. (2004). Raised parenchymal interleukin-6 levels correlate with improved outcome after traumatic brain injury. *Brain, 127,* 315–320.

Yoles, E., Hauben, E., Palgi, O., Agranov, E., Gothilf, A., Cohen, A., et al. (2001). Protective autoimmunity is a physiological response to CNS trauma. *Journal of Neuroscience, 21,* 3740–3748.

Young, M. R., Matthews, J. P., Kanabrocki, E. L., Sothern, R. B., Roitman-Johnson, B., & Scheving, L. E. (1995). Circadian rhythmometry of serum interleukin-2, interleukin-10, tumor necrosis factor- and granulocyte-macrophage colony-stimulating factor in men. *Chronobiology International, 12,* 19–27.

# PART IV

Research in
Reducing Health
Disparities Among
Vulnerable
Populations

# Chapter 9

## HIV Symptoms

Carmen J. Portillo, William L. Holzemer,
and Fang-Yu Chou

### ABSTRACT

*People with HIV/AIDS are a vulnerable group whose symptoms can seriously affect their quality of life. HIV/AIDS symptoms can result from the disease itself, from secondary complications of the disease, or from side-effects of highly active antiretroviral therapy (HAART) and other medications related to comorbidities. HIV symptoms are the single most important indicators for patients and practitioners. Symptoms prompt patients to seek medical attention and provide health care providers with essential clues about changes in health status and quality of life. Despite increased recognition of the importance of addressing symptoms among people with HIV/AIDS, few studies have examined the management of HIV symptoms. This chapter introduces HIV symptoms, reports on the methods of review, provides an overview of contextual issues including the literature on symptoms, issues related to symptom measures, theoretical foundations on symptom management, HIV-specific measures, non-HIV-specific measures, translation of findings into practice, and implications for future research and policy.*

Keywords: HIV/AIDS; HIV/AIDS symptoms; HIV/AIDS
symptom measures

# INTRODUCTION

At the 2005 National HIV Prevention Conference in Atlanta, the Centers for Disease Control and Prevention (CDC) reported an estimated 1.1 million people living in the United States with HIV (Henry J. Kaiser Family Foundation, 2005). This is the highest number of cases ever recorded in the nation, and almost half (47%) are among African Americans. Of these HIV-infected persons, an estimated 25% are unaware of their HIV-positive status. AIDS diagnoses increased 7% between 1998 and 2000 for women, while it decreased 5% for men (CDC, 2002). The overall increase of the prevalence of HIV reflects the growing number of people living longer because of current antiretroviral treatment, but also reflects our failure to develop adequate prevention interventions.

HIV/AIDS, once a fatal disease, has now become a reversible chronic disease, with the possibility of long-term survival for many. People with HIV/AIDS are vulnerable and experience symptoms arising from the disease progression itself, from secondary complications of AIDS, and from side-effects of highly active antiretroviral therapy (HAART) and other medications. While preventing the progression of HIV and minimizing secondary complications continue to be primary goals of care, managing symptoms associated with HIV has emerged as essential for improving quality of life. A person's experience of HIV symptoms can affect health-seeking behaviors, adherence to medications, perception of illness and coping responses, and ultimately health status and quality of life. For health care providers, symptoms serve to define a differential diagnosis as prognostic factors, and as outcome variables to evaluate treatment effectiveness.

Like other chronic diseases, HIV/AIDS affects both the physiological and psychological aspects of health. Physiologically, HIV infection not only allows for opportunistic infections to take hold, but also influences the functions of multiple organ systems. Psychologically, the unpredictable course of sudden exacerbations of illness interspersed with long periods of relative wellness promotes the onset of psychological distress (Holzemer, 1997). People living with HIV/AIDS encounter many physiological, psychological, and cognitive symptoms, such as pain, diarrhea, fever, fatigue, depression, memory loss, and balance and walking problems. These symptoms may significantly restrict a person's quality of life. Managing multiple symptoms and maintaining optimal quality of life have, therefore, become major daily tasks for people living with HIV/AIDS (Bedell, 2000; Hench, Anderson, Grady, & Ropka, 1995; Zeller, Swanson, & Cohen, 1993).

Since the beginning of the epidemic, nurse clinicians and researchers have recognized the importance of assessing and managing HIV/AIDS-related symptoms.

Zeller, Swanson, and Cohen (1993) provided suggestions for advancing research in symptom management. These authors recommended that research studies should focus on five areas: (a) respiratory symptoms, (b) malnutrition and gastro-intestinal symptoms, (c) neurological symptoms, (d) opportunistic and nosocomial infections, and (e) pain.

A number of recent seminal published works have provided needed exper-tise in this area. For example, Ropka and Williams (1998) published a compen-dium entitled "HIV Nursing and Symptom Management."

Clinical practice guideline articles that focus upon the management of specific symptoms also have been developed (Coyne, Lyne, & Watson, 2002). Further, summary articles have provided evidence-based guidelines for symp-tom management (Holzemer, 2002). Most recently, Ferri (2004) clarified the importance of symptom management in the age of antiretroviral therapy. As symptom management or symptom relief has always been a central focus of nursing care, understanding the symptom experience must begin from the client's perspective. This chapter explores the research on HIV symptom measures.

## Methods of Review

The HIV/AIDS symptom literature from the past 20 years is extensive. This review focuses on U.S. literature about HIV/AIDS care symptoms, excluding studies where symptoms were conceptualized solely as side effects of a drug trial or where the discussion of symptoms focused primarily upon palliative, end-of-life care. Because of the vast amount of literature available on individual HIV/AIDS-related symptoms such as fatigue, sleep, and depression, these areas are not covered in this review. Rather, the focus of this literature review is on the HIV/AIDS-related symptoms of HIV/AIDS clients being cared for primarily in outpatient settings.

PubMed and the Cumulative Index to Nursing & Allied Health Literature were searched for databased articles from 1998 to 2005 related to HIV/AIDS symptom assessment, prevalence, correlates, and management. The search was limited to articles concerning adult patients, as well as articles written in Eng-lish. Use of the search term *HIV symptoms* resulted in 9,403 retrievals. Further limits applied to include an abstract resulted in 471 retrievals. Changes to the term to reflect *HIV symptom* resulted in 283 retrievals. Similarly, when the terms *HIV symptom* and *measures* were combined, this resulted in 90 retrievals. The combination of the terms *HIV symptom* and *assessment* resulted in 68 retriev-als. The studies identified in the two searches were compared and contrasted to obtain the final sample of 47 studies reviewed in this chapter.

# OVERVIEW OF CONTEXTUAL ISSUES

## Symptom Literature

People living with HIV/AIDS face multiple problems related to the symptoms that accompany the progression of HIV disease and the current combination therapies. Studies have shown that patients in the stages of symptomatic HIV disease and AIDS can experience on average more than 10 different physical and psychological symptoms concurrently (Mathews et al., 2000; Reilly et al., 1997; Vogl et al., 1999). Although there is a clinically asymptomatic state in the initial HIV infection stage for most patients, the current antiretroviral agents have brought a variety of symptoms that patients may experience due to the adverse effects of medication (Andrews, 1998). Because of the variability in the severity of symptoms and the progression of HIV disease, appropriate symptom assessment is essential in HIV clinical management and research.

Evidence exists to suggest that there is poor agreement on symptom reports between nurses and patients (Reilly et al., 1997), and that medical providers often underestimate and under-treat symptoms (Breitbart, Rosenfeld, et al., 1996; Larue et al., 1994). Evaluation of symptom reports from patients and nurses showed that there was poor agreement between patients' and nurses' ratings of HIV-related signs and symptoms (Reilly et al., 1997). Those symptoms included: shortness of breath with activity, shortness of breath at rest, fatigue, cough, weakness, dry mouth, insomnia, lack of appetite, concern over weight loss, and headaches. Medications for AIDS patients experiencing pain, diarrhea, nausea, and vomiting are often underprescribed; 85% of patients who reported pain were receiving inadequate analgesia (Breitbart, Rosenfeld, et al., 1996).

HIV/AIDS is a disease that disproportionately affects socially marginalized populations (e.g., racial and ethnic minorities, low socioeconomic groups), and the disparities do not stop with HIV/AIDS diagnosis. Some evidence suggests that among HIV-positive populations, those with low socioeconomic status, members of minority populations, and women have poorer quality of life as measured by symptom status. In comparison to other groups, minority populations and women more often report symptoms of depression (Anastos et al., 2005; Hudson, Lee, & Portillo, 2003; Moneyham, Sowell, Seals, & Demi, 2000), which has also been shown to correlate with quality of life and functional status (Hudson, Kirksey, & Holzemer, 2004; Vidrine, Amick, Gritz, & Arduino, 2003) and increased risk of mortality (Cook et al., 2004). The Institute of Medicine Report (IOM) entitled, *Unequal Treatment: Confronting Racial and Ethnic Disparities in Health Care* (IOM, 2003), concluded that there is clear and convincing evidence for racial disparities in health care in the United States (Smedley, Stith, & Nelson, 2003). Some of this disparity may be attributable to communication and patient-provider relationship; in the United States, Whites are half as likely as Latinos and one-third less likely than African Americans to perceive difficulty communicating with their provider (Davis, Schoenbaum, Collins, Tenney, & Hughes, 2002).

It is virtually impossible for anyone to remain 100% adherent to a medical regimen to treat HIV disease, albeit the reasons for non-adherence may not always be completely clear. Symptom prevalence has been related to patients' reported treatment adherence. One study reported HIV patients who had higher symptom scores, especially depression, were less likely to adhere to medications regimens, to follow providers' advice, and to attend their medical appointments (Holzemer, Corless, et al., 1999). This finding is consistent with the results of a meta-analysis of 12 studies conducted with chronically ill patients; indicating that the odds were three times greater for the depressed patients to be non-compliant with medical treatment than were non-depressed patients (DiMatteo, Lepper, & Croghan, 2000).

Research on the relationship of symptoms and physiological parameters warrants further investigation. Although immune status is a known predictor of future disease progression and functional deterioration (Marder et al., 1995), no association has been observed between symptoms and immune status (Vlahov et al., 1994; Vogl et al., 1999). One study, for example, found no difference by CD4 cell count for diarrhea, fatigue, weight loss, shortness of breath, or enlarged posterior cervical lymph nodes (Vlahov et al., 1994), and two other studies found no relationship between depression or psychological distress and immune status (Rabkin, Rabkin, Wagner, 1994; Rabkin, Wagner, & Rabkin, 1994).

## Theoretical Foundations on Symptom Management

Theoretical foundations based on models developed by Wilson and Cleary (1995) and the University of California San Francisco (UCSF) Symptom Management Model (Dodd et al., 2001; Larson et al., 1994) have guided this review. Wilson and Cleary (1995) suggested a model for linking clinical variables to quality of life. The authors posit that there is relatively little empirical research that shows clinicians how to translate quality of life diagnoses into clinical therapies. Further, to more consistently improve patients' quality of life, clinicians need to accurately assess health-related quality of life, and know which clinical parameters are both strongly related to variations in health-related qualify of life. As a first step toward understanding those relations, the authors identify five sets of variables in the model, including physiological and biological factors, symptoms status, functional status, general health perceptions, and overall quality of life. Individual and environmental characteristics are said to comprise clusters of variables that have the potential to impact all five levels. They assert that general health perceptions are the best predictors of use of general medical and mental health services and a strong predictor of mortality. This assertion supports the value of thorough history taking. Finally, there is need to test causal models that explore relationships among different measures of health status in an attempt to bring to light the pathogenesis of disorders of health related quality of life. Until we as nurses and physicians and health care systems, understand more about the determinants of poor health status and mechanisms by which they occurs interventions at multiple points can be made possible, and better management of symptoms realistic.

The UCSF Symptom Management Model is depicted in Figure 9.1 as a dynamic picture of the nature of symptoms and the challenges of understanding the symptom experience, interventions, and outcomes. The model has three interacting circles: (a) symptom experience or the input circle (number of symptoms, symptom intensity, symptom distress, and depressive symptoms); (b) symptom management or the process circle (self-care strategies); and (c) symptom outcomes or the output circle (controlled symptoms, quality-of-life, and adherence). This interdependent process is embedded within three domains of nursing that interact with each other and the input-process-output components. The person system represents all the individual variables that influence symptom management; the environment system represents all the social and cultural variable; and finally, the health and illness system represents the risk factors, such as injury or infection. The model is based on six assumptions: (a) The gold standard is the patient's self-report of symptom experiences; (b) The presence of a symptom is not required for the applicability of the mode; (c) The risk for developing a symptom is a reason for the initiation of interventions before individual symptoms can be experienced; (d) Non-verbal patients experience symptoms, and symptom interpretations by family members and caregivers are assumed to be accurate information for symptom management; (e) Management strategies can be targeted toward the individual, groups, a family, or the work environment; (f) Symptom management is a dynamic process, which is modified by individual outcomes and influences.

The nurse researchers who developed the UCSF Symptom Management Model do not describe a methodical process to test the model. Hence, the model has not been tested, but rather used as a guiding framework in research (Hudson, Lee, & Portillo, 2003; Humphreys, Lee, Neylan, & Marmar, 1999; Miles et al., 2003; Nokes & Kendrew, 2001; Voss, 2005) to better understand symptoms, management strategies and the evaluation of outcomes.

## Critical Issues Related to Symptom Measures

This review of the literature identified several valid and reliable scales available to measure HIV symptoms. When selecting an instrument to measure

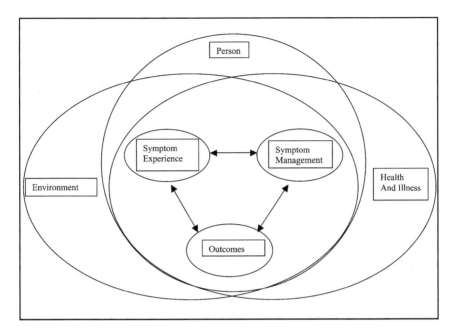

**FIGURE 9.1**    UCSF Symptom Management Model.

symptoms, several issues must be addressed: (a) self-report versus observational assessment of symptoms; (b) response formats; and (c) conceptual and methodological issues.

## Self-Report Versus Observational Assessment of Symptoms

Symptoms are assessed through self-report, provider observation, and caregiver or family observation. There is consensus in the literature that the patient is the gold standard for understanding his or her own symptom experience and this can only be assessed through self-report (Holzemer, 2002; Hughes, 2004; Osoba, 1993; Wu et al., 2004). Rather than thinking about self-reported symptoms as subjective, care providers are advised to listen to self-reports of symptoms as one kind of evidence that documents the patient's current status or severity of illness from their perspective.

There are advantages and disadvantages to both the self-report and observer-rated approaches to reporting symptoms. Self-report of symptoms includes the symptom status from patients' perspectives and avoids of observers' biases. Some patients, however, may overreport their symptoms. Others may be unable to self-report their symptoms because of their psychomotor conditions or severity of illness, or may need assistance self-reporting their symptoms due to low levels of literacy, eyesight problems, or attention deficits. Observer-rated symptom assessment may yield benefits in reducing missing data and non-response rates. Nonetheless, the training and reliability of observers may hinder accuracy in reporting patient symptom status (McCorkle, 1987; Pasacreta, 1997).

Studies comparing patient symptom self-reports and provider symptom assessments have reported incongruence. It has been reported that physicians tend to underestimate symptoms compared to the patient's report (Vogl et al., 1999). A French study of AIDS patients and their physicians concluded that doctors poorly estimate symptom prevalence and under-prescribe symptomatic treatment, especially for pain, diarrhea, nausea, and vomiting (Larue et al., 1994). Studies have also reported that for most symptoms, nurses tend to underestimate symptom distress (Larson, Viele, Coleman, Dibble, & Cebulski, 1993; Tangue, Evers, & Paridaens, 1998), symptom intensity, and symptom frequency relative to patients (Justice et al., 2001; Justice, Rabeneck, Hays, Wu & Bozzette, 1999; Reilly et al., 1997). Camp (1988) also reported that nursing clinical notes lacked documentation of patients' perception of pain.

## Response Formats

HIV symptom assessment instruments can be classified as open-ended or closed-ended. Open-ended questions such as "How would you describe your symptoms?" have no specified response format, and the respondent is free to provide any answer. Open-ended questions are easier to construct and can cause respondents to provide more information in their own words. The major disadvantage to open-ended questions, however, is that the data are often difficult to code and interpret when large samples are involved. Closed-ended questions offer specified responses from which the participants can choose. They are more difficult to construct, but have better uniformity and reliability; they are also easier to code and interpret. Participants' responses, however, are limited to the range of information or scaling assigned by the investigators (Cummings, Strull, Nevitt, & Hulley, 1988; Waltz, Strickland, & Lenz, 1991).

## Conceptual and Methodological Issues

Research on measuring and improving the symptom experience of HIV/AIDS patients faces several conceptual issues. First, it has long been recognized that symptoms can be temporary, vary over time, or be chronically present. This makes symptom control outcome studies a particular challenge. Second, growing evidence supports the fact that symptoms occur in clusters and not as isolated events. As such, intervention studies are challenged to disentangle symptoms that often appear together, such as fatigue and depression (Dodd, Miaskowski, & Lee, 2004; Gift, Stommel, Jablonski, & Given, 2003). Third, there is the assumption that physiological markers or biomarkers correspond with the symptom experience, which is often not the case (Holzemer, 2002). One study found that no statistical relationship between physiological markers and the symptom experience (Cosby, Holzemer, Henry, & Portillo, 2000). Fourth, depending how symptoms are conceptualized, whether as measures of severity of illness, moderators of outcomes such as medication adherence or quality of life, or as outcome, measures need to be clarified at the onset of any study. Finally, the various symptom assessment inventories do not use the same response time frames. For example, the Hopkins Symptom Check List (HSCL) asks people to respond thinking about the past 7 days whereas the Revised Sign and Symptom Check-List for HIV (SSC-HIVrev) asks the person to rate the symptoms they are experiencing today. The kind, type, and severity of symptoms experienced only for 1 day or 1 week has significant implications for developing appropriate intervention strategies.

## Measures of HIV/AIDS Symptoms

The measures of HIV/AIDS-related symptoms that have been assessed in multiple studies can be separated into two groups: (a) scales developed specifically for assessing HIV symptoms; and (b) scales initially developed for other conditions and later applied to HIV. Scales that have been used in only one study are not reviewed here. Table 9.1 presents the instruments, the number of items in each of the instruments, and the primary references for each instrument.

## HIV-SPECIFIC MEASURES

## ACTG-HIV: AIDS Clinical Trials Group HIV Symptom Index

The ACTG HIV Symptom Index is a checklist that measures the intensity and bothersomeness of commonly occurring HIV symptoms (Justice et al., 2001). An earlier version of this instrument included 12 symptoms independently determined to be the most common and bothersome for people with advanced HIV disease. The set of symptoms was used to assess relative frequencies of self-report and provider-report symptoms and the sensitivity and specificity of provider-report for self-report symptoms. Mean values were calculated by summing the

**TABLE 9.1**    Instruments Used in Research to Assess HIV/AIDS-Related Symptoms

| Name of Measure | Number of Items | Primary Reference |
|---|---|---|
| **HIV specific measures** | | |
| ACTG-HIV Symptom Index. AIDS Clinical Trials Group HIV Symptom Index | 20 | Justice et al., 2001; Justice, Rabeneck, Hays, Wu, & Bozzette, 1999 |
| HCSUS Symptom Measure. The HIV Cost and Services Utilization Study | 14 | Mathews et al., 2000 |
| HIV Symptom Index | 12 | Whalen, Antani, Carey, & Landefeld, 1994 |
| MOS-HIV. Medical Outcome Study – HIV (modeled after the MOS-SF36) | 34 | Wu, Hays, Kelly, Malitz, & Bozzette, 1997; Wu, Revicki, Jacobson, & Malitz, 1997 |
| SSC-HIVrev. Revised Sign and Symptom Check-List for HIV | 72 | Holzemer, Hudson, Kirksey, Hamilton, & Bakken, 2001 |
| **Non-HIV specific measures** | | |
| HSCL. Hopkins Symptom Check List | 58 | Derogatis, Lipman, Rickels, Uhlenhuth, & Covi, 1974a |
| SCL-90-R. Symptom Checklist-90 Revised | 90 | Derogatis, 1983 |
| BSI. Brief Symptom Inventory | 53 | Derogatis, 1993 |
| MSAS-SF. Memorial Symptom Assessment Scale – Short Form | 32 | Portenoy, et al., 1994; Chang, Hwang, Feuerman, Kasimis, & Thaler, 2000 |

symptom scores and dividing by 12. The mean for self-report was 5.2, whereas a mean of 1.3 symptoms was reported using provider-report ($p < .0001$). These same symptoms were also used to test inter site variation and test-retest reliability (8 weeks interval).

The more current version includes 20 symptoms developed from input from the Outcomes Committee of the AACTG, based upon prior studies of HIV symptoms and expert opinion. The first validation was conducted with 73 HIV-positive volunteers from 7 Adult AIDS Clinical Trial Group sites (Justice et al., 2001) (see Table 9.2). Participants were asked to remember their symptoms over the previous 4 weeks, along with additional questions regarding the comprehensiveness and comprehensibility of the instrument. Participants reported that the index required less than 5 minutes to complete, and felt that it was understandable and covered most of the common and bothersome symptoms associated with HIV infection. The second validation process focused on conducting a cross-sectional construct validity. This validation process used a consecutive sample of 113 HIV patients from one site. In addition to patients completing the symptom index, they also completed an HIV-specific measure of health-related to quality of life (MOS-HIV). The sample was predominantly male (95%), non-White (62%), with a mean age of 44. When symptom counts were compared with counts restricted to bothersome symptoms, the two were strongly correlated (p = .85). The median number of symptoms was 15. The most common symptoms were fatigue (81%), diarrhea (77%), anxiety (77%), sadness (76%), and difficulty sleeping (76%). Fatigue was also the most common bothersome symptom (77%). Anxiety, sadness, and difficulty sleeping were the next most common bothersome symptoms (respectively 68, 67, and 66%). The subscores on mental health and physical health were consistently associated with both symptom frequency and bother. This instrument is unique in that it includes the concept of bothersomeness. Participants are asked, "How much you have been bothered by each symptom?" Bothersomeness is measured on a 4-point Likert scale from "it doesn't bother me" to "it bothers me a lot." The authors note that they were unable to make a conclusive statement about the reliability of the instrument, although symptoms reported by patients or their providers are associated with functional status, global quality of life, and survival (Justice et al., 1999). The ACTG-HIV is a convenient self-report scale that has demonstrated construct validity and offers a simple approach to measuring HIV symptoms.

## HCSUS Symptom Scale: The HIV Cost and Services Utilization Study

The HIV Cost and Services Utilization Study (HCSUS) symptom scale assesses the presence and bothersomeness of 14 symptoms experienced during the preceding six months (Mathews et al., 2000). The instrument was tested with a national probability sample of 4,042 people from the HCSUS study cohort (see Table 9.2). Participants in this study were predominantly White men, who were receiving care from providers. The authors report adequate reliability with a coefficient of reliability for the 14-item scale of 0.75. Support for construct validity was demonstrated when compared with other measures of disease severity, such as CD4 lymphocyte count, year of HIV diagnosis, and disability status. After adjustment for CD4 count, both symptom number and bothersomeness varied significantly ($P < 0.05$) by teaching status of care setting, exposure/risk group,

**TABLE 9.2** Selected Research Articles Reviewed on HIV-Related Measures

| Measure | Author(s) | Method | Selected Findings |
|---|---|---|---|
| MOS-HIV | Bozzette, S . A., Kanouse, D. E., Berry, S., Duan, N. (1995) | *Design:* Randomized controlled trial. *Sample:* Open-label clinical trial of 843 HIV-infected patients. | Captured decline in health before end-points reached in standard time-to-event analyses. Effect sizes were substantially larger than those for conventional endpoints, and are evident for disability indicators. |
| SSC-HIVrev | Corless, I. B., Bakken, S., Nicholas, P. K., Holzemer, W. L., McGibbon, C. A., Inouye, J., Nokes, K. M., Turner, J. G., Powell-Cope, G. M., Brown, M. A., & Portillo, C. J. (2000) | *Design:* Descriptive, correlational *Sample:* 728 HIV/AIDS patients receiving care from seven clinical sites in the United States; predominantly White males. | Using hierarchical multiple regression analysis, symptom status explained the largest amount of variance in cognitive functioning. |
| SSC-HIVrev | Holzemer, W. L., Hudson, A., Kirksey, K. M., Hamilton, J. J., & Bakken, S. (2001) | *Design:* Methodological. *Sample:* 372 adults from an HIV/AIDS outpatient clinic in Harris County, TX; 118 women and 250 men; 271 African Americans. | Three parts resulted: Part 1 consists of 45 items that clustered into 11 factors, with reliability estimates ranging from 0.76 to 0.91; Part 2 consists of 19 HIV-related symptoms that did not cluster into factor scores but are interesting from a clinical point; and Part 3 consists of 8 items related to gynecological symptoms. |

| | | | |
|---|---|---|---|
| ACTG-HIV Symptom Index | Justice, A. C., Holmes, W., Gifford, A. L., Rabeneck, L., Zackin, R., Sinclair, G., Weissman, S., Neidig, J., Marcus, C., Chesney, M., Cohn, S. E., & Wu, A. W. (2001) | *Design:* Multistage quantitative review of existing literature, qualitative and quantitative analyses of pilot data, and quantitative analyses of a prospective sample. *Sample:* 73 adults from a multisite convenience sample within the AIDS Clinical Trials Group; and 115 patients from a prospective sample from the Cleveland Veterans Affairs Medical Center, who were predominantly male (95%) and non-White (62%). | Two levels of validation were conducted. First validation process of the 18-item index required less than 5 minutes to complete for a convenience sample, and was deemed comprehensive and comprehensible. The second construct validation process with 20 items using a cross-sectional prospective sample demonstrated strong associations with physical and mental health summary scores with disease severity. |
| HCSUS Symptom | Mathews, W. C., McCutchan, J. A., Asch, S., Turner, B. J., Gifford, A. L., Kuromiya, K., Brown, J., Shapiro, M. F., Bozzette, S. A. (2000) | *Design:* Multistage national probability sample (N = 4,042) to select study cohort. *Sample:* 76% of 4,042 baseline interviews from patients, predominantly White men, who were receiving care from 145 providers in 28 metropolitan areas and 51 providers in 25 rural areas. | Prevalence of symptoms was substantial for most of the categories. Aggregate measures of symptom number and bothersomeness had adequate internal consistency (0.75) and construct validity (compared with CD4 lymphocyte count, year of HIV diagnosis, and disability status). Cronbach's alpha for the bothersomeness index was 0.80. Symptoms were greater in women, injection drug users, and people with lower educational levels, lower income, and enrolled in Medicare or who were followed up at teaching hospitals; 51.1% of sample reported fever/night sweats as the most prevalent symptom. |

*(Continued)*

**TABLE 9.2** Selected Research Articles Reviewed on HIV-Related Measures (*Continued*)

| Measure | Author(s) | Method | Selected Findings |
|---------|-----------|--------|-------------------|
| BSI: Depression Subscale | Moneyham, L., Sowell, R., Seals, B., & Demi, A. (2000) | *Design:* Secondary analysis *Sample:* 152 women, primarily single, African American. | Coefficient alpha was reported as 0.85. Mean depressive symptoms score for subsample of African Americans was considerably higher than published means for normative samples. |
| SCL-90-R | Pergami, A., Gala, C., Burgess, A., Durbano, F., Zanello, D., Riccio, M., Invernizzi, G., & Catalan, J. (1993) | *Design:* Cross-sectional controlled *Sample:* 80 women; 57 were HIV seropositive and 23 were HIV seronegative from an outpatient clinic in Milan, Italy. | Significant differences between HIV + and HIV- women on 6 subscales (global severity index, hostility, paranoid ideation, interpersonal sensitivity, depression, and anxiety). HIV- women were predominantly injection drug users; therefore, may perceive themselves at risk for HIV, in turn affecting their psychological status. |
| SSC-HIV | Reilly, C., Holzemer, W. L., Henry, S. B., Slaughter, R. E., & Portillo, C. J. (1997) | Design: Repeated measures Sample: 207 patients; 103 nurses. | Ten symptoms were reported by 50% or more of the patients; mean patient intensity ratings for all signs and symptoms, except anxiety, were higher for patients than nurses. |
| ACTG Symptom Distress; MOS-HIV | Reynolds, N. R., Testa, M. A., Marc, L. G., Chesney, M. A., Neidig, J. L., Smith, S. R., Vella, S. & Robbins, G. K. (2004) | Design: Cross-sectional. Sample: 980 participants from ACTG 384; primarily men; ethnically diverse, with 47% While, 35% Black, and 17% Hispanic. | Personal and situational factors, such as depressive symptoms, perceived stress, and lower education, were associated with less certainty about one's perceived ability to adhere to therapy. |

| | | |
|---|---|---|
| MSAS-SF | Vogl, D., Rosenfeld, B., Breitbart, W., Thaler, H., Passik, S., McDonald, M. & Portenoy, R. K. (1999) | Design: Cross-sectional survey. Sample: 504 ambulatory patients; African Americans, Whites, Hispanics from three New York hospitals. Measure: MSAS-SF | Most prevalent symptoms were worrying, fatigue, sadness, and pain. The number of symptoms and symptom distress were highly associated with psychological distress and poorer quality of life. |
| HIV Symptom Index | Whalen, C. C., Antani, M., Carey, J. & Landefeld, C. S. (1994) | Design: Prospective, cohort. Sample: 148 randomly selected HIV-infected outpatients from a university hospital in northeast Ohio; 89% were male; 65% White or Hispanic; 35% Black. | Scores were higher in patients with more advanced disease and in patients who were functionally impaired. The Index was responsive to changes in health as the disease progressed. |

273

educational achievement, sex, annual income, employment, and insurance category. However, the magnitude was quite small. Symptoms were greatest in women and injection drug users, as well as in persons with lower educational levels, lower income, and Medicare enrollment or those who were followed up at teaching hospitals.

## HIV Symptom Index

The Whalen HIV Symptom Index assesses the frequency of 12 common HIV symptoms (Whalen, Antani, Carey, & Landefeld, 1994). This measure was tested on 148 randomly selected outpatients (predominantly homosexual men) from one HIV community specialty clinic. The HIV Symptom Index Scale sums the frequency ratings for 12 symptoms resulting in a range of scores from 0 to 31. The test-retest reliability was high (intraclass correlation coefficient = 0.92), as was the internal consistency (Cronbach's alpha = 0.79). Content and construct validity were established, as well as the stability and responsiveness of the instrument. The HIV Symptom Index has been used as a guideline to develop other HIV symptom indices (Gifford et al., 2000; Mathews et al., 2000) and as an index for testing validity of quality of life instruments (Revicki, Sorensen, & Wu, 1998; Smith, Avis, Mayer, & Swislow, 1997).

## MOS-HIV: Medical Outcomes Study–HIV

Wu, Hays, Kelly, Malitz, and Bozzette (1997) report on the modification of the Medical Outcomes Study-Short Form 36 (MOS-SF36) to create the MOS-HIV for people living with HIV/AIDS. It is a 30-item instrument that measures 10 of the factors from the MOS-SF36, including physical functioning, role function, disability days, pain, social functioning, emotional well-being, energy/fatigue, general health, overall quality of life, and overall health. Each scale has a different number of items and is converted to a 0–100 score, where 100 is the most positive response. The MOS-HIV has been used extensively in HIV clinical trials and observational studies (Bozzette, Kanouse, Berry, & Duan, 1995; Carretero, Burgess, Soler, Soler, & Catalan, 1996; Revicki, Wu, & Murray, 1995; Wu, Revicki, Jacobson, Malitz, 1997). The MOS-HIV serves as a measure of quality of life and includes various symptoms as part of its conceptualization of quality of life. Demonstrated measures of internal consistency with a Cronbach's alpha have been consistently above 0.75. Bozzette and colleagues (1995) conducted a study using the MOS-HIV with a sample of 624 individuals with HIV/AIDS who were predominantly White males with approximately 28% diagnosed with AIDS. The MOS-HIV measure was sensitive in functional measures, such as physical functioning, energy/fatigue, mental well-being, social functioning, and others (see Table 9.2). The scale scores for the MOS-HIV have been shown to correlate with health care utilization and with clinical and physiological status in AIDS (Bozzette et al., 1995). Construct validity has been demonstrated using multi method multi trait analyses.

## SSC-HIVrev: The Revised Sign and Symptom Checklist for HIV

The Sign and Symptom Checklist for Persons with HIV Disease (SSC-HIV) was initially developed as a 41-item instrument to capture the intensity and frequency of commonly reported signs and symptoms experienced by HIV/AIDS patients (Holzemer, Henry, et al., 1999). The checklist covers a variety of physical and psychological symptoms, such as diarrhea, lack of appetite, fatigue, or depression. The 41 items were selected based on HIV/AIDS literature and nursing care plans. Signs or symptoms are rated on a 3-point severity scale. After the scale was submitted to a principal components factor analysis with a Varimax rotation, a new version with a 26-item checklist in six symptom clusters (factors) was proposed. Internal consistency, construct validity, and concurrent validity were established from two HIV/AIDS study samples. The checklist's sensitivity to change over time was also supported (Holzemer, Henry, et al., 1999).

The SSC-HIV was later utilized to compare the symptom ratings reported by HIV-positive patients and nurses. Content validity was supported by the patient sample in this study (Reilly, Holzemer, Henry, Slaughter, & Portillo, 1997). Selected symptoms of this checklist were used as predictors of HIV patients' medication adherence in which satisfactory reliabilities (.79–.90) were reported (Holzemer, Corless, et al., 1999). In addition, the checklist was applied to compare the symptom status of people living with HIV/AIDS who were younger than age 50 with people living with HIV/AIDS who are older than age 50 (Nokes et al., 2000). The checklist was also used to find the average number of symptoms reported in African Americans living with HIV disease (Coleman & Holzemer, 1999). Seven symptoms were selected to predict HIV patients' cognitive functioning in a study conducted by Corless et al. (2000) (see Table 9.2).

More recently, the SSC-HIV was further revised and validated in a sample of HIV-positive persons (Holzemer, Hudson, Kirksey, Hamilton, & Bakken, 2001). The revised scale (SSC-HIVrev) includes items to measure gynecological symptoms and the impact of lipodystrophy (body fat redistribution) due to anti-retroviral therapy on patient's symptom experience. A principal component factor analysis with Varimax rotation determined an 11-factor solution that explained 73.3% of the variance (see Table 9.2). The SSC-HIVrev has three parts. Part I consists of 45 items and 11 factor scores, along with a total score, with reliability estimates ranging from 0.76–0.91. Part II consists of 19 HIV-related symptoms that do not cluster into factor scores but may be of interest from a clinical perspective. Part III consists of eight items related to gynecological symptoms for women. Of the measures described herein, the SSC-HIVrev is the only measure that includes specific gynecological symptoms for women.

In summary, the five measures are related to HIV and used in HIV studies, but clearly the MOS-HIV may be more of an exception than the other four measures. Whereas the purpose of the ACTG, HCSUS, HIV Symptom Index and SSC-HIVrev is to measure symptoms, the purpose of the MOS-HIV is to summarize the effect of an individual's health on the quality of their existence from the individual's perspective. In contrast, the other four measures identify and to some extent, describe specific symptoms that may reflect underlying clinical phenomenon for the purposes of targeted intervention.

## NON-HIV-SPECIFIC MEASURES

### HSCL: Hopkins Symptom Checklist

HSCL is a 58-item self-report instrument that consists of five primary symptom constructs. It was first utilized as a criterion measure in psychotropic drug trials (Derogatis, 1983; Derogatis et al., 1974b). It was then revised to reflect the psychological symptom patterns of medical patients, psychiatric patients, and community respondents (The Symptom Checklist-90-Revised [SCL-90-R]). The Brief Symptom Inventory (BSI) was later designed as a short version of SCL-90-R (Derogatis & Melisaratos, 1983). It is comprised of 53 items with the same nine subscales found in SCL-90-R. The reliability and validity of the HSCL, SCL-90-R, and BSI have been well documented in several clinical populations. Reliability was established by measuring internal consistency using Cronbach alpha coefficient and test-retest measures of 1–2 week intervals. The Cronbach alpha coefficients for the HSCL subscales ranged from 0.84 to 0.87 (Derogatis et al., 1974a; Derogatis et al., 1974b); SCL-90 ranged from 0.77 to 0.90 (Derogatis, 1977; Derogatis, Rickels, & Rock, 1976); and BSI subscales ranged from 0.71 to 0.85 (Derogatis & Melisaratos, 1983). The test-retest correlation coefficients for HSCL subscales ranged from 0.75 to 0.84 with 1-week interval (Derogatis, 1974b); SCL-90 subscales ranged from 0.75 to 0.84 with no interval reported (Derogatis, 1977; Derogatis, Rickels, & Rock, 1976); and BSI subscales ranged from 0.68 to 0.90 with a 2-week interval (Derogatis & Melisaratos, 1983). Validity evidence for these measures included convergent and discriminant validity; convergent validity was established for the SCL-90 by using the MMPI clinical scales and Tryon cluster scales with correlations ranging from 0.57 to 0.75; excellent convergent scores (coefficients > 0.30) between the BSI and clinical scales of the MMPI, Wiggins Content Scales of the MMPI, and the Tryon Cluster Scores (Derogatis & Melisaratos, 1983).

All three checklists have been applied in assessing HIV/AIDS patients' psychological distress. The HSCL was used in the Multicenter AIDS Cohort Study to evaluate depression and psychological functioning in a cohort of gay men who were predominantly White, well-educated, and fairly affluent. The Cronbach alpha coefficient for the HSCL subscales ranged from 0.79 to 0.91 (Joseph et al., 1990). Mean scores for the HSCL depression and anxiety suggested that the levels were higher than in the general population, but lower than those observed in psychiatric outpatients. The depression and anxiety mean scores of HIV-positive gay men were consistently higher than those found in general population surveys but lower than those observed in psychiatric outpatients. The depression subscale was also found to correlate consistently with the Center for Epidemiologic Studies–Depression (CES-D) scale over time (Joseph et al., 1990). The Multicenter AIDS Cohort and the Coping and Change Study also utilized the HSCL. The Cronbach alpha coefficient for the HSCL subscales ranged from 0.83 to 0.91 (Lackner, Joseph, Ostrow, & Eshleman, 1993). The HSCL detected higher level of general distress in HIV seropositive men who reported low levels of subjective social support. The SCL-90-R was applied in HIV studies related to women (Peragallo, 1996; Pergami et al., 1993), and male injecting drug users (Davis et al., 1995). No particular validity or reliability testing was performed in these HIV patient groups. The study results showed, however, that SCL-90-R is able to detect the changes in psychological symptomatology among HIV-positive and HIV-negative groups in women (Pergami et al., 1993) (see Table 9.2) and in male injection drug users over time (Davis et al., 1995).

## BSI: Brief Symptom Index

The BSI is a shorter version of the SCL-90-R, with nine psychological symptom categories. Items on the BSI are rated on a 5-point Likert scale from 0 (not at all) to 4 (extremely) for a time frame covers the "past week and today" (Derogatis, 1993).

Several studies were found using the BSI. Among HIV-related participants, the BSI has been used to evaluate outcomes of treatments and interventions, such as depressive drug trials (Rabkin, Rabkin, & Wagner, 1994; Rabkin, Wagner, & Rabkin, 1994), chemotherapy (Remick et al., 1993), acupuncture therapy (Beal & Nield-Anderson, 2000), and exercise and testosterone treatment (Wagner, Rabkin, & Rabkin, 1998). The BSI scores were also used to evaluate the change in level of psychological distress over time (Rabkin, Ferrando, Jacobsberg, & Fishman, 1997), and to determine participants associated with psychopathology (Perry et al., 1990; Perry et al., 1993). Among the BSI dimensions, it was found that females have higher scores than males on every dimension (Kennedy, Skurnick, Foley, & Louria, 1995), and HIV patients who had more pain complaints had significantly higher mean BSI depression scores (Singer et al., 1993). High internal consistency reliability was reported in the whole scale in HIV-related patients and caregivers; the overall alpha for the 53-item scales was 0.97 (McShane, Bumbalo, & Patsdaughter, 1994). In a secondary analysis of data collected from HIV-positive African American women, the BSI-depression scale had a reported internal consistency of 0.85 (Moneyham et al., 2000) (see Table 9.2). Higher levels of depressive symptoms were associated with lower levels of self-esteem, family cohesion, and quality of life, and higher levels of HIV symptoms. Differences in depressive symptoms according to different levels of demographic variables were assessed using analysis of variance.

## Memorial Symptom Assessment Scale-Short Form (MSAS-SF)

The Memorial Symptom Assessment Scale (MSAS) is a multidimensional symptom assessment checklist that evaluates patient-rated severity, frequency, and distress related to 32 physical and psychological symptoms (Portenoy, Thaler, Kornblith, Lepore, Friedlander-Klar, Coyle, et al., 1994; Portenoy, Thaler, Kornblith, Lepore, Friedlander-Klar, Kiyasu et al., 1994). The short form (MSAS-SF) assesses only the frequency of these 32 symptoms (Chang, Hwang, Feuerman, Kasimis, & Thaler, 2000). Validity and reliability of both forms have been reported in cancer populations of males and females; no ethnic background identifiers were noted. A factor analysis of the MSAS yielded two factors that distinguished three major symptom groups and several subgroups. The major groups were comprised of psychological symptoms, high prevalence physical symptoms, and low prevalence physical symptoms. The Cronbach alpha coefficient ranged from 0.58 (low prevalence physical symptoms) to 0.88 (high prevalence physical symptoms). Convergent and discriminant validity of the MSAS was demonstrated by correlating its various potential subscale scores with the scores on the validation measures (Revised Rand Mental Health Inventory, Symptom Distress Scale, Functional Living Index-Cancer, Karnofsky Performance Status Scale, and Mood Visual Analogue Scale). The analyses resulted with highly significant associations between the MSAS or MSAS subscales and the validation measures. The strongest association was between the MSAS and Functional Living Index-Cancer (–0.78) (Portenoy, Thaler, Kornblith, Lepore, Friedlander-Klar, Kiyasu et al., 1994).

The MSAS-SF also performed well in a population of cancer patients at the Veterans Administration Hospital. Participants in this study completed the MSAS-SF and Functional Assessment Cancer Therapy (FACT-G). Summary scores for the MSAS-SF and FACT-G were significant for inpatients who had higher symptom distress scores on the subscale of the MSAS-SF: physical distress

(P < .02); global distress index (P < .03); total symptom distress (P < .02); and number of symptoms (P < .046). The mean number of symptoms reported by all of the patients was 10.5 (SD = 5.7; range 0–26), and the most reported symptoms included pain (72%), lack of energy (70%), and dry mouth (55%). The Cronbach alpha coefficient ranged from 0.76 to 0.87. The MSAS-SF subscales showed convergent validity with FACT subscales. Correlation coefficients were –0.74 (P < .001) for the physical and FACT-G physical well-being subscales, and –0.68 (P < .001) for the psychological and FACT emotional well-being subscales, and –0.70 (P < .001) for global distress index and FACT summary of quality of life subscales. The MSAS-SF subscales demonstrated convergent validity with performance status, inpatient status, and extent of disease. The test-retest correlation coefficients for the MSAS-SF subscales ranged from 0.86 to 0.94 at 1 day and from 0.40 to 0.84 at 1 week. In addition to information about symptom prevalence and characteristics, both versions generate a global symptom distress index and two subscales that characterize physical symptom distress and psychological distress. MSAS-SF was used to characterize symptom prevalence and distress of AIDS patients at outpatient settings (Vogl et al., 1999); the number of symptoms experienced by AIDS patients (Breitbart, Passik et al., 1998); level of physical symptom distress of AIDS patients (Breitbart, McDonald et al., 1996); and absence or presence of fatigue in AIDS patients (Breitbart, McDonald, Rosenfeld, Monkman, & Passik, 1998). Adequate internal consistency reliability was reported in Vogl et al.'s study (1999). Worrying was the most prevalent symptom in AIDS patients, but difficulty sleeping was rated as most distressful (Vogl et al., 1999). The reviewed articles that utilized the above instruments are listed in Table 9.2 by author(s), method, and results.

In summary, the five HIV specific measures are relatively new indices that have great potential on advancing the science on HIV symptoms. In general, the instruments have been deemed comprehensive and comprehensible, and can be self-administered except for the HIV Symptom Index. Reliability and validity levels have been demonstrated in most, but their responsiveness to changes in clinical status with longitudinal data has yet to be documented.

Four out of the five measures are brief, while the SSC-HIVrev is the most substantially complete with 72 items, and 8 of those symptoms are specifically related to women's gynecological problems. This is a unique feature of the SSC-HIVrev. The time frame for reporting the symptoms is not consistent across the HIV specific measures. The ACTG asks about symptoms in the past 4 weeks; HCSUS asks about symptoms during the preceding 6 months; and the SSC-HIVrev asks about symptoms the patient is experiencing on the day they are filling out the survey. The HIV Symptom Index and the MOS-HIV were the two surveys that ask about symptoms from the previous 2 weeks.

The four non-HIV specific measures are much more developed as far as their psychometric properties. Over the years there has been a growing appreciation of the complex ways in which the HIV/AIDS epidemic has influenced the lives of those affected; these effects include quality of life, psychological well-being, mood states, or social functioning;. In assessing the consequences of the HIV disease, it has been important to not just focus on the specific effects of HIV and AIDS, but on the overall impact of the multiple and complex changes created by the epidemic.

Overall, the review revealed several gaps and limitations within this body of research that was not exclusively within nursing. Included among them were gaps in definitions of what constitutes an HIV symptom; the measurement of frequency, bothersomeness, or intensity of HIV symptoms; the lack of measuring HIV symptoms in ethnic and racial communities; information on women living with HIV/AIDs; and limitations relative to research design, sampling, and instrumentation. In addition, the paucity of studies reported in the nursing literature was somewhat surprising, especially in light of the fact that both the National Institute of Nursing Research and National Institutes of Health state that the goal of symptom management is critical to nursing. Of the sample of 47 studies included in this review, only 10 were conducted by nurse researchers. One might expect that the literature base would have been more robust, but the opposite was true. It only revealed the work that needs to be accomplished.

A commonly reported outcome in these studies was the influence of symptoms on quality of life. In one study of a sample of 118 women, symptom intensity, as measured by the SSC-HIVrev, was significantly related to role and physical functioning among the women as measured by the MOS-SF36. Zingmond et al. (2003) demonstrated differences in the symptom experience, as measured by HCSUS, between younger and older HIV patients. Older non-Whites were less likely to report experiencing symptoms than younger Whites. Hudson, Lee, and Portillo (2003) demonstrated a link between depressive symptoms, as measured by the CES-D and functional status in a sample of 104 HIV-positive women. Burgoyne, Rourke, Behrens, and Salit (2004) studied changes in virological markers, quality of life, and symptom profiles over time and reported that quality of life was less sensitive to immunological or virological changes compared to responsiveness to symptoms. Cook et al. (2004) demonstrated in a sample of 1,716 HIV-positive women that, after controlling for medications and other variables, depressive symptoms correlated with increased risk of mortality. These studies continue to document the importance of the relationship between symptoms and quality of life for people living with HIV disease.

The association between symptoms and psychological distress was also noted in the reported studies. The result of a patient experiencing symptoms and also being psychologically distressed may cause the patients to delay or reduce appropriate treatment. Patients' interpretations of the absence and presence of HIV-related physical symptoms were found to influence their intentions to seek medical care (Siegel, Schrimshaw, & Dean, 1999). Symptom prevalence has also been related to patients' reported treatment adherence. In a regression analysis (n = 420), HIV-positive patients who had higher symptom scores, especially depression, were less likely to adhere to medication regimens, to follow providers' advice, and to attend their medical appointments (Holzemer, Corless et al., 1999). This finding is consistent with the results of one meta-analysis of 12 studies in chronically ill patients, which indicated that the odds were three times greater for the depressed patients to be noncompliant with medical treatment than the patients who were not depressed (DiMatteo et al., 2000).

Another important concept related to symptoms is adherence. Understanding the factors related to adherence in highly active antiretroviral therapy (HAART) is critical to the completion of this treatment regimen. Symptoms are beginning to be investigated as the factors that influence adherence to HAART. Spire et al. (2000) examined the effect of the number of symptoms on HIV-infected patients' adherence (n = 336). The findings from the logistic regression analysis indicated that people who reported more than four symptoms in the first month after HAART initiation were more likely to be nonadherent at the fourth month after the treatment started. Holzemer, Henry, Portillo, and Miramontes (2000) reported on a pilot study of a tailored nurse intervention designed to enhance adherence to medications. One component of the intervention is to assess symptoms related to side effects of medication and to provide assistance in finding strategies to alleviate those side effect symptoms.

## TRANSLATING FINDINGS INTO PRACTICE

Evidence-based practice guidelines are increasingly used by health care professionals to guide patient care and affect positive patient outcomes. The practice of evidence-based care means integrating individual clinical expertise with the best available external clinical evidence from systematic research (Sackett, Richardson, Rosenberg, & Haynes, 1998). Evidence is considered to be clinically meaningful and trustworthy, or in other words, evidence is information that is relevant to the treatment-related issue at hand. There are three types of sources to form evidence-based guidelines: clinical expertise or clinician experience, patient preferences, and scientific findings. The sources below are in the form of all three; however none of the guidelines have been explored for their effectiveness in assisting either providers or patients in managing HIV symptoms.

Selected guidelines or manuals available for health care providers and persons living with HIV/AIDS to assist them in managing their symptoms include: (a) *Symptom Management Strategies: A Manual for People Living With HIV/AIDS* (2004), available in several languages at http://www.ucsf.edu/aidsnursing; (b) *HIV Symptom Management* (Association of Nurses in AIDS Care, 2004), available for purchase at https://secure.ar51.net/anacnet/

orderform.htm; (c) *HIV Patient Manual Symptom Management* (Davis, 2000), available at http://www.vh.org/adult/patient/internalmedicine/hivmanual/08symptommanagement.html; (d) *HIV Nursing Secrets* (Shaw & Mahoney, 2002), available only in print form; (e) *Symptom Management Guidelines* (Capaldini, 2004) HIV Insite, available at http://hivinsite.ucsf.edu; and (f) *The Guide to Living With HIV Infection* (Barlett & Finkbeiner, 2001), written by the Director of Infectious Disease Division at Johns Hopkins Hospital is available only in print form.

## IMPLICATIONS FOR FUTURE RESEARCH AND POLICY

### Research Implications

This review provided an opportunity to analyze and critique key HIV symptom research with regard to assessing patient symptomatology. Symptoms are the major reason for patients to seek out health care. Nurses and health care providers have the difficult and ongoing challenge of addressing the complicated nature of patients' symptoms. Focusing on patients' reports about their symptoms provides a theoretical advantage in that it can guide the process of care by identifying symptoms that are particularly burdensome for a given patient. It also directs the attention to aspects of the disease and care that are most salient to the patient. When treatment is not curative, capturing symptoms that impacts the patient's daily life is crucial to the patient's needs. Relieving symptoms can affect simple functional outcomes, complements knowledge on the relative physiological and clinical effects of drugs, and can potentially affect the disease process.

While the HIV symptom literature suggests that patients' reports about symptoms are reliable and a better predictor of outcomes than reports from a nurse or physician, a so-called double-edge syndrome exists. Self-report of symptoms includes the perception of the symptom status from patients' perspectives and avoids observers' biases. Some patients, however, may overreport their symptoms, or highlight some symptoms and not others. On the other hand, there are other patients that may not be able to self-report symptoms or may need assistance self-reporting their symptoms, due to low levels of literacy, eyesight problems, attention deficits, or cultural customs related to reporting symptoms. As symptom research continues to progress in the United States, patient self-report of symptoms will take on a different meaning as research is conducted in international settings.

A significant proportion of the studies included in the review involved racially and ethnically defined minority populations as participants. However, data analyses revealed that there was not reasonable representation of all the major racially and ethnically defined minority population groups. Moreover, none of the studies reported or compared the study findings within and between the ethnic and racial groups. A number of the studies reported on subpopulations who may be somewhat more symptomatic even after adjustment for degree of immunosuppression: women, patients care for at teaching hospitals, those with low income and lower educational levels, those who acquired HIV through injection drug use. However, to demonstrate the clinical importance of the relatively small observed differences in symptom scores among these groups, prospective comparisons to changes in accepted indicators of health status will be required.

There is reason to believe that symptoms may not act congruently. Some symptoms may be more pronounced among healthy patients because the symptoms are associated with effective antiviral therapy or because healthier patients may be more bothered by or sensitive to the symptom (e.g., gas and bloating). Still other symptoms may be more associated with greater disease severity (e.g., wasting, hand or foot pain) or with psychiatric comorbidity (e.g., sadness). Further, these associations may vary, depending upon the population under study.

Another implication for future research is the issue of understanding the synergistic effect of symptoms that constitute symptom clustering. None of the studies reviewed in this chapter examined symptom clustering. Further symptom research could explore the following questions: What are the possible symptom clusters in our ongoing scientific work? What is the relationship between the symptoms? and, What happens when one symptom is more severe than the other(s)?

The ultimate goal of assessing and managing symptoms is to improve quality of life for people living with HIV/AIDS. Research on symptom assessment requires greater emphasis on intervention models that use a standardized symptom assessment among all levels of providers in which a symptom-based guideline is tested to determine its effects on quality of life. Likewise, nursing research can make a contribution to the understanding of the relationship between symptom experience, symptom management strategies, and symptom outcomes. Further development and use of symptom-based guidelines and quality measures, which are not well captured by more conventional quality measures, are warranted and could help improve nursing care.

Finally, symptom management plays an important role in effective HIV/AIDS care, and includes the prevention, assessment, and treatment of symptoms. The goal of symptom management is to avert or delay a negative outcome through biomedical, professional, and self-care strategies (Group, UCSF School of Nursing Symptom Management, 1994). Effective symptom management requires the collaboration of health care professionals and the patient. Teaching HIV/AIDS patients how to manage their own symptoms is part of the health care professional's role. It is also the best intervention that nurses can provide in the long course of disease progression (Lietzau, 1996). Although patients can obtain symptom management advice from professionals, the actual tasks of daily management of those complex and unpredictable symptoms (e.g., assessment, evaluation, and alleviation) still needs to be carried out by themselves, their partners, or their friends (Siegel & Krauss, 1991).

## Policy Implications

In 2004 The Henry J. Kaiser Family Foundation issued a policy brief entitled, "Financing HIV/AIDS Care: A Quilt With Many Holes" (Henry J. Kaiser Family Foundation [HKFF], 2004). As exemplified in the report, of those who are insured and in the health care system, most are covered by the public sector insurance program. However, the uninsured and the underinsured rely on array of safety net programs including the Ryan White Comprehensive AIDS Resources Emergency Act, community and migrant health centers, private so-called free clinics, and public hospitals. "As such, the current system of financing for HIV care represents a complex patchwork that leaves some outside the system and presents others with financial barriers to access needed care" (HKFF, p. 1). Policymakers face the challenge of searching for ways to improve access, which cuts across multiple sources of financing and care that are needed for people with HIV/AIDS. In turn, as researchers, we face the obligation of working with policymakers on advocating for our patients and communities and educating policymakers on the health challenges, such as the multiple symptoms and effects on their daily lives, that people with HIV/AIDS face.

Equally, public policy barely recognizes the enormous needs in the area of mental health, alcohol and drug rehabilitation, and social services needed by people with HIV/AIDS and their families. Although the majority of funding is directed to primary care, policy needs to be developed that would increase funding allocation to those areas mentioned and blend federal funding streams, which would result in better coordination of care. This would aid a significant proportion of people with HIV/AIDS who are most likely to be members of already disadvantaged groups and who are more likely to rely on the public sector for health care.

In conclusion, the ongoing work of HIV symptom assessment is a long-term endeavor. This review provides an important contribution to knowledge about HIV symptom assessment but there are still many important areas to be addressed. In addition to learning more about symptom assessment, we need to know more about effective symptom management strategies, programs, and guidelines. Failure to understand patients' self-care abilities and what they actually do to manage symptoms could impede any practical intervention. Because of nursing's focus on symptoms, nursing is positioned to lead the development of symptom assessment and management.

ACKNOWLEDGMENTS

The authors would like to acknowledge Emily Huang and Yvette Cuca for their valuable contributions of literature review and critical eyes.

## REFERENCES

Anastos, K., Schneider, M. F., Gange, S. J., Minkoff, H., Greenblatt, R. M., Feldman, J., et al. (2005). The association of race, sociodemographic, and behavioral characteristics with response to highly active antiretroviral therapy in women. *Journal of Acquired Immune Deficiency Syndromes, 39*(5), 537–544.

Andrews, L. (1998). *The pathogenesis of HIV infection.* Sudbury, MA: Jones and Bartlett.

Association of Nurses in AIDS Care. (2004). 2004 HIV symptom management booklet. Akron, OH: ANAC. Retrieved from https://secure.ar51.net/anacnet/orderform.htm

Barlett, J. G., & Finkbeiner, A. K. (2001). *The guide to living with HIV infection* (5th ed.). Baltimore, MD: The Johns Hopkins University Press.

Beal, M. W., & Nield-Anderson, L. (2000). Acupuncture for symptom relief in HIV-positive adults: Lessons learned from a pilot study. *Alternative Therapies in Health and Medicine, 6*(5), 33–42.

Bedell, G. (2000). Daily life for eight urban gay men with HIV/AIDS. *American Journal of Occupational Therapy, 54*(2), 197–206.

Bozzette, S. A., Kanouse, D. E., Berry, S., & Duan, N. (1995). Health status and function with zidovudine or zalcitabine as initial therapy for AIDS. A randomized controlled trial. Roche 3300/ACTG 114 Study Group. *Journal of the American Medical Association, 273*(4), 295–301.

Breitbart, W., McDonald, M. V., Rosenfeld, B., Monkman, N. D., & Passik, S. (1998). Fatigue in ambulatory AIDS patients. *Journal of Pain Symptom Management, 15*(3), 159–167.

Breitbart, W., McDonald, M. V., Rosenfeld, B., Passik, S. D., Hewitt, D., Thaler, H., et al. (1996). Pain in ambulatory AIDS patients: Pain characteristics and medical correlates. *Pain, 68*(2–3), 315–321.

Breitbart, W., Passik, S., McDonald, M. V., Rosenfeld, B., Smith, M., Kaim, M., et al. (1998). Patient-related barriers to pain management in ambulatory AIDS patients. *Pain, 76*(1–2), 9–16.

Breitbart, W., Rosenfeld, B. D., Passik, S. D., McDonald, M. V., Thaler, H., & Portenoy, R. K. (1996). The undertreatment of pain in ambulatory AIDS patients. *Pain, 65*(2–3), 243–249.

Burgoyne, R. W., Rourke, S. B., Behrens, D. M., & Salit, I. E. (2004). Long-term quality-of-life outcomes among adults living with HIV in the HAART era: The interplay of changes in clinical factors and symptom profile. *AIDS Behavior, 8*(2), 151–163.

Camp, L. D. (1988). A comparison of nurses' recorded assessments of pain with perceptions of pain as described by cancer patients. *Cancer Nursing, 11*(4), 237–243.

Capaldini, L. (2004). *Symptom management guidelines. HIV InSite knowledge base chapter.* HIV InSite. Retrieved January 20, 2005, from http://hivinsite.ucsf.edu/InSite?page=kb-03&doc=kb-03-01-06

Carretero, M. D., Burgess, A. P., Soler, P., Soler, M., & Catalan, J. (1996). Reliability and validity of an HIV-specific health-related quality-of-life measure for use with injecting drug users. *AIDS, 10*(14), 1699–1705.

Centers for Disease Control and Prevention. (2002). *Commentary. CDC-NCHSTP DHAP: HIV/AIDS Surveillance Supplemental Report, 8*(2), Retrieved July 5, 2005, from http://www.cdc.gov/hiv/stats/hasrsupp2082/commentary.htm

Chang, V. T., Hwang, S. S., Feuerman, M., Kasimis, B. S., & Thaler, H. T. (2000). The memorial symptom assessment scale short form (MSAS-SF). *Cancer, 89*(5), 1162–1171.

Coleman, C. L., & Holzemer, W. L. (1999). Spirituality, psychological well-being, and HIV symptoms for African Americans living with HIV disease. *Journal of the Association of Nurses in AIDS Care, 10*(1), 42–50.

Cook, J. A., Grey, D., Burke, J., Cohen, M. H., Gurtman, A. C., Richardson, J. L., et al. (2004). Depressive symptoms and AIDS-related mortality among a multisite cohort of HIV-positive women. *American Journal of Public Health, 94*(7), 1133–1140.

Corless, I. B., Bakken, S., Nicholas, P. K., Holzemer, W. L., McGibbon, C. A., Inouye, J., et al. (2000). Predictors of perception of cognitive functioning in HIV/AIDS. *Journal of the Association of Nurses in AIDS Care, 11*(3), 19–26.

Cosby, C., Holzemer, W. L., Henry, S. B., & Portillo, C. J. (2000). Hematological complications and quality of life in hospitalized AIDS patients. *AIDS Patient Care and STDs, 14*(5), 269–279.

Coyne, P. J., Lyne, M. E., & Watson, A. C. (2002). Symptom management in people with AIDS. *American Journal of Nursing, 102*(9), 48–56; quiz 57.

Cummings, S. R., Strull, W., Nevitt, M. C., & Hulley, S. B. (1988). *Planning the measurements: Questionnaires.* Baltimore: Williams & Wilkins.

Davis, K. (2000). Symptom management. HIV Patient. Manual Virtual Hospital. Retrieved January 20, 2005, from http://www.vh.org/adult/patient/internalmedicine/hivmanual/08symptommanagement.html.

Davis, K., Schoenbaum, S., Collins, K. S., Tenney, K., & Hughes, D. L. (2002). *Room for improvement: Patients report on the quality of their health care.* New York: The Commonwealth Fund.

Davis, R. F., Metzger, D. S., Meyers, K., McLellan, A. T., Mulvaney, F. D., Navaline, H. A., et al. (1995). Long-term changes in psychological symptomatology associated with HIV serostatus among male injecting drug users. *AIDS, 9*(1), 73–79.

Derogatis, L. R. (1977). *The SCL-90 Manual I: Scoring, administration and procedures for the SCL-90.* Clinical Psychometric: Baltimore, MD.

Derogatis, L. R. (1983). Misuse of the symptom checklist 90. *Archives of General Psychiatry, 40*(10), 1152–1153.

Derogatis, L. R. (1993). *BSI brief symptom inventory.* Minneapolis, MN: National Computer Systems, Inc.

Derogatis, L. R., Lipman, R. S., Rickels, K., Uhlenhuth, E. H., & Covi, L. (1974a). The Hopkins Symptom Checklist (HSCL): A self-report symptom inventory. *Behavioral Science, 19*(1), 1–15.

Derogatis, L. R., Lipman, R. S., Rickels, K., Uhlenhuth, E. H., & Covi, L. (1974b). The Hopkins Symptom Checklist (HSCL). A measure of primary symptom dimensions. *Modern Problems of Pharmacopsychiatry, 7*(0), 79–110.

Derogatis, L. R., & Melisaratos, N. (1983). The Brief Symptom Inventory: An introductory report. *Psychological Medicine, 13*(3), 595–605.

Derogatis, L. R., Rickels, K., & Rock, A. F. (1976). The SCL-90 and the MMPI: A step in the validation of a new self-report scale. *British Journal of Psychiatry, 128*, 280–289.

DiMatteo, M. R., Lepper, H. S., & Croghan, T. W. (2000). Depression is a risk factor for noncompliance with medical treatment: Meta-analysis of the effects of anxiety and depression on patient adherence. *Archives of Internal Medicine, 160*(14), 2101–2107.

Dodd, M., Janson, S., Facione, N., Faucett, J., Froelicher, E. S., Humphreys, J., et al. (2001). Advancing the science of symptom management. *Journal of Advanced Nursing, 33*(5), 668–676.

Dodd, M. J., Miaskowski, C., & Lee, K. A. (2004). Occurrence of symptom clusters. *Journal of the National Cancer Institute. Monographs* (32), 76–78.

Ferri, R. S. (2004). Symptom management in the age of highly active antiretroviral therapy. *Journal of the Association of Nurses in AIDS Care, 15*(5 Suppl), 5S-6S.

Gifford, A. L., Bormann, J. E., Shively, M. J., Wright, B.C., Richman, D. D., & Bozzette, S. A. (2000). Predictors of self-reported adherence and plasma HIV concentrations in patients on multidrug antiretroviral regimens. *Journal of Acquired Immune Deficiency Syndromes, 23*(5), 386–395.

Gift, A. G., Stommel, M., Jablonski, A., & Given, W. (2003). A cluster of symptoms over time in patients with lung cancer. *Nursing Research, 52*(6), 393–400.

Group, UCSF, School of Nursing Symptom Management. (1994). A model for symptom management. The University of California, San Francisco School of Nursing Symptom Management Faculty Group. *Image—The Journal of Nursing Scholarship, 26*(4), 272–276.

Hench, K., Anderson, R., Grady, C., & Ropka, M. (1995). Investigating chronic symptoms in HIV: An opportunity for collaborative nursing research. *Journal of the Association of Nurses in AIDS Care, 6*(3), 13–17.

Henry J. Kaiser Family Foundation. (2004). *HIV/AIDS Policy Issue Brief. Financing HIV/AIDS Care: A quilt with many holes.* Retrieved August 31, 2005, from http://www.kff.org/hivaids/upload/Financing-HIV-AIDS-Care-A-Quilt-with-Many-Holes.pdf

Henry J. Kaiser Family Foundation. (2005). *Daily HIV/AIDS Report. Across the nation more than 1M HIV-positive people living in United States.* Retrieved July 12, 2005, from http://www.kaisernetwork.org/daily_reports/rep_index.cfm?DR_ID = 30727

Holzemer, W. L. (1997). Post-Vancouver: Implications for nursing practice and nursing research. *Journal of the Association of Nurses in AIDS Care, 8*(4), 62–66.

Holzemer, W. L. (2002). HIV and AIDS: The symptom experience. What cell counts and viral loads won't tell you. *American Journal of Nursing, 102*(4), 48–52.

Holzemer, W. L., Corless, I. B., Nokes, K. M., Turner, J. G., Brown, M. A., Powell-Cope, G. M., et al. (1999). Predictors of self-reported adherence in persons living with HIV disease. *AIDS Patient Care and STDs, 13*(3), 185–197.

Holzemer, W. L., Henry, S. B., Nokes, K. M., Corless, I. B., Brown, M. A., Powell-Cope, G. M., et al. (1999). Validation of the Sign and Symptom Check-List for Persons with HIV Disease (SSC-HIV). *Journal of Advanced Nursing, 30*(5), 1041–1049.

Holzemer, W. L., Henry, S. B., Portillo, C. J., & Miramontes, H. (2000). The Client Adherence Profiling-Intervention Tailoring (CAP-IT) intervention for enhancing adherence to HIV/AIDS medications: A pilot study. *Journal of the Association of Nurses in AIDS Care*, *11*(1), 36–44.

Holzemer, W. L., Hudson, A., Kirksey, K. M., Hamilton, M. J., & Bakken, S. (2001). The revised Sign and Symptom Check-List for HIV (SSC-HIVrev). *Journal of the Association of Nurses in AIDS Care*, *12*(5), 60–70.

Hudson, A., Kirksey, K., & Holzemer, W. (2004). The influence of symptoms on quality of life among HIV-infected women. *Western Journal of Nursing Research*, *26*(1), 9–23; discussion 24–30.

Hudson, A. L., Lee, K. A., & Portillo, C. J. (2003). Symptom experience and functional status among HIV-infected women. *AIDS Care*, *15*(4), 483–492.

Hughes, A. (2004). Symptom management in HIV-infected patients. *Journal of the Association of Nurses in AIDS Care*, *15*(5 Suppl), 7S-13S.

Humphreys, J. C., Lee, K. A., Neylan, T. C., & Marmar, C. R. (1999). Sleep patterns of sheltered battered women. *Image—The Journal of Nursing Scholarship*, *31*(2), 139–43.

Institute of Medicine. (IOM). (2003). *Unequal treatment. Confronting racial and ethnic disparities in healthcare*. Washington, DC: Institute of Medicine of the National Academies.

Joseph, J. G., Caumartin, S. M., Tal, M., Kirscht, J. P., Kessler, R. C., Ostrow, D. G., et al. (1990). Psychological functioning in a cohort of gay men at risk for AIDS. A three-year descriptive study. *Journal of Nervous and Mental Disease*, *178*(10), 607–615.

Justice, A. C., Holmes, W., Gifford, A. L., Rabeneck, L., Zackin, R., Sinclair, G., et al. (2001). Development and validation of a self-completed HIV symptom index. *Journal of Clinical Epidemiology*, *54 (Suppl) 1*, S77–90.

Justice, A. C., Rabeneck, L., Hays, R. D., Wu, A. W., & Bozzette, S. A. (1999). Sensitivity, specificity, reliability, and clinical validity of provider-reported symptoms: A comparison with self-reported symptoms. Outcomes Committee of the AIDS Clinical Trials Group. *Journal of Acquired Immune Deficiency Syndromes*, *21*(2), 126–133.

Kennedy, C. A., Skurnick, J. H., Foley, M., & Louria, D. B. (1995). Gender differences in HIV-related psychological distress in heterosexual couples. *AIDS Care*, *7 (Suppl) 1*, S33–38.

Lackner, J. B., Joseph, J. G., Ostrow, D. G., & Eshleman, S. (1993). The effects of social support on Hopkins Symptom Checklist-assessed depression and distress in a cohort of human immunodeficiency virus-positive and -negative gay men. A longitudinal study at six time points. *Journal of Nervous and Mental Disease*, *181*(10), 632–638.

Larson, P. J., Carrieri-Kohlman, V., Dodd, M. J., Douglas, M., Faucett, J., Froehlicher, E., et al. (1994). A model on symptom management. *Image—Journal of Nursing Scholarship*, *26*, 272–276.

Larson, P. J., Viele, C. S., Coleman, S., Dibble, S. L., & Cebulski, C. (1993). Comparison of perceived symptoms of patients undergoing bone marrow transplant and the nurses caring for them. *Oncology Nursing Forum*, *20*(1), 81–87; discussion 87–88.

Larue, F., Brasseur, L. K., Musseault, P., Demeulemeester, R., Bonifassi, L., & Bez, G. (1994). Pain and symptoms in HIV disease: A national survey in France (abstract). *Journal of Palliative Care*, *10*, 95.

Lietzau, J. (1996). Teaching symptom management of HIV/AIDS using algorithms. *Cancer Nursing*, *19*(4), 263–268.

Marder, K., Liu, X., Stern, Y., Dooneief, G., Bell, K., Schofield, P., et al. (1995). Neurologic signs and symptoms in a cohort of homosexual men followed for 4.5 years. *Neurology*, *45*(2), 261–267.

Mathews, W. C., McCutchan, J. A., Asch, S., Turner, B. J., Gifford, A. L., Kuromiya, K., et al. (2000). National estimates of HIV-related symptom prevalence from the HIV Cost and Services Utilization Study. *Medical Care, 38*(7), 750–762.

McCorkle, R. (1987). The measurement of symptom distress. *Seminars in Oncology Nursing, 3*(4), 248–256.

McShane, R. E., Bumbalo, J. A., & Patsdaughter, C. A. (1994). Psychological distress in family members living with human immunodeficiency virus/acquired immune deficiency syndrome. *Archives of Psychiatric Nursing, 8*(1), 53–61.

Miles, M. S., Holdtich-Davis, D., Eron, J., Black, B. P., Pedersen, C., & Harris, D. A. (2003). An HIV self-care symptom management intervention for African American mothers. *Nursing Research, 52*(6), 350–360.

Moneyham, L., Sowell, R., Seals, B., & Demi, A. (2000). Depressive symptoms among African American women with HIV disease. *Scholarly Inquiry for Nursing Practice, 14*(1), 9–39; discussion 41–36.

Nokes, K. M., Holzemer, W. L., Corless, I. B., Bakken, S., Brown, M. A., Inouye, J., et al. (2000, May). Health-related quality of life in persons younger and older than 50 who are living with HIV/AIDS. *Research on Aging, 22*(3), 290–310.

Nokes, K. M., & Kendrew, J. (2001). Correlates of sleep quality in persons with HIV disease. *Journal of the Association of Nurses in AIDS Care, 12*(1), 17–22.

Osoba, D. (1993). Self-rating symptom checklists: A simple method for recording and evaluating symptom control in oncology. *Cancer Treatment Reviews, 19 (Suppl A)* 43–51.

Pasacreta, J. V. (1997). Depressive phenomena, physical symptom distress, and functional status among women with breast cancer. *Nursing Research, 46*(4), 214–221.

Peragallo, N. (1996). Latino women and AIDS risk. *Public Health Nursing, 13*(3), 217–222.

Pergami, A., Gala, C., Burgess, A., Durbano, F., Zanello, D., Riccio, M., et al. (1993). The psychosocial impact of HIV infection in women. *Journal of Psychosomatic Research, 37*(7), 687–696.

Perry, S., Jacobsberg, L., Card, C. A., Ashman, T., Frances, A., & Fishman, B. (1993). Severity of psychiatric symptoms after HIV testing. *American Journal of Psychiatry, 150*(5), 775–779.

Perry, S. W., Jacobsberg, L. B., Fishman, B., Weiler, P. H., Gold, J. W., & Frances, A. J. (1990). Psychological responses to serological testing for HIV. *AIDS, 4*(2), 145–152.

Portenoy, R. K., Thaler, H. T., Kornblith, A. B., Lepore, J. M., Friedlander-Klar, H., Coyle, N., et al. (1994). Symptom prevalence, characteristics and distress in a cancer population. *Quality of Life Research, 3*(3), 183–189.

Portenoy, R. K., Thaler, H. T., Kornblith, A. B., Lepore, J. M., Friedlander-Klar, H., Kiyasu, E., et al. (1994). The Memorial Symptom Assessment Scale: An instrument for the evaluation of symptom prevalence, characteristics and distress. *European Journal of Cancer, 30A*(9), 1326–1336.

Rabkin, J. G., Ferrando, S. J., Jacobsberg, L. B., & Fishman, B. (1997). Prevalence of axis I disorders in an AIDS cohort: A cross-sectional, controlled study. *Comprehensive Psychiatry, 38*(3), 146–154.

Rabkin, J. G., Rabkin, R., & Wagner, G. (1994). Effects of fluoxetine on mood and immune status in depressed patients with HIV illness. *Journal of Clinical Psychiatry, 55*(3), 92–97.

Rabkin, J. G., Wagner, G., & Rabkin, R. (1994). Effects of sertraline on mood and immune status in patients with major depression and HIV illness: An open trial. *Journal of Clinical Psychiatry, 55*(10), 433–439.

Reilly, C. A., Holzemer, W. L., Henry, S. B., Slaughter, R. E., & Portillo, C. J. (1997). A comparison of patient and nurse ratings of human immunodeficiency virus-related signs and symptoms. *Nursing Research, 46*(6), 318–323.

Remick, S. C., McSharry, J. J., Wolf, B.C., Blanchard, C. G., Eastman, A. Y., Wagner, H., et al. (1993). Novel oral combination chemotherapy in the treatment of intermediate-grade and high-grade AIDS-related non-Hodgkin's lymphoma. *Journal of Clinical Oncology, 11*(9), 1691–1702.

Revicki, D. A., Sorensen, S., & Wu, A. W. (1998). Reliability and validity of physical and mental health summary scores from the Medical Outcomes Study HIV Health Survey. *Medical Care, 36*(2), 126–137.

Revicki, D. A., Wu, A. W., & Murray, M. I. (1995). Change in clinical status, health status, and health utility outcomes in HIV-infected patients. *Medical Care, 33*(4 Suppl), AS173–182.

Ropka, M., & Williams, A. (1998). *HIV nursing and symptom management.* Sudbury, MA: Jones and Bartlett.

Sackett, D. L., Richardson, W. S., Rosenberg, W., & Haynes, R. B. (1998). *Evidence-based medicine: How to practice and teach EBM.* Edinburgh: Churchill Livingston.

Shaw, J., & Mahoney, E. (2002). *HIV/AIDS nursing secrets.* Philadelphia: Hanley and Belfus Medical Publishers.

Siegel, K., & Krauss, B. J. (1991). Living with HIV infection: Adaptive tasks of seropositive gay men. *Journal of Health and Social Behavior, 32*(1), 17–32.

Siegel, K., Schrimshaw, E. W., & Dean, L. (1999). Symptom interpretation: Implications for delay in HIV testing and care among HIV-infected late middle-aged and older adults. *AIDS Care, 11*(5), 525–535.

Singer, E. J., Zorilla, C., Fahy-Chandon, B., Chi, S., Syndulko, K., & Tourtellotte, W. W. (1993). Painful symptoms reported by ambulatory HIV-infected men in a longitudinal study. *Pain, 54*(1), 15–19.

Smedley, B. D., Stith, A. Y., & Nelson, A. R. (Eds.). (2003). *Unequal treatment: Confronting racial and ethnic disparities in health care.* Washington, DC: National Academies Press.

Smith, K. W., Avis, N. E., Mayer, K. H., & Swislow, L. (1997). Use of the MQoL-HIV with asymptomatic HIV-positive patients. *Quality of Life Research, 6*(6), 555–560.

Spire, B., Duran, S., Raffi, F., Sobel, A., Souala, F., Journot, V., et al. (2000). *A high number of self-reported symptoms following HAART initiation is predictive of poor adherence at 4 months of treatment in HIV-infected patients.* Paper presented at the XIII International AIDS Conference, Durban, South Africa.

*Symptom management strategies: A manual for people living with HIV/AIDS.* (2004). Retrieved from http://www.ucsf.edu/aidsnursing

Tangue, A., Evers, G., & Paridaens, R. (1998). Nurses' assessment of symptom occurrence and symptom distress in chemotherapy patients. *European Journal of Oncology Nursing, 2*(1), 14–26.

Vidrine, D. J., Amick, B.C., Gritz, E. R., & Arduino, R. C. (2003). Functional status and overall quality of life in a multiethnic HIV-positive population. *AIDS Patient Care and STDs, 17*(4), 187–197.

Vlahov, D., Munoz, A., Solomon, L., Astemborski, J., Lindsay, A., Anderson, J., et al. (1994). Comparison of clinical manifestations of HIV infection between male and female injecting drug users. *AIDS*, 8(6), 819–823.

Vogl, D., Rosenfeld, B., Breitbart, W., Thaler, H., Passik, S., McDonald, M., et al. (1999). Symptom prevalence, characteristics, and distress in AIDS outpatients. *Journal of Pain and Symptom Management, 18*(4), 253–262.

Voss, J. G. (2005). Predictors and correlates of fatigue in HIV/AIDS. *Journal of Pain and Symptom Management, 29*(2), 173–84.

Wagner, G., Rabkin, J., & Rabkin, R. (1998). Exercise as a mediator of psychological and nutritional effects of testosterone therapy in HIV+ men. *Medicine and Science in Sports and Exercise, 30*(6), 811–817.

Waltz, C. F., Strickland, O. L., & Lenz, E. R. (1991). *Measurement in nursing research* (2nd ed.). Philadelphia: F. A. Davis.

Whalen, C. C., Antani, M., Carey, J., & Landefeld, C. S. (1994). An index of symptoms for infection with human immunodeficiency virus: Reliability and validity. *Journal of Clinical Epidemiology, 47*(5), 537–546.

Wilson, I. B., & Cleary, P. D. (1995). Linking clinical variables with health-related quality of life. A conceptual model of patient outcomes. *Journal of the American Medical Association, 273*(1), 59–65.

Wu, A. W., Dave, N. B., Diener-West, M., Sorensen, S., Huang, I. C., & Revicki, D. A. (2004). Measuring validity of self-reported symptoms among people with HIV. *AIDS Care, 16*(7), 876–881.

Wu, A. W., Hays, R. D., Kelly, S., Malitz, F., & Bozzette, S. A. (1997). Applications of the Medical Outcomes Study health-related quality of life measures in HIV/AIDS. *Quality of Life Research, 6*(6), 531–554.

Wu, A. W., Revicki, D. A., Jacobson, D., & Malitz, F. E. (1997). Evidence for reliability, validity and usefulness of the Medical Outcomes Study HIV Health Survey (MOS-HIV). *Quality of Life Research, 6*(6), 481–493.

Zeller, J. M., Swanson, B., & Cohen, F. L. (1993). Suggestions for clinical nursing research: symptom management in AIDS patients. *Journal of the Association of Nurses AIDS Care, 4*(3), 13–17.

Zingmond, D. S., Kilbourne, A.M., Justice, A. C., Wenger, N. S., Rodriguez-Barradas, M., Rabeneck, L., et al. (2003). Differences in symptom expression in older HIV-positive patients: The Veterans Aging Cohort 3 Site Study and HIV Cost and Service Utilization Study experience. *Journal of Acquired Immune Deficiency Syndromes, 33*(2), S84–S92.

# Chapter 10

## Promoting Culturally Appropriate Interventions Among Vulnerable Populations

Joyce Newman Giger and Ruth Davidhizar

## ABSTRACT

*Evidence-based practice is critical for the improvement of interventions for culturally diverse and disadvantaged groups in the community. Nurses are strategically located in the line of patient care and must be grounded in knowledge related to the delivery of culturally appropriate intervention strategies. Although many of the health care disciplines have failed to conduct or disseminate culturally competent interventions among vulnerable populations, it is important to note that nursing has long been engaged in such activities. Clearly, all health care professionals must be provided with the tools that they need to give appropriate and effective care to patients and to conduct and disseminate relevant research about vulnerable populations. This chapter focuses on culturally competent interventions for ethnic and racial minority groups, women, and the mentally ill.*

Keywords: culturally competent; interventions; ethnic minorities; women; mentally ill

# INTRODUCTION

Over the last several decades, there have been numerous attempts to define the term *vulnerable population*. Heretofore, a vulnerable population was thought to represent very different groups. Stevens (1990) described vulnerability as the experience of being exposed to or unprotected from health damaging environments. Today, the term vulnerable has come to refer to populations who experience social or economic hardships and include groups such as unwanted children, unwed mothers, widows, the elderly, the impoverished, and various racial and ethnic groups that suffer from greater risks of morbidity and mortality than do their more privileged or wealthier counterparts (International Union for the Scientific Study of Population, 2005). Vulnerable populations face increased risks due in part to lack of access to health care and inadequate health care services. This problem is dramatically illustrated by statistics revealing that poor people have twice the death rates of those with incomes above the poverty level. In fact, poverty is a predisposing factor to traumatic injuries, violence, and homicide. Moreover, higher rates of infant deaths, premature births, and low birth weights frequently accompany social and economic inequities (Vezeau, Peterson, Nakao, & Ersek, 1998).

## Purpose and Scope of Review With Criteria for Selection of Studies

The purpose of this chapter is to focus on research promoting culturally appropriate interventions among vulnerable populations. To accomplish this task, we conducted literature searches between 1995 and 2005 via PubMed, Medline, World CAT, and Cumulative Index on Nursing and Allied Health. Specifically, we searched for a variety of disease categories and clinical services where culturally appropriate interventions were applied to vulnerable populations. The search terms included *culturally competent interventions*, *vulnerable populations*, and *culturally sensitive intervention*. The aforementioned search terms were applied across the broad categories recognized as vulnerable populations, which included women, ethnic and racial minorities, and the mentally ill.

## Research Reviewed

Over 200 articles were identified from the search. Articles were deemed relevant for the chapter if they included culturally competent and appropriate interventions. A number of research articles (n = 17) that related to interventions in the community with vulnerable populations were reviewed and are subsequently summarized and highlighted in Table 10.1. Included in this review are a few non-intervention studies that are particularly relevant to the development of culturally competent research interventions with vulnerable populations.

**TABLE 10.1** Culturally Competant Research With Vulnerable Populations

| Citation | Sample Size | Ethnicity | Design | Intervention | Outcome Variable | Results |
|---|---|---|---|---|---|---|
| **Intervention with Women** | | | | | | |
| Wechsberg, Lam, Zule, & Bobashev (2004) | 620 women | African American women | Randomized field experiment with four modules of two individual and two group sessions (women-focused, standard NIH intervention and pure control) | Women – focused intervention of culturally enriched content grounded in empowerment theory and feminism/skills training relative to HIV risk for crack users versus a standard NIDA intervention and control group | Crack cocaine use; Engagement in unprotected sex choices. | All groups decreased crack use; decrease in unprotected sex and improvement in housing and employment status among participants in the women focused intervention |
| Nyamathi, Flaskerud, Keenan & Leake (1998) | 241 women | African American and Latina | Site randomized into two programs (Traditional and Specialized) with further randomization into women alone or woman with supportive person (SP) | The Traditional program provided in small group format a culturally sensitive program detailing factual AIDS risk information, including the provision of condoms and bleach kits over a 7-week period with 45-minute weekly. The Specialized participants were provided a culturally sensitive comprehensive program of eight weekly sessions of 2 hours duration. | Concerns, threat appraisal, AIDS knowledge, depression, coping, and risk behavior. | Significant improvement at both the 6- and 12-month follow-up for both groups in all risk behaviors, and cognitive and psychosocial functioning except active coping. Women in the Specialized group improved to a greater extent on AIDS knowledge and reduction in non-injection drug use than did their counterparts in the Traditional program. |

*(Continued)*

**TABLE 10.1** Culturally Competant Research with Vulnerable Populations (*Continued*)

| Citation | Sample Size | Ethnicity | Design | Intervention | Outcome Variable | Results |
|---|---|---|---|---|---|---|
| Norr, et al. (2003) | 588 women | 406 African Americans And 182 Mexican Americans | Randomized clinical trial | Reach-Futures program was composed of three integrated perspectives that included: (a) The WHO Primary Health Care Model, (b) the ecological model of child development, and (c) the previous experience of the researchers. | Rate of repeat pregnancy; parenting attitudes; infant health outcomes; communication life skills | Parenting attitudes for both African American (AA) and Mexican American (MA) mothers became more positive over time; MAs had more negative scores on the empathy subscale and more positive scores on the avoidance of punishment subscale of the parenting attitudes scale at 12 months than did the AAs; the incidence of repeat pregnancy did not vary by ethnic groups; MAs in the Reach-Future group had significantly higher CLSS than did their controls at 12 months; for the infants, there were no significant differences between the ethnic groups or between the treatment and control groups for any health problem variables. |

| Author (Year) | Sample | Population | Design | Method | Variable | Findings |
|---|---|---|---|---|---|---|
| Mezey, Bacchus, Bewley, & White (2005) | N = 200 | White British women | Cross sectional | Women receiving post-natal and prenatal care at one maternity service were screened for lifetime experiences of trauma and domestic violence. Women completed the Edinburgh post natal depression scale and the post traumatic diagnostic history | Domestic violence | Awareness of impact of trauma and abuse on psychological health can enable more appropriate assessment and support during maternity care. |
| Wood, Duffy, Morris, & Carnes (2002) | 326 Women | Primarily African American | Quasi-experimental, pre and post-test, dual site, community based study; two groups | Practice with sensitive self-monitored video breast health kit | Knowledge about breast cancer risk and screening and breast self-examination (BSC) proficiency. | Intervention group had significantly higher BSE skill scores than that of control group. |
| Erwin, Spatz, Stotts, & Hollenberg (1999) | N=206 in intervention group and 204 in control group | African American women | Intervention and control group delivery | Educational program promoting early detection, self-breast examination, and mammography | Practice of BSE and obtaining mammography | Intervention participants significantly increased in BSE and mammography |

*(Continued)*

**TABLE 10.1** Culturally Competant Research With Vulnerable Populations (*Continued*)

| Citation | Sample Size | Ethnicity | Design | Intervention | Outcome Variable | Results |
|---|---|---|---|---|---|---|
| **Health related intervention in ethnic and racial minorities** | | | | | | |
| Holkup, Tripp-Reimer, Salois, & Weinert (2004) | One family | Native American | Phase 1 of a planned experimental design using a Family Care Conference | Use family group model and family unity model principles to solve problems of Native American families | Acceptable problem solutions | A model was designed on which to base further research |
| Linnan et al. (2005) | All customers in two beauty salons for a period of 1 year | One shop served African Americans one served Whites. | Experimental design with 4-hr. workshop for licensed cosmetologists | 7-week pilot intervention with educational displays and communication with customers | Self-reported change in health status, patient satisfaction, readiness to change | 55% of customers reported changes in health status. 81% of customers continued to read educational displays, 86% to talk with cosmetologists about project. |
| The Diabetes Prevention Program Research Group (2002) | $N = 1,079$ | African Americans 20% Hispanic Americans 16% American Indian 5% Asian Americans 4% | Intervention was consistently administered in 27 centers. This group was randomized to lifestyle intervention from a larger group of 3,234 who were part of other intervention strategies. | A comprehensive life style protocol was implemented | Incidence rate of diabetes | 58% reduction in incidence of rate of diabetes in the randomized experimental group |

| Piette, Weinberger, McPhee, et al. (2000) | N = 280 with 137 in the intervention group | English and Spanish speaking participants in two medical clinics in California | Randomized controlled trial with 12 months of follow up | Automatic telephone assessment and education with nurse follow up. The message included health tips, an education module focusing on diet and weight control, and tailored education and advice on glucose self-monitoring, foot care, and medication adherence. | Self care and glycaemic control of patients with diabetes | Patients who received the intervention had better perceived glycaemic control; more frequent glucose monitoring, weight monitoring, fewer problems with medication adherence and diabetic symptoms; a higher probability of having normal HbA concentration, and a lower mean serum glucose concentration than those who received usual care. The groups did not differ for mean HbA concentration. |
|---|---|---|---|---|---|---|
| Nyamathi, Stein, & Schumann (in press) | 494 homeless men and women | Primarily African American | Experimental site randomized clinical trial | Latent Tuberculosis Infection (LTBI) completion program including nurse case management, incentives, directly observed preventive therapy (DOPT), education and skills training, and a tracking protocol versus a usual care program, which included a brief TB prevention education session, as well as DOPT and incentive. | Completion of treatment and predictors including TB knowledge, depression, attitudes about treatment completion, ease of treatment, satisfaction with care | Participants in the Specialized program were significantly more likely to complete LTBI treatment than those in the usual care program. Greater depression, alcohol use, and prior negative attitudes about health care did not predict less treatment completion. These participants also reported higher TB knowledge, greater ease of treatment, and less dissatisfaction with care |

(Continued)

**TABLE 10.1** Culturally Competent Research With Vulnerable Populations (*Continued*)

| Citation | Sample Size | Ethnicity | Design | Intervention | Outcome Variable | Results |
|---|---|---|---|---|---|---|
| Orleans, Boyd, Binger, et al. (1998) | $N = 1,422$ in 14 communities with 63.6% females | African Americans | Random assignment to standard quit smoking counseling and guide or tailored to the quitting needs and barriers of African American smokers | Tailored intervention included Pathways-to-Freedom guide, which is tailored to quitting needs and barriers of African American smokers | Attempts to quit, use of prequitting strategies, 1 week abstinence and quitting success rates. | In the 6-month follow-up, 893 participants in the Tailored program showed significantly more quit attempts ($p = 0.002$) and greater use of prequitting strategies ($p = < 0.05$) than among Standard participants. No differences in self-reported, 1-week abstinence were found. In the 12-month follow-up, a significantly higher quit rate was found among participants receiving the Tailored group as compared with Standard participants (25% vs. 15%, respectively, $p = 0.034$). |
| Resnicow, Vaughan, Futterman et al. (1997) | African Americans were recruited from health care facilities, | African American | Randomized control trial | The intervention group received a printed guide, video, telephone booster call; control group received health education materials not related to tobacco use | Short-term smoking cessation | There was more benefit from the culturally appropriate materials plus a phone contact in terms of short-term cessation. However, 10–30% of the low-income minority |

| | | | | | | |
|---|---|---|---|---|---|---|
| | housing developments, and churches. Of these, 3,000 were African American smokers: 1,244 completed the home interview and were included in the study (703 intervention; 541 comparison) | | | | | households did not have a telephone. |

## Intervention with the mentally ill

| | | | | | | |
|---|---|---|---|---|---|---|
| Toro, Passero Rabideau, Bellavia, Daeschler, Wall, Thomas, et al. (1997) | 202 cases (213 adults; 70 children) | 54% were African American | Experimental design whereby intervention clients received a minimum of 41 staff contacts over a 4-to-8-month period. | Intensive case management offered persons in the intervention group access and linkage services | Experience of homelessness, physical health, and life in stressful events. | Adult participants improved dramatically in terms of their experience of homelessness, and stressful life events, physical health. |

*(Continued)*

**TABLE 10.1** Culturally Competant Research With Vulnerable Populations (*Continued*)

| Citation | Sample Size | Ethnicity | Design | Intervention | Outcome Variable | Results |
|---|---|---|---|---|---|---|
| Miranda Azocar, Organista, Dwyer, & Areane (2003) | N = 199 | 39%; African American 54% White 7% other | A randomized clinical trial | Comparison of cognitive-behavioral group psychotherapy along with the same therapy supplemented by clinical case management | Symptoms and functioning | Supplemental case management (SCM) was found to be related to a greater improvement in symptoms and functioning than cognitive-behavioral therapy (CBT) among Spanish-speaking patients (N=77). It was less effective for English-speaking persons (N=122). For Spanish-speaking patients the more culturally appropriate intervention was SCM rather than group psychotherapy by itself |
| Dixon, Stewart, Krauss, Robbins, Hackman, & Lehman (1998) | N = 77 | 59% African American 2% Hispanic | Experimental design with intervention. Use of a family outreach worker (FOW) 12 hrs. a week to work with patients, families, and team members | The FOW interacted with staff provided the family perspective, education, and made RX suggestions. The FOW designed a family consent form and expressed motherly concern. She provided support to families and education | Interactions of clients with their families stable housing | 73% of clients had contact with their families. Family contact was related to an increase in stable housing |

# INTERVENTIONS WITH WOMEN

## HIV, Drug Use, and Women

Today, African American women have the highest HIV prevalence rates, which range from approximately 1.7% among non-injecting drug users with no sex trading history to 54% among homeless women, who are more likely than not to trade sex for drugs (Tortu et al., 2000; Metsch, McCoy, McCoy, et al., 1995; Wechsberg et al., 2003). It is interesting to note that whereas the Centers for Disease Control and Prevention (CDC) do not track the relationship between crack use and HIV prevention, research findings indicate that crack cocaine use is often associated with increased sexual activity, acts involving sex craving, engaging in sex with multiple partners, and engaging in unprotected sex (Baseman, Ross, & Williams, 1998; Booth, Kwiatkowski, & Chitwood, 2000; Falck, Wang, Carlson, & Siegal, 1997; Tortu, McCoy, Beardsley, Deren, & McCoy, 1998; Nyamathi et al., 1999; Nyamathi, Stein, Dixon, Longshore, & Galaif, 2003; Wingood & DiClemente, 1998). Women who use crack and other drugs may place themselves at a high risk for HIV/AIDS by engaging in high risk sexual behaviors. Further, many of these women are impoverished, live in crime ridden environments, and face other social challenges (e.g., unemployment, homelessness, low educational attainment) that increase their vulnerability.

Wechsberg, Lam, Zule, and Bobashev (2004) conducted a study assessing risk behavior, employment, and housing status of out-of-drug-treatment African American women who used crack (n = 620). The women were randomly assigned to one of three study conditions. These study conditions included (a) the Women-Focused Intervention (WFI), (b) a revised intervention modeled on the National Institute of Drug Abuse standard (ST) group, and (c) a delayed treatment control (DTC) group. Group 1 and Group 2 were expected to complete four modules that included two individual and two group sessions. This culturally competent innovative study utilized African American crack users to inform and shape the intervention in focus groups and to deliver the intervention. Specific barriers facing African American women and how these barriers often affect daily experiences and choices were addressed in the culturally appropriate curriculum. Consequently, the content presented was culturally enriched as well as grounded in empowerment theory and African American feminism (Brunswick & Flory, 1998).

Focus group findings indicated that the women viewed drug dependence as a form of bondage; consequently, the WFI group was designed to facilitate greater independence, to increase feelings of personal power, and to teach control over behavioral choices. It also provided psychosocial educational information and skills training relative to HIV risk and drug use. The resultant material was presented within the context of the African American women's lived experiences. Women in the ST group received similar content as did women in the WFI group. However, the modules did not incorporate gender or culture-specific empowerment approaches to develop life skills or change social contexts. Women in the WFI and ST groups all completed at least one intervention session, with 67% of WFI and 65% of the ST group completing all four intervention sessions. The third group received no intervention during the first 6 months of the study enrollment.

Findings from this study indicate that all three groups reported significant decreases in the number of days of crack use at 3-month and 6-month follow-ups. Using a regression model which adjusted for crack use at baseline, days of crack use in both the WFI and ST groups were significantly lower than in the DTC group; with WFI participants actually reporting the greatest reduction of crack use.

In a 5-year National Institute on Drug Abuse–funded investigation, Nyamathi et al. (1998) placed 241 homeless and drug-addicted women and their supportive person (spouse, close friend, or family member) into one of two culturally sensitive programs aimed at reducing substance use and unprotected sexual activity. The women came from homeless shelters and drug recovery programs. These programs were developed with the feedback of the targeted community as provided by early qualitative focus group data (Nyamathi & Bennett, 1997) and community advisory group feedback.

The traditional program provided a culturally sensitive program in small group format. Run by trained nurses and outreach workers, the program detailed factual AIDS risk information, as well as how to use condoms and bleach kits. Over a 7-week period, 45-minute weekly sessions continued with participants randomized to receiving the education alone or with their supportive person. Booster sessions were provided at 6 and 12 months.

The specialized participants were provided a culturally sensitive comprehensive program of eight weekly sessions of 2 hours duration. Specifically, the same factual information as the traditional program provided was as well as: (a) demonstration and return demonstration of risk-reducing behaviors, such as placement of condoms on models, and needle and syringe disinfections; (b) discussion of problem-focused coping responses in dealing with concerns experienced; and (c) instruction in techniques for enhancing self-esteem and feelings of control. These sessions were also provided to participants alone or with their supportive person. Outcome variables included concerns, threat appraisal, AIDS knowledge, depression, coping, and risk behavior.

Findings revealed significant improvement at both the 6- and 12-month follow-up for both groups in all risk behaviors, and cognitive and psychosocial functioning except active coping. Moreover, women in the specialized group improved to a greater extent on AIDS knowledge and reduction in non-injection drug use than did their counterparts in the traditional program. Whereas supportive persons also demonstrated improvement, the women were not impacted by their presence in the group session. These findings provide evidence that culturally sensitive programs may be sufficient to produce improvement in a variety of cognitive, behavioral, and psychosocial measures; however, a more intensive program is needed to reduce risk behaviors in persons at greater risk for HIV/AIDS.

The impact of a nurse-led team of trained community residents on infant mortality was evaluated in a randomized clinical trial conducted by Norr and colleagues (2003). The sample was composed of self-identified African American (n = 406) and Mexican American (n = 182) low-income, inner-city women recruited from two university prenatal clinics in Chicago. Due to differences in baseline characteristics between the African Americans and Mexican Americans  the intervention and control groups were offered separately for each subgroup, with participants assigned to one of four groups: the Reach-Futures Intervention delivered separately for Mexican Americans and African Americans.

The Reach-Futures program was composed of three integrated perspectives that included: (a) The World Health Organization (WHO) Primary Health Care Model, (b) the ecological model of child development, and (c) the previous experience of these researchers working with mothers and infants in an inner-city environment. To enhance cultural sensitivity, a team composed of community workers (advocates) led by a nurse was formed; thus, combining the health knowledge of the nurse with the advocates' understanding of the social reality of the community. The team assigned to Mexican Americans was bilingual in English and Spanish.

During the intervention, the families were contacted once a month or more often if necessary. The first home visit was conducted within 2 weeks after delivery. At 2 months, when the advocates determined the mother-child dyad was doing well, telephone conversations were offered as an option for alternate monthly home visits. During the home visits, information was presented on the infant's health status, growth and development, parenting strategies, nutrition, signs of illness and appropriate responses, and preventive health care. The control group received routine child visits at the clinic or standard care with the provider of their choice.

The outcome measures in this study provided evaluations of maternal well-being and the parenting environment; these included rates of repeat pregnancy between birth and 12-month interview, community life skills measured by the Community Life Scales Skills (CLSS; Barnard, 1991), parenting attitudes assessed with the Adult-Adolescent Parenting Inventory (AAPI; Bavolek, 1984), cognitive growth stimulation of the parenting environment evaluated using the Home Observation for the Measurement of Environment (HOME; Caldwell & Bradley, 1984), and home safety hazards. Measures of infant outcomes at 12 months included maternal recall of illness and injury episodes, immunization rates, nurse-assessed mental and motor developmental status, and reported child abuse or neglect.

Findings from this study showed improvement over time in parenting attitudes of both African American and Mexican American mothers; however, Mexican Americans had lower scores on the empathy subscale and more positive scores on the avoidance of punishment subscale of the AAPI and the HOME scales at 12 months than African American mothers. Mexican Americans in the Reach-Futures group had significantly higher CLSS scores than did their controls at 12 months after birth, even after an adjustment for higher income was made. The incidence of repeat pregnancy did not vary by ethnic groups. No significant group differences were found for any of the infant health variables between ethnic or treatment groups.

Another major maternal health concern during pregnancy and early motherhood addressed by nurse scientists is domestic violence. Campbell et al. (1999) noted that domestic violence often starts or intensifies during pregnancy. Bacchus, Mezey, and Bewley (2002) concluded that screening for domestic violence by health care professionals is very likely to increase identification and disclosure of abuse. Further support for the importance of screening for domestic violence is provided by findings from a cross-sectional study conducted by Mezey, Bacchus, Bewley, and White (2005) in South London Hospital maternity services.

In this study, 200 women receiving postnatal or antenatal care were screened for lifetime experiences of trauma and domestic violence. Women completed the Edinburgh Postnatal Depression Scale and the Posttraumatic Diagnostic Scale. Findings revealed that 121 (61%) of the women reported at least one traumatic event and two-thirds of these had experienced multiple traumatic events. The most frequent traumatic event (34%) was witnessing or experiencing physical assault by a family member; however, nearly one quarter of the women (24%) experienced domestic violence.

The investigators also noted that childhood abuse creates a vulnerability to retraumatization in adulthood and therefore puts these women at higher risk. Awareness of the impact of trauma and abuse on psychological health can enable care providers to render more appropriate clinical services and support for women receiving maternity care. Data from this cross-sectional study and similar investigations may provide important foundations for development of culturally appropriate interventions for the treatment of domestic violence.

## Breast Health Care and Women

Wood, Duffy, Morris, and Carnes (2002) conducted a quasi-experimental, pre- and posttest, dual-site, community-based study in the northeast and the southeast of the United States to promote breast self-examination in older

African American and Caucasian women. The purpose of this study was to test the efficacy of an innovative, age- and race-sensitive self-monitored video breast health kit on increasing knowledge about breast cancer risk and screening and breast self-examination proficiency. The sample consisted of 328 women (206 in the intervention group; 122 in the control group). The women were primarily African American (77%), over 60 years of age, with a mean education of 11 years, and an annual income <$10,000 per year (50%).

All participants including those in the control group received standard information on breast cancer risks and the benefits of screening. However, those in the intervention group received education using the ethnically appropriate video breast health kits. The Breast Self Examination (BSE) rating instrument (Wood, 1999) was administered. Information in Medicare coverage and BSE procedures was also obtained. Ten items were designed to measure BSE inspection and palpitation skills of women demonstrating BSE on a simulated breast models with seven imbedded lumps. The alpha coefficients for this instrument was 0.85 in this study (Wood et al., 2002).

Findings from this study suggest statistically significant differences in the outcome variables of increased knowledge about breast cancer risk and screening and BSE proficiency between the intervention and the control groups. Analysis of the data indicated that after removing the influence of age, education, cognitive ability based on the Mini Mental Status Exam, pretest knowledge scores, and pretest lump detection scores, participants in the intervention group had a significantly higher knowledge score, higher BSE skills, and higher lump detection scores than their counterparts in the control group.

In another study of rural underserved African American women, Erwin, Spatz, Stotts, and Hollenberg (1999) examined the effectiveness of the Witness Project, a culturally competent, community-based, cancer education program to train cancer survivors to promote early cancer detection and to increase breast self-examination and mammography. The setting of the study was the African American church and included surveys of 206 women in an intervention group and 204 in a control group, wherein no intervention was provided. The intervention involved seven local African American women who had survived breast or cervical cancer; these women spoke to groups of two to five persons each at local churches and community organization meetings. The groups were presented as part of the scheduled activity of the church or community event.

Findings from this study suggested that this culturally competent intervention had a profound effect on the study participants in that a significant number of these vulnerable women increased the practice of self-breast examination (p = < .0001) and underwent more frequent mammography (p = <.005) when compared to the control group.

## Health-Related Interventions Among Ethnic and Racial Minorities

The next section features a wide array of studies, involving everything from general health promotion interventions to culturally sensitive programs related to diabetes, tuberculosis, and smoking cessation. A number of these innovative and efficacious intervention studies among ethnic and racial minorities use community-based participatory research (CBPR), in which an emphasis is placed on joining the researcher with the community as full and equal partners in every phase of the research process. Because of the emphasis on participatory research for conducting intervention studies, CBPR is an appealing model for use with vulnerable populations.

Holkup, Tripp-Reimer, Salois, and Weinert (2004) used a CBPR approach to conduct an intervention study in a Native American community. The two-phase pilot study of the Caring for Native Elders project involved utilization of a Native American woman on the research team. The first phase which is reported here was designed to provide background and contextual data for the second phase involving implementation and evaluation of a family conference intervention methodology. Core elements of the Family Group Model (American Humane Association, 2001; Pennel & Burford, 2000) and the Family Unit Model (Rodgers, 2001) were adapted to integrate the strengths of both into a strategy called the Family Care Conference, which addressed the cultural needs of elder Native American adults. Four guidelines from Harrison (2001) were utilized by the researchers including: (a) flexibility and self-awareness, (b) collaboration, (c) attention to ethical issues, and (d) applying the concept of culture in everyday working relationships. The evaluation criteria were designed to include issues of methodological soundness and community participation described by Guba and Lincoln (1989) as well as issues of acceptable problem solution and feasibility of project sustainability. These foundational concepts were later applied to a second phase of the study.

Linnan et al. (2005) conducted a pilot study using a CBPR approach to recruit and train licensed cosmetologists from beauty salons in a select area to deliver relevant health promotion messages to the customers they served. The participants were expected to attend a 4-hour workshop to assist them in delivering health promotion messages to their customers. In this creative design, the researchers also used educational displays in the salon to enforce targeted messages promoting cancer prevention. Each display included targeted cancer prevention messages, brochures, BEAUTY Project promotional items, and a "due to action" message that encouraged customers to "Ask Your Cosmetologist" for more information. Both qualitative and quantitative methodological approaches were used to ascertain information about participant satisfaction, readiness to change, and self-reported health behavior changes in customers immediately post-intervention and at 12 months.

Findings from this study revealed that when participants were adequately trained to deliver these messages, they reported an intent to deliver these messages even after the completion of the study. In fact, after the 7-week pilot intervention, 81% of customers continued to read the educational displays, and 86% of customers continued to talk with their cosmetologist about the project. At 12 months, 55% of the customers reported making changes in their health status, primarily as a result of their ongoing conversations with their cosmetologists. As women are likely to visit cosmetologists, it is plausible to assume that training cosmetologists to deliver tailored health messages is an effective way to intervene to promote health among all populations, and in particular, vulnerable populations.

It is significant to note that whereas empirical support exists for the effectiveness of lifestyle interventions with type 2 diabetes mellitus, some 60% of visits to a physician's office result in a prescription (Schappert, 1998). For lifestyle interventions to be effective, an intervention shift must occur both among clients and care providers. Pharmaceutical interventions for chronic health conditions are appealing and easy to implement, whereas lifestyle changes are much more complicated and require more resources and support, and present a significant challenge to care providers (Smith, Freeland, Heffler, & McKusick, 1998).

The Diabetes Prevention Program (DPP) Research Group (2002) provided a detailed description of a highly successful lifestyle intervention which was administered to 1,079 individuals, of which 45% were racial and ethnic minority individuals. The intervention program was directed at obtaining two goals: (a) weight loss (minimum of 7%) and weight maintenance, and (b) a minimum of 150 minutes per week of physical activity. The methods used to obtain these lifestyle goals included a multifaceted approach involving: (a) individual case managers or so-called lifestyle coaches, (b) frequent contact with participants, (c) a structured, state-of-the-art, 16-session core-curriculum teaching behavioral self-management strategies for weight loss and physical activity, (d) supervised physical activity sessions, (e) a more flexible maintenance intervention, combining group and individual approaches, motivational campaigns, and restarts, (f) individualization through a "toolbox" of adherence strategies, (g) tailoring of materials and strategies to address ethnic diversity, and (h) an extensive network of training, feedback, and clinical support. The DPP lifestyle intervention program was based on a review of the literature on nutrition, exercise, and behavioral weight control applied to the prevention of type 2 diabetes among diverse ethnic groups. The outcome of the intervention resulted in a 58% reduction in the incidence rate of diabetes in the experimental group. The significant reduction of incidence of diabetes suggests that this was a highly effective multifaceted approach.

Piette et al. (2000) conducted an intervention study with persons with low income, little formal education, and psychosocial problems that complicated their diabetes care. Their study was a randomized controlled trial with 12-month follow-up evaluations and involved two general medical clinics in California. The sample included 280 English- or Spanish- speaking adults under 75 years of age who had diabetes for less than 6 months and were using hypoglycemic medication; 137 of the participants received the intervention and 143 received usual care.

The intervention consisted of usual care plus biweekly automated tele-phone assessment and self-care education calls with telephone follow-up by a nurse educator. The automatic calls were available in Spanish or English and lasted between 5 and 8 minutes. The message included health tips, an education module focusing on diet and weight control, and tailored education and advice on glucose self-monitoring, foot care, and medication adherence. The follow-up by the nurse included more education and time to address problems reported in the assessments. The self-reported outcomes were perceived glycemic control, glucose monitoring, foot inspection, weight monitoring; problems with medica-tion adherence, and symptoms of poor glycemic control.

Over the 1-year period, participants in the intervention group had a mean of 1.4 automated assessment and self-education calls each month as well as 6 minutes of personal nurse contact per telephone conversations each month. Intervention participants reported significantly better self-care glucose monitor-ing, foot inspection, and weight monitoring than did their counterparts in the control group. They were less likely to report problems with adherence than the control group (p < .003). Moreover, the intervention participants decreased their serum glucose levels by 41 mg/dL (p = .002) as well as improved their self-reported glycemic control (p = .005).

Findings from this study demonstrate the exciting possibilities that advance-ments in technology can have for diabetes education among vulnerable popu-lations. This knowledge may enable diabetes education programs to prioritize patient contacts and focus on reducing patient frustration with diabetes control by relatively inexpensive and brief technologically advanced patient contacts.

In a NIH-funded study of 494 primarily African American homeless men and women, Nyamathi, Stein, Schumann, and Tyler (in press) assessed predic-tors of Latent Tuberculosis Infection (LTBI) completion, comparing a culturally sensitive program including nurse case management, incentives, directly observed preventive therapy (DOPT), education and skills training, and a tracking protocol versus a usual care control program on completion of a 6-month LTBI chemopro-phylaxis treatment with isoniazid (INH). The usual care group received a brief TB prevention education session, as well as DOPT and incentive. Participants were site randomized into one of two programs. Outcome variables included completion of treatment and predictors including TB knowledge, depression, attitudes about treatment completion, ease of treatment, and satisfaction with care.

Findings revealed participants in the specialized program were significantly more likely to complete LTBI treatment than their counterparts in the usual care program. Interestingly, greater depression, alcohol use, and prior negative attitudes about health care did not predict less treatment completion. These participants also reported higher TB knowledge, greater ease of treatment, and less dissatisfaction with care; thus demonstrating a portable program for increasing compliance that can be adapted to various difficult populations and a variety of treatment areas.

## Smoking Interventions and Ethnic Minorities

A self-help intervention was conducted by Orleans et al. (1998) for African American smokers. In spite of having the highest smoking rates of all U.S. adult groups, African Americans remain a critically underserved population for smoking cessation interventions. This two-year study addressed this area of health disparity by evaluating the effectiveness of a tailored, culturally sensitive intervention for African American smokers (n = 1,422) in 14 communities. Participants were randomly assigned to a standard quit smoking counseling and guide (Clearing the Air) or to counseling and a guide (Pathways to Freedom), tailored to the quitting needs and barriers of African American smokers. The results were impressive in that in the 6-month follow-up, 893 participants in the Tailored program showed significantly more quit attempts (p = 0.002) and greater use of prequitting strategies (p = < .05) than among standard participants. No differences in self-reported, 1-week abstinence were found. However, in the 12-month follow-up, a significantly higher quit rate was found among participants receiving the tailored group as compared with standard participants (25% vs. 15%, respectively, p < .04). The culturally sensitive materials revealed promise of boosting efforts to quit smoking and success rates among African American smokers.

Similarly, Resnicow et al. (1997) tested a culturally sensitive, smoking cessation intervention for 1,244 African American smokers in Harlem who completed the home interview and were randomly assigned to receive either a multi component smoking cessation intervention comprising a printed guide, a video, and a telephone booster call versus health education materials not directly addressing tobacco use (703 intervention; 541 comparison). The study results were mixed. There was more benefit from the culturally appropriate materials plus a phone contact in terms of short-term cessation. However, 10%–30% of the low-income minority households did not have a telephone.

## INTERVENTIONS WITH MENTALLY ILL

Interventions with the mentally ill in the community have been a subject of a number of research studies. Poverty has been shown to increase the risk of common mental disorders (Kessler et al., 1994). It is commonly accepted that interventions for persons who are mentally ill, homeless, and impoverished should take into account the beliefs, values, and social conditions of those being served (Miranda, Azocar, Organista, Dwyer, & Areane, 2003). Thus, interventions for mental illness should be considered from a cultural perspective if a positive outcome is to be obtained.

In a study evaluating the effectiveness of an intensive case intervention among 202 homeless persons, participants were randomly assigned to either the control or the intervention group (Toro et al., 1997). Whereas most existing services for the homeless population are emergency oriented, this intervention took a holistic approach that combined services concerned with home training placement and locating permanent housing and support services. Intensive case management with persons in the intervention group (a median of 41 staff contacts over a 4-to-8 month period) offered access and linkage services.

Findings revealed that 19% of the group had major affective disorder, 46% alcohol abuse, and 38% drug abuse or dependence. A total of 54% were African American and 42% were women. Intervention results yielded three statistically significant linear time effects among the intervention participants, indicating general changes across the follow-up period. Adult participants improved dramatically in terms of their experience of homelessness (F $[1,102]$ = 9.46, p < .01). Similar improvements were seen on physical health (F $[1,102]$ = 14.51, p < .01) and fewer stressful life events. Attending to the long-term needs of the homeless adults was seen as crucial to the success of intervention strategies with this cultural group.

In a randomized control trial, Miranda and colleagues (2003) compared cognitive-behavioral (CB) group psychotherapy (n = 103) versus CB group therapy supplemented by clinical case management with ethnically diverse, impoverished medical outpatients (N = 96). Participants were 39% African American, 54% White, and 7% other. Findings revealed that participants who received supplemental case management had lower dropout rates than those who received CB group therapy alone. Supplemental case management was also found to be related to a greater improvement in symptoms and functioning than CB group therapy alone for patients whose first language was Spanish (N = 77), but was less effective for individuals in the group whose first language was English (N = 122). These investigators noted that for Spanish-speaking patients, the more culturally appropriate intervention was supplemental case management rather than CB therapy by itself.

Dixon et al. (1998) conducted a study on the use of a family outreach worker with homeless persons with severe mental illness and their families. The study was conducted as part of a larger randomized study comparing the efficacy of a variety of services in the care of homeless persons (Lehman, Dixon, Kernan, Deforge, & Postrado, 1997). The sample consisted of 67 individuals who met strict criteria for homelessness. Sixty-five percent of the participants were men, 59% were African American, and 2% were Hispanic. The principal psychiatric diagnoses were schizophrenic disorder (69%), affective disorder (19%), substance abuse disorder (11%), and anxiety disorder (1%). A total of 47 participants (71%) had a lifetime history of substance use. Mothers and siblings were the most frequent participants in treatment.

Findings revealed that the use of a family outreach worker appeared to result in increased family contact, which in turn increased client days in stable housing ($p < .05$). There was an increase in satisfaction levels with family relations and housing. Moreover, 73% of intervention participants had contact with their families. In particular, the family outreach worker interacted with staff, provided the family perspective, education and treatment suggestions, and designed a family consent form. The team's ratings of the frequency and importance of contacts with clients and their families were related to patient satisfaction with family relations, housing, and hospitalization outcomes.

## SUMMARY

Evidence-based practice is critical for the improvement of interventions for culturally diverse and disadvantaged groups in the community. Findings from culturally competent and culturally sensitive intervention studies clearly illustrate the significance of such interventions in improving outcomes in vulnerable populations. It is plausible to assume that when intervention strategies are crafted in a culturally and linguistically appropriate manner for the population to which they are intended, more compliance with the research protocols is likely on the part of the participants. Clearly, findings from the studies presented here suggest that intervention participants were more likely to have positive outcomes than their counterparts and see a change in health status as a result of such interventions. Health care researchers must heed the clarion call to conduct culturally competent interventions if a new body of knowledge is to be added that ultimately assists in improving the overall health status of vulnerable populations.

## REFERENCES

American Humane Association. (2001). *Family group decision making project*. Retrieved June 2001, from http://www.americanhuman.org/default.asp

Bacchus, L., Mezey, G., & Bewley, S. (2002). Women's perceptions and experiences of routine questioning for domestic violence in a maternity setting. *BJOC: An International Journal of Obstetrics and Gynecology, 109*, 9–16.

Barnard, K. (1991). *Community life skills scale*. Seattle, WA: Nursing Child Assessment Satellite Training.

Baseman, J., Ross, M., & Williams, M. (1998). Sale of sex for drugs and drugs for sex: An economic context of sexual risk behavior for STDs. *Sexually Transmitted Disease, 26,* 444–449.

Bavolek, S. J. (1984). *Handbook for the AAPI: Adult-adolescent parenting inventory.* Eau Claire, WI: Family Development Resources, Inc.

Booth, R. R., Kwiatkowski, C., & Chitwood, D. (2000). Sex-related HIV risk behaviors differential risks among injection drug users, crack smokers, and injection drug users who smoke crack. *Drug Alcohol Dependence, 58,* 219–226.

Brunswick, A. F., & Flory, M. J. (1998). Changing HIV infection rates and risk in an African-American community cohort. *AIDS Care, 10,* 267–281.

Campbell, J., Torres, S., Ryan, J., King, C. Campbell, D. Stallings, R., et al. (1999). Physical and non-physical partner abuse and other risk factors for low birth weight among full term and preterm babies: a multi-ethnic case-control study. *American Journal of Epidemiology, 150,* 714–726.

Caldwell, B. M., & Bradley, R. H. (1984). *Administration manual: Home observation for measurement of the environment.* (Revised Ed.). Little Rock: University of Arkansas at Little Rock.

Dixon, L., Stewart, B., Krauss, N., Robbins, J., Hackman, A., & Lehman, A. (1998). The participation of families of homeless persons with severe mental illness in an outreach intervention. *Community Mental Health, 34*(3), 251–259.

Erwin, D., Spatz, T. Stotts, R., & Hollenberg, J. (1999). Increasing mammography practice by African American women. *Cancer Practice, 7*(2), 78–85

Falck, R. S., Wang, J., Carlson, R. G., & Siegal, H. A. (1997). Factors influencing condom use among heterosexual users of injection drugs and crack cocaine. *Sexually Transmitted Disease, 24,* 191–204.

Guba, E., & Lincoln, Y. (1989). *Fourth generation tradition.* Newbury Park, CA: Sage.

Harrison, B. (2001). *Collaborative programs in indigenous communities: From fieldwork to practice.* Walnut Creek, CA: Altamira Press.

Holkup, P. A., Tripp-Reimer, T., Salois, E. M., & Weinert, C. (2004). Community-based participatory research: an approach to intervention research with a Native American community. *Advances in Nursing Science 27,* 162–175.

International Union for the Scientific Study of Population. (2005). XXV International population conference, Session 25, vulnerable populations, Français, Tours, France, July 18–23, 2005. Retrieved from http://iussp2005.princeton.edu/default.aspx#

Kessler, R., McGonagle, K., Zhao, S., Nelson, C. B., Hughes, M., Eshleman, S., et al. (1994). Lifetime and 12 month prevalence of DSM-III-R psychiatric disorders in the United States. *Archives of General Psychiatry, 51*(1), 8–17.

Lehman, A. F., Dixon, L. B., Kernan, E., DeForge, B. R., & Postrado, L. T. (1997). A randomized trial of assertive community treatment for homeless persons with severe mental illness. *Archives of General Psychiatry, 54*(11), 1038–1043.

Linnan, L. A., Ferguson, Y. O., Wasilewski, Y., Lee, A. M., Yang, J., Solomon, F., et al. (2005) Using community-based participatory research methods to reach women with health messages: Results from the North Carolina Beauty and health pilot project. *Health Promotion Practice, 6*(2), 164–173.

Metsch, L. R., McCoy, C. B., McCoy, H. V., Shultz, J. M., Lai, S., Weatherby, N. L., et al. (1995). HIV-related risk behaviors and seropositivity among homeless drug-abusing women in Miami, Florida. *Journal of Psychoactive Drugs, 27,* 435–446.

Mezey, G., Bacchus, L., Bewley, S., & White, S. (2005). Domestic violence, lifetime trauma and psychological health of childbearing women. *BJOG, An International Journal of Obstetrics and Gynaecology, 112(2),* 197–204.

Miranda, J., Azocar, F., Organista, K. C., Dwyer, E., & Areane, P. (2003). Treatment of depression among impoverished primary care patients from ethnic minority groups. *Psychiatric Services, 54(2),* 219–225.

Norr, K. F., Crittenden, K. S., Lehrer, E. L., Reyes, O., Boyd, C. B., Nacion, K. W., et al. (2003). Maternal and infant outcomes at one year for a nurse-health advocate home visiting program serving African Americans and Mexican Americans. *Public Health Nursing, 20(3),* 190–203.

Nyamathi, A., Bayley, L., Anderson, N., Keenan, C., & Leake, B. (1999). Perceived factors influencing the initiation of drug and alcohol use among homeless women and reported consequences of use. *Women and Health, 29,* 99–114.

Nyamathi, A., & Bennett, C. (1997). Visual coping scenarios: To facilitate discussion of coping responses with impoverished women at risk for AIDS. *Journal of Psychosocial Nursing and Mental Health Characteristics, 35,* 17–23.

Nyamathi, A., Flaskerud, J., Keenan, C., & Leake, B. (1998). Effectiveness of a specialized vs. traditional AIDS education program attended by homeless and drug-addicted women alone or with supportive persons. *AIDS Education & Prevention, 10,* 433–446.

Nyamathi, A., Stein, J., Dixon, E., Longshore, D., & Galaif, E. (2003). Predicting positive attitudes about quitting drug and alcohol use among homeless women. *Psychology of Addictive Behaviors, 17,* 32–41.

Nyamathi, A., Stein, J. A., Schumann, A., & Tyler, D. (in press). Latent variable assessment of outcomes in a nurse case managed intervention to increase latent tuberculosis treatment completion in homeless adults. *Health Psychology.*

Orleans, C., Boyd, N., Binger, R., Sutton C., Fairclaugh, D., Heller, D., et al. (1998). A self-help intervention for African American smokers: Tailoring cancer information service counseling for a special population. *Prevention Medicine, 27,* S61–S70.

Pennell, J., & Burford, G. (2000). Family group decision-making: Protecting children and women. *Child Welfare, 79(2),* 131–158.

Piette, J., Weinberger, M., McPhee, S., Mah, C., Kraemer, F., & Crapo, L. (2000) Do automatic calls with nurse follow up improved self care and glycemic control in patients with diabetes. *American Journal of Medicine, 108(1),* 20–27.

Resnicow, K. Vaughan, R., Futterman, R., Weston, R., Royce, J., Parms, C., et al. (1997). A self-help smoking cessation program for inner-city African Americans: Results from the Harlem health connection project. *Health Education and Behavior, 24(2),* 201–217.

Rodgers, A. (2001). Family decision meetings: A profile of average use in Oregon's Child Welfare Agency: Final report. Retrieved from http://www.ahafgdm.org

Schappert, S. (1998). Ambulatory care visits to physician offices, hospital outpatient departments, and emergency departments: United States, 1996. *Vital Health Statistics, 13(1),* 1–37.

Smith, S., Freeland, M., Heffler, S., & McKusick, D. (1998). The next ten years of health spending: What does the future hold? The Health Expenditures Project Team. *Health Affairs (Millwood)*, 17, 128–140.

Stevens, P. (1990). A critical social reconceptualization of environment in nursing: Implications for methodology. *Advances in Nursing Science*, 11(4), 56–68.

The Diabetes Prevention Program Research Group. (2002). The diabetes prevention program: Description of lifestyle intervention. *Diabetes Care*, 25(12), 2165–2171.

Toro, P. A., Passero Rabideau, J. M., Bellavia, C. W., Daeschler, C.V., Wall, D. D, Thomas, D. M. et al. (1997). Evaluating an intervention for homeless persons: Results of a field experiment. *Journal of Consulting & Clinical Psychology*, 65(3), 476–484.

Tortu, S., Beardsley, M., Deren, S., Williams, M., McCoy, H. V., Stark, M., et al. (2000). HIV infection and patterns of risk among women drug injectors and crack users in low and high sero-prevalence sites. *AIDS Care*, 12(1), 65–76.

Tortu, S., McCoy, H. V., Beardsley, M., Deren, S., & McCoy, C. B. (1998). Predictors of HIV infection among women drug users in New York and Miami. *Women & Health*, 27(1–2), 191–204.

Vezeau, T., Peterson, J., Nakao, C. & Ersek, M. (1998). Education of advanced practice nurses serving vulnerable populations. *Nursing and Health Care Perspectives*, 19(3), 124–131.

Wechsberg, W. M., Lam, W. K., Zule, W. A., & Bobashev, G. (2004). Efficacy of a woman-focused intervention to reduce HIV risk and increase self-sufficiency among African American crack abusers. *American Journal of Public Health*, 94(7), 1165–1173.

Wechsberg, W. M., Lam, W. K., Zule, W. A., Hall, G., Middlesteadt, R., & Edwards, J. (2003). Violence, homelessness, and HIV risk among crack-using African-American women. *Substance Use and Misuse*, 38, 671–701.

Wingood, G., & DiClemente, R. (1998). The influence of psychosocial factors, alcohol, drug use on African-American women's high-risk sexual behavior. *American Journal of Preventive Medicine*, 15, 54–59.

Wood R. (1999). Breast self-examination proficiency in older women: Measuring the efficacy of video self-instruction kits. *Cancer Nursing*, 19(6), 429–436.

Wood, R., Duffy, M., Morris, S., & Carnes, J. (2002). The effect of an educational intervention on promoting breast self-examination in older African American and Caucasian women. *Oncology Nurses Forum*, 29(7), 1081–1090.

# Chapter 11

## Community-Academic Research Partnerships With Vulnerable Populations

Janna Lesser and Manuel Angel Oscós-Sánchez

### ABSTRACT

*Community-academic research partnerships have evolved as a multidisciplinary approach to involve those communities experiencing health disparities in the development, implementation, and evaluation of health interventions. Community-academic partnerships are intended to bring together academic researchers and communities to share power, establish trust, foster colearning, enhance strengths and resources, build community capacity, and address community-identified needs and health problems. The purpose of this chapter is to review the current state of community-academic research partnerships in the United States and Canada. We discuss contextual issues; present a review of the current literature; identify the major strengths, challenges, and lessons learned that have emerged during the course of these research collaborations; and explore implications for future research and policy.*

Keywords: community-academic partnerships; community capacity building; health disparities; vulnerable populations

# INTRODUCTION

## Purpose

Nursing, through community health nursing, has been involved in the effort to improve the health of vulnerable and at-risk communities in the United States since the late 1800s (Portillo & Waters, 2004). Involving the community as an active partner in its own health promotion and disease prevention has been recognized as an important model in community health nursing since the later part of the 20th century and continues to be a core component of most undergraduate nursing education curriculums. More recently, community-academic research partnerships, also known as Community-Based Participatory Research (CBPR), have evolved as a multidisciplinary approach to involve communities in the development, implementation, and evaluation of health interventions. Recognition of the relevance of this approach to research can be found in the increasing number of participatory research courses taught in schools of nursing, public health, sociology, social work, and psychology (Israel, Eng, Schulz, & Parker, 2005).

Research-based intervention programs that are thought to be well-constructed and carefully implemented usually have very little impact if they are not culturally sensitive and specific to the target population's needs and life concerns. The inclusion of communities helps to develop more effective and culturally relevant health interventions for vulnerable populations, which experience a myriad of health disparities. Community-academic research partnerships have the potential to address many of the shortcomings of solely academic based research. As marginalized and disenfranchised groups have multiple reasons to mistrust academic health researchers and their interventions, community-academic research partnerships have emerged as a viable method to promote equality and trust among partners throughout the research process. Ideally such partnerships combine the knowledge base and skills of academic researchers, practitioners, and community residents; as a result, CBPR research partnerships have the potential to overcome existing mistrust within various vulnerable populations. Furthermore, knowledge acquired through these partnership projects is delivered back to the community in meaningful ways (Perera et al., 2002). Through collaborative efforts, community-academic research partnerships have generated positive health outcomes while building the capacity of communities to promote health and prevent disease (Galea et al., 2001).

The purpose of this chapter is to review the current state of multidisciplinary community-academic research partnerships in the United States and Canada. We discuss contextual issues; present a review of the current literature; identify the major strengths, challenges, and lessons learned, which have emerged during the course of these research collaborations; and explore implications for future research and policy.

## Scope of Review

The following approach was used to identify research publications on community-academic partnerships. A computerized keyword search of Medline citations for *community-academic partnership* resulted in 107 citations, and for *community-academic collaboration* resulted in 77 citations. Perhaps because community-academic collaborative research is still an emerging field, publications of this kind of research are more often focused on partnership structures and process methods, rather than on research outcomes. Many of the articles are theoretical, describing a model approach or guideline for development of a community-academic partnership. Only articles published between 1999 and 2005 that described actual collaborative case studies were included for this review. In addition, one article that was in press at the time of the writing of this chapter was included. Wallerstein and colleagues (2005) speak to the growing recognition of culturally supported interventions. They also find that the indigenous theories and practices, which have emerged organically from communities, have in general not been formally studied or evaluated to any great extent. This collaborative case study represents the use of this type of culturally supported intervention. The final sample, therefore, consisted of 25 citations as depicted in Table 11.1. We acknowledge that important publications may have been inadvertently overlooked; we are hopeful that those included provide a representative sample of current approaches.

## Overview of Contextual Issues

The goal, theoretical underpinnings, key elements, and cultural stance of community-academic research partnerships are discussed in this section.

Community-academic partnerships emerged as an approach to address health disparities as recognition grew that inequities in health status were associated with social, political, and economic issues such as poverty, inadequate housing, unemployment, racism, and lack of access to resources necessary to maintain health (Israel, Schulz, Parker, & Becker, 1998). Community-academic partnerships are intended to bring together academic researchers and communities to share power, establish trust, foster colearning, enhance strengths and resources, build community capacity, and address community-identified needs and health problems (Israel et al., 2005). This approach differs radically from the more traditional research methods in community and public health that focus

**TABLE 11.1** Community-Academic Partnerships by Form of Control

| Authors | Members of Partnership | Area of Focus | Health Issue | Target Population |
|---|---|---|---|---|
| **Academic researcher controlled form** | | | | |
| Cotter, Welleford, Vesley-Massey, & Thurston (2003) | Department of Gerontology, School of Allied Health Professions, Virginia Commonwealth University and Area Agency on Aging | Increasing health care utilization | Long-term care | Older persons with Alzheimer's disease and related disorders |
| Crist & Escandon-Dominguez (2003) | University of Arizona and the Elders' Use of Services Community Advisory Council | Increasing health care utilization | In-home community services | Hispanic elders |
| DeMarco & Johnsen (2003) | Boston College School of Nursing, a CBO, and women living with HIV/AIDS | Risk reduction, prevention, or treatment of a specific disease | HIV/AIDS | Women of color living with HIV/AIDS |
| Erwin, Blumenthal, Chapel, & Allwood (2004) | Six institutions of higher learning, an urban school system, two CBOs, and two private enterprises | Health care work-force issues | Increasing representation of minorities in the health profession | African American youth |
| Forti & Koerber (2002) | Medical University of South Carolina, a federally qualified community health center, and a rural health clinic | Increasing health care utilization | Improving access to and utilization of health care and social services | Older African Americans in rural South Carolina. |
| Levine, Bone, Hill, et al. (2003) | Johns Hopkins University and a CAB with members from CBOs, health departments, social service agencies, and community residents | Risk reduction, prevention, or treatment of a specific disease | Hypertension | Urban African Americans |

| Parra-Medina, D'Antonio, Smith, et al. (2004) | Norman J. Arnold School of Public Health, University of South Carolina and South Carolina Primary Health Care Association | Risk reduction, prevention, or treatment of a specific disease | Weight management for people living with diabetes | People with diabetes living in rural, medically underserved counties of South Carolina |
|---|---|---|---|---|
| Perera, Illman, Kinney, et al. (2002) | The Columbia Center for Children's Environmental Health in Washington Heights and 10 community-based health and environmental advocacy organizations | Health promotion or disease prevention related to social and environmental risk factors | Environmentally related diseases in young children | African American and Latino children living in Washington Heights, Harlem, and the South Bronx |
| Taylor, Turner, Davis, et al. (2001) | Lombardi Cancer Center of Georgetown University and the Most Worshipful Prince Hall Grad Lodge | Risk reduction, prevention, or treatment of a specific disease | Prostate cancer | African American men |

**Partnership controlled form in which academic researchers partnered with a community-based organization**

| Anderko & Uscian (2002) | A rural nursing center, a community college, a local county health department, and a state-university nursing school | Risk reduction, prevention, or treatment of a specific disease | Sexually transmitted infections | Rural college-age students |
|---|---|---|---|---|
| Caldwell, Zimmerman, & Isichei (2001) | University of Michigan School of Public Health, the Genesee County Health Department, and eight CBOs | Risk reduction, prevention, or treatment of a specific disease | Substance use, violence, early initiation of sexual activity | African American nonresidential fathers and their sons |
| Galea, Factor, Bonner, et al. (2001) | Center for Urban Epidemiological Studies (CUES), a research center that works collaboratively with the community | Risk reduction, prevention, or treatment of a specific disease | Substance use, infectious disease, and asthma | Community members of Harlem, NYC |

*(Continued)*

**TABLE 11.1** Community-Academic Partnerships by Form of Control (*Continued*)

| Authors | Members of partnership | Area of focus | Health issue | Target population |
|---|---|---|---|---|
| Grinstead, Zack, & Faigeles (1999) | The Center for AIDS Prevention Studies at the University of California, San Francisco, a CBO (Centerforce) and staff and inmate peer educators inside a state prison | Risk reduction, prevention, or treatment of a specific disease | HIV | Male prison inmates and their female partners |
| Haire-Joshu, Brownson, Schechtman, Nanney, Houston, & Auslander (2001) | Saint Louis University School of Public Health, Washington University at St. Louis, and Parents as Teachers (PAT), a national organization | Health promotion or disease prevention related to social and environmental risk factors | Cancer and other chronic diseases due to dietary patterns | African Americans |
| Lesser, Verdugo, Koniak-Griffin, et al. (2005) | UCLA School of Nursing and the Bien-venidos Family Services National Latino Fatherhood and Family Institute (NLFFI) | Risk reduction, prevention, or treatment of a specific disease | HIV | Latino adolescent parents |
| Maciak, Guzman, Santiago, et al. (1999) | The Detroit Community-Academic Urban Research Center (URC) | Risk reduction, prevention, or treatment of a specific disease | Intimate partner violence | Latina women |
| Meade & Calvo (2001) | H. Lee Moffitt Cancer Research Center, Research Institute at the University of South Florida in Tampa, and Suncoast Community Health Center | Risk reduction, prevention, or treatment of a specific disease | Breast cancer | Rural Hispanic migrant and seasonal farmworker women |
| Parker, Israel, Williams, et al. (2003) | The Detroit Community-Academic Urban Research Center (URC) | Health promotion or disease prevention related to social and environmental risk factors | Effects of outdoor and indoor air quality on exacerbation of childhood asthma | Community in Detroit, Michigan |

| Citation | Partnership | Purpose | Topic | Population |
|---|---|---|---|---|
| Quand, Arcury, & Pell (2001) | Wake Forest University School of Medicine, University of North Carolina at Chapel Hill, & the North Carolina Farmworkers' Project (NCFP) | Health promotion or disease prevention related to social and environmental risk factors | Pesticide exposure | Farmworkers in North Carolina |
| Schulz, Israel, Parker, et al. (2001) | The Detroit Community-Academic Urban Research Center (URC) | Health promotion or disease prevention related to social and environmental risk factors | To address the social determinants of health using a lay health advisor intervention | Residents of Detroit's east side |
| VanDevanter, Hennessy, Howard, et al. (2002) | Mailman School of Public Health, Columbia University, New York City Department of Health, and the community of Central Harlem, NYC | Risk reduction, prevention, or treatment of a specific disease | Sexually transmitted infections | Community members in Central Harlem, NYC |

**Partnership controlled form in which academic researchers partnered directly with members of the community**

| Citation | Partnership | Purpose | Topic | Population |
|---|---|---|---|---|
| Angell, Kreshka, McCoy, et al. (2003) | The Sierra-Stanford Partnership, a group of rural breast cancer patients, medical and social work professionals in Nevada City, CA, and psychosocial oncology researchers from Stanford University School of Medicine | Risk reduction, prevention, or treatment of a specific disease | Rural women with breast cancer | Impoverished women in a rural California community |
| Hackbarth, Shnopp-Wyatt, Katz, et al. (2001) | Loyola University Chicago, the American Lung Association of Metropolitan Chicago, and Community Activists | Health promotion or disease prevention related to social and environmental risk factors | Alcohol and tobacco use | African American and Hispanic neighborhoods in Chicago |

*(Continued)*

**TABLE 11.1** Community-Academic Partnerships by Form of Control (*Continued*)

| Authors | Members of Partnership | Area of Focus | Health Issue | Target Population |
|---|---|---|---|---|
| Northridge, Vallone, Merzel, et al. (2000) | Joseph L. Mailman School of Public Health of Columbia University and West Harlem Environmental Action (WE ACT) | Health promotion or disease prevention related to social and environmental risk factors | Environmental projects | Community of Harlem, NYC |
| **Community controlled form** | | | | |
| O'Neil, Elias, & Wastesicoot (2005) | Manitoba First Nations and the Department of Community Health Sciences at the University of Manitoba | Health promotion or disease prevention related to social and environmental risk factors | Identification of determinants of health. Provision of community- and university-based education and training in health research | First Nations and aboriginal communities |

on activities for the community rather than of or by the community (Minkler & Wallerstein, 2003).

Critical social theory underpins the development of community-academic partnerships (Crist & Escandon-Dominguez, 2003). Power inequities, which influence the health and well-being of groups, need to be identified and approached through cooperative methods (Crist & Escandon-Dominguez, 2003). Critical social theory puts forward the notion of a critical and normative framework that is committed to emancipation from all forms of oppression. In this research model, academic researchers and community members work together to meet community-identified goals and to find solutions to community-identified problems. If emancipation from oppression underpins the process of a community-academic collaboration, as is implicit in the perspective of critical social theory, then collaboration should help the community experiencing the health disparities, as well the researchers themselves, become more knowledgeable and empowered. A major aim of this research is to integrate knowledge with action in the form of community interventions, policy development, and social change. In addition, an increase in community participation and community membership is more likely to lead to relevant, sustainable, or institutionalized interventions (VanDevanter et al., 2002).

Israel and colleagues (1998) in their review of community-based research, identified a set of eight key elements of "community-centered research." These key elements include (a) recognizing the community as a unit of identity, (b) building on strengths and resources within the community, (c) facilitating collaborative partnerships in all phases of the research, (d) integrating knowledge and action for mutual benefit of all partners, (e) promoting a colearning and empowering process that attends to social inequalities, (f) involving a cyclical and iterative process, (g) addressing health from both positive and ecological perspectives, and (h) disseminating findings and knowledge gained to all partners.

A final contextual issue of importance is that academic researchers are most often from outside the community of interest, and are frequently different from the members of the community in class, ethnicity, and culture. To develop meaningful partnerships, these differences need to be acknowledged and addressed. The concepts of cultural humility and cultural safety are fundamental to researchers' ability to work effectively in cultures different than their own (Israel et al., 2005). The concepts of cultural humility, originating in medical education, and cultural safety, stemming from nursing education, are goals that health professionals working in community-academic partnerships should continually strive to achieve. Cultural humility refers to a process that requires a commitment to ongoing self-reflection and self-critique, including the identification and examination of one's own unintentional and intentional racism and classism. The concept of cultural safety extends that of cultural humility to include the acknowledgment that differences in language and worldview, as well as the social, economic, political, and historical determinants of health disparities, have a major influence on relationships between professionals and communities (Israel et al., 2005).

## Review of the Literature

This review of the current community-academic research partnerships literature is organized along three major areas: (a) health disparity issues being addressed, (b) forms of community-academic research partnerships, and (c) lessons learned.

## Health Disparity Issues Being Addressed

The kinds of health disparity issues that have been addressed by the community-academic collaborations and described in the 25 publications reviewed in this chapter can be categorized into four major foci. These foci include: (a) risk reduction, prevention, or treatment of a specific disease (Anderko & Uscian, 2002; Angell et al., 2003; Caldwell, Zimmerman, & Isichei, 2001; DeMarco & Johnsen, 2003; Galea et al., 2001; Grinstead, Zack, & Faigeles, 1999; Lesser et al., 2005; Levine et al., 2003; Maciak, Guzman, Santiago, Villalobos, & Israel, 1999; Meade & Calvo, 2001; Parra-Medina et al., 2004; Taylor et al, 2001; VanDevanter et al., 2002); (b) health promotion or disease prevention related to social and environmental risk factors (Hackbarth et al., 2001; Haire-Joshu et al., 2001; O'Neil, Elias, & Wastesicoot, 2005, Perera et al., 2002; Northridge et al., 2000; Parker et al., 2003; Schulz et al., 2001; Quandt, Arcury, & Pell, 2001); (c) increasing health care utilization (Cotter, Welleford, Vesley-Massey & Thurston, 2003; Crist & Escandon-Dominguez, 2003; Forti & Koerber, 2002); and (d) health care work-force issues (Erwin, Blumenthal, Chapel, & Allwood, 2004; O'Neil et al., 2005) (see Table 11.1).

## Forms of Community-Academic Research Partnerships

Four different types of community-academic partnerships were described in this literature: an academic researcher-controlled form; a partnership-controlled form in which academic researchers partnered with a community-based organization (CBO); a partnership-controlled one in which researchers partnered directly with members of the community; and a community-controlled form (see Table 11.1). In reality, most collaborative research projects do not fall precisely into one category. Community advisory boards (CABs) may be a component of any form of community-based collaboration. The purpose of the CABs is to incorporate the community's knowledge and ideas into the development of the research project, including but not limited to interventions, thus helping to ensure relevance and acceptability (VanDevanter et al., 2002).

## Academic Researcher-Controlled Form

A common form of community-academic research partnership found in publications is one describing the process of research projects initiated and controlled by the academic researcher. In these partnerships, the researcher comes to the community of interest with an identified research question and asks for help from the community with implementing a study. The community input helps to insure that the study is successfully conducted, most often being instrumental in providing access to the target population and advising on appropriate and culturally-sensitive recruitment and retention strategies. Nine of the 25 articles represented this form of partnership (Cotter et al., 2003; Crist & Escandon-Dominguez, 2003; DeMarco & Johnsen, 2003; Erwin, Blumenthal, Chapel, & Allwood, 2004; Forti & Koerber, 2002; Levine et al., 2003; Parra-Medina et al., 2004; Perera et al., 2002; Taylor et al., 2001). All three of the partnerships addressing issues of health care utilization were academic researcher-controlled (Cotter et al., 2003; Crist & Escandon-Dominguez, 2003; Forti & Koerber, 2002). One researcher-controlled partnership addressed issues related to health care work-force (Erwin et al., 2004). The remainder addressed either health promotion or disease prevention related to social and environmental risk factors (Perera, Illman, Kinney, et al., 2002) or prevention or treatment of a specific disease entity or risk behavior related to specific diseases (DeMarco & Johnsen, 2003; Levine et al., 2003; Parra-Medina et al., 2004; Taylor et al., 2001). Perera and colleagues (2002) addressed a variety of environmentally related diseases in young children living in New York City. Specific disease entities addressed by this form of partnership included HIV/AIDS, weight management in persons living with diabetes, and prostate cancer.

The following case study highlights an academic researcher-controlled partnership between six institutions of higher learning, an urban school system, two CBOs, and two private enterprises built to address health disparities by increasing minority representation in the health profession workforce (Erwin et al., 2004). Although this kind of partnership, particularly with public school systems, is not uncommon in efforts to increase minority representation in the field of medicine, few evaluations of the partnerships have been published in the literature. The paper presents an evaluation of a health career pipeline created to stimulate the interest of African American students in health careers and to facilitate entry into professional schools. A major contribution to the literature by these authors is their reporting on tensions commonly experienced among such partners and methods to resolve tensions. The partnering program directors completed questionnaires regarding a sense of common mission, vision, coordination, and collaboration three times during the 3-year project. The sense of common mission and vision was strong throughout the project. By addressing tensions among partners head on, the program directors were able to better identify the problems and work toward their resolution. The fear of loss of autonomy was identified as one of the major factors that threatened collaboration among partners. Through a process of building trust, the perception of coordination and collaboration was improved.

## Partnership-Controlled Form With a Community-Based Organization

In the partnership-controlled forms, the partners share power, status, and decision making. The research projects in this model are motivated by the community's identification of problems and concerns, the community's ability to work alongside the researchers, and the community and researchers' ability to share in the benefits of the research.

Academic researcher partnerships with CBOs were described in 12 of the publications (Anderko & Uscian, 2002; Caldwell et al., 2001; Galea et al., 2001; Grinstead et al., 1999; Haire-Joshu et al., 2001; Lesser et al., 2005; Maciak et al., 1999; Meade & Calvo, 2001; Parker et al., 2003; Quandt et al., 2001; Schulz et al., 2001; VanDevanter et al., 2002). Of these 12 publications, three of the partnerships addressed health promotion or disease prevention related to social and environmental risk factors; eight partnerships addressed prevention or treatment of a specific disease entity or risk behavior related to specific diseases; and one partnership addressed both these kinds of health disparity issues.

The three case studies that follow highlight academic researcher partnerships with CBOs; one specifically addressed health promotion or disease prevention related to social and environmental risk factors, one addressed prevention or treatment of a specific disease entity, and one addressed both of these health disparity issues simultaneously.

Quandt et al. (2001) described a 4-year project formed to investigate migrant and seasonal farmworker exposure to pesticides in North Carolina and to develop effective interventions to reduce exposure. The PACE (Preventing Agricultural Chemical Exposure in North Carolina Farmworkers) was a partnership between academic researchers (from Wake Forest University, School of Medicine and University of North Carolina at Chapel Hill) and a CBO (the North Carolina Farmworkers' Project), which provide services and advocacy for farmworkers throughout the state. The PACE project began with a year of formative research to understand farmworker and grower beliefs and attitudes concerning the use of pesticides and their health effects. Based on this formative research, a health education intervention for farmworkers was constructed. This intervention was tested using a randomized group trial. The focus and strength of this article, however, was the assessment of the structure of the partnership. The article identified the barriers impeding the progress of the project, as well as the types of actions that were fundamental to overcoming barriers and moving toward successful collaboration (Quandt et al., 2001).

The case study that follows highlights the use of a culturally supported intervention to prevent HIV. Lesser and colleagues (2005) described a two-phase community and academic collaboration, funded by the California Collaborative Research Initiative of the Universitywide AIDS Research Program, in which the partners developed and tested the feasibility of an HIV prevention program relevant to the needs of a population of inner-city Latino teen parenting couples. The partnership involved the University of California Los Angeles (UCLA) School of Nursing and a CBO already successful in providing innovative services to adolescent fathers, the Bienvenidos Family Services National Latino Fatherhood and Family Institute. The intervention development was guided by the "Healing the Wounded Spirit" framework (Tello, 1998). Curriculums developed with the "Healing the Wounded Spirit" framework are based on culturally rooted concepts and on the values of the indigenous teachings and writing of the ancestors of many Chicano, Latino, Hispanic, and Native American people. This publication describes the identification of special issues that needed to be addressed before the formation of a productive partnership could proceed. The first phase of the project, focus groups and individual interviews with members of the target population, informed the intervention development. Findings of the intervention pilot study illustrate participants' responses to the curriculum, and the feasibility of program implementation and evaluation in a community setting, including recruitment and retention challenges and descriptive findings.

In their publication examining the partnership process of a CBPR project, the Community Action Against Action (CAAA) project, Parker and colleagues (2003) described a process evaluation of the community-academic partnership. The CAAA project addressed the outdoor and indoor environmental factors that exacerbate asthma in children by designing and implementing a household- and neighborhood-level intervention aimed at reducing exposure to environmental asthma triggers in neighborhoods in eastside and southwest Detroit. Representatives of CBOs, the University of Michigan Schools of Public Health and Medicine, and the Detroit Health Department, designed and implemented the project. The process evaluation identified partnership accomplishments including: the successful implementation of a complex project, the identification of children with previously undiagnosed asthma, and diverse participation and community influence in decision making.

## Partnership-Controlled Form With Members of the Community

Partnerships with CBOs differ from partnerships with members of the target population or so-called community of identity. Israel and colleagues (1998) define the concept of community, central to community-based research, as an aspect of collective and individual identity. In this sense, community is characterized by a sense of identification and connection to other members, not necessarily sharing a geographic area (Israel et al., 1998). Community-academic collaborative projects that involve partnership and shared power directly with the community of identity are found far less often in the literature than are partnerships with CBOs. Partnerships with CBOs may include input from community members (for example, as members of the CAB, as employees of the CBO, or through data collected with participatory action methods): however, rarely do these community members share equally in power, status, and decision making. Only 3 of the 25 published articles represented partnerships where the academic researchers partnered directly with the target population. Two of these partnerships addressed health promotion or disease prevention related to social and environmental risk factors (Hackbarth et al., 2001; Northridge et al., 2000), and one partnership addressed prevention or treatment of a specific disease entity (Angell et al., 2003).

Hackbarth and colleagues (2001) describe a collaborative research and action partnership between Loyola University Chicago, the American Lung Association of Metropolitan Chicago (ALAMC), and a group of community activists from a predominantly African American church, St. Sabina Parish. Whereas this collaborative partnership has been in place for over 10 years, the research and action plan described in this paper involves a cross-sectional prevalence survey of alcohol and tobacco outdoor advertising. This study revealed that African American and Hispanic neighborhoods were disproportionately targeted for outdoor advertising of alcohol and tobacco. This data was used to convince the Chicago City Council to pass one of the nation's toughest anti-alcohol and anti-tobacco billboard ordinances, demonstrating the importance of linkages among academia, health organizations, and grassroots community groups in working together to change policy related to social determinants of health disparities.

Northridge and colleagues (2000) describe a community academic partnership initiated by community members. Community activists at West Harlem Environmental Action (WE ACT) partnered with researchers at the Joseph L. Mailman School of Public Health of Columbia University to advance the health of their community challenged by grave social, structural, and physical environmental inequities. This paper highlights a partnership in which "all partners establish their own power and legitimacy" (Northridge et al., p. 54). WE ACT, a community-based environmental advocacy group founded in 1988 to promote environmentally sound planning and practices in northern Manhattan, reached an unprecedented settlement agreement with the city of New York that provided relief from the adverse environmental impacts of the North River Water Pollution Control Plant on the banks of the Hudson in West Harlem. This settlement enabled WE ACT to have the resources needed to contract for scientific expertise (Northridge et al., 2000).

Lastly, a group of breast cancer survivors living in a rural community in California, initiated a partnership with academic researchers to develop and evaluate a low-cost, community-based Workbook-Journal (WBJ), designed to improve psychosocial functioning in geographically and economically isolated women with primary breast cancer (Angell et al., 2003). A randomized controlled trial was used to compare the WBJ intervention plus educational materials to educational materials alone (usual care). Community partners took the lead in developing the recruitment procedures, recruiting participants, conducting assessments, and designing strategies to reduce rural women's fears about participating in a research study. Although there were no main effects for the WBJ, three significant interactions suggested that women who received usual care reported decreased fighting spirit, increased emotional venting, and posttraumatic stress disorder. In addition, 74% of the women who received the WBJ reported feeling emotionally supported.

## Community-Controlled Form

Infrequently seen in the literature, the fourth form is a partnership that is controlled almost entirely by the community. Only one publication included in this chapter described this form of partnership. In their paper, O'Neil, Elias, and Wastesicoot (2005) described a partnership between Manitoba First Nations and researchers in the Department of Community Health Sciences at the University of Manitoba. This is significant as it advanced self-government in the First Nations context. At a time when Aboriginal communities were highly skeptical of the value of academic research, this partnership resulted in the development of the Manitoba First Nations Centre for Aboriginal Health Research; its mission to initiate, coordinate, and support research activities was designed to assist First Nations and Aboriginal communities in their efforts to promote wellness in their communities. The mission and objectives of this unit were as follows: to initiate and conduct research projects determined as relevant by the northern communities; to ensure that the research projects were sensitive and responsive to community needs and were supported by the communities; to encourage research training of northern persons; and to expose these communities to university research methods and results, thus increasing their awareness and assisting them in setting their own research priorities. In this partnership, the Aboriginal peoples controlled all aspects of the studies.

## Lessons Learned

Two major areas of lessons learned emerged in the articles written by investigators involved in community-academic research partnerships: (a) relationship issues between the partners; and (b) impact of the collaboration on the conduct of research.

## Relationship Issues

Critical to each case example reviewed was the development of meaningful relationships. The establishment of mutual respect and trust between the academic researchers and the community collaborators was cited as paramount to the success in all four forms of these partnerships (Angell et al., 2003; Erwin et al., 2004; Grinstead et al., 1999; Lesser et al., 2005; Northridge et al., 2000; O'Neil et al., 2005; VanDevanter et al., 2002). Another universal lesson learned was that it took time to develop functional community-academic partnerships. Extended periods of time were needed to develop the basic mutual respect and trust. Many of the academic investigators had a prolonged engagement with the communities with which they worked; the relationships had evolved over long periods of time (Caldwell et al., 2001; Cotter, et al., 2003; Northridge et al., 2000; O'Neil et al., 2005; VanDevanter et al., 2002). Investigators commented on the intensive time needed to overcome the established mistrust, which came out of past research having been conducted on communities rather than with communities.

During the time that relationships were developing, it was crucial to have clear, open, and ongoing communication (Haire-Joshu et al., 2001; Meade & Calvo, 2001; VanDevanter et al., 2002), with careful attention being paid to creating cultural sensitivity (Caldwell et al., 2001; Levine et al., 2003; Parra-Medina et al., 2004; Quandt et al., 2001). As academic researchers and community members had differing priorities, these discrepancies needed to be discussed and acknowledged up-front (Haire-Joshu, et al., 2001; Grinstead et al., 1999; Quandt et al., 2001). Successful partnerships were established only when a mutual commitment to a common goal was clearly established (Erwin et al., 2004; Northridge et al., 2000; Quandt et al., 2001; VanDevanter et al., 2002). Taking time to define and refine both the goals and roles of the each partner had long-term benefits (Cotter et al., 2003).

Equity among partners was another critical goal. The need to establish processes of decision making so that power and control of research projects was shared was a recurrent theme throughout these articles (Erwin et al., 2004; Grinstead et al., 1999; Haire-Joshu et al., 2001; O'Neil et al., 2005; Quandt et al., 2001). A commonly cited challenge in the implementation of the projects was the inequity between the amount of resources available to the academic researchers and to the community partners (Caldwell, et al., 2001; Grinstead et al., 1999; Quandt et al., 2001; VanDevanter et al., 2002). Because of traditional power differentials and hierarchical relationships, it worked best to make sure that the involvement of the community partners at all stages was stressed. Throughout the partnerships, both parties must perceive that they are mutually receiving tangible benefits from the relationship (Caldwell et al., 2001; Erwin et al., 2004)

## Impact on Research

The second area of lessons learned centered on the impact of the collaborations on the conduct of research itself. Overwhelmingly the effects of the partnership on the research process and products were experienced as positive. Community partners helped to refine the appropriateness of the research questions being asked (Angell et al., 2003; Schulz et al., 2001). The community partners helped to develop theoretical frameworks that were context specific. More effective interventions and instruments were developed (Caldwell et al., 2001; DeMarco & Johnsen, 2003; Lesser et al., 2005; Schulz et al., 2001). Recruitment of community participants was facilitated (Angell et al., 2003; Lesser et al., 2005). The partnerships increased the feasibility of project implementation (Cotter, et al., 2003; DeMarco & Johnsen, 2003; Grinstead et al., 1999; Perera et al., 2002). The partnerships also helped with data interpretation and dissemination of findings (Schulz et al., 2001).

One recurrent challenge addressed was the need to modify traditionally rigorous research designs, such as random assignment to control and experimental groups, which from the community perspective can interfere with the more important priority of service provision (Angell et al., 2003; Caldwell et al., 2001; Cotter et al., 2003; Haire-Joshu et al., 2001; Lesser et al., 2005). Lesser and colleagues (2005) described how their partnering CBO members felt strongly that their agency's honor and reputation would be compromised if any of their clients were assigned to a control group. Ultimately the experimental design needed to be modified in order for the partnership, and the project, to be successful.

## Implications for Future Research and Policy

In the foreword to the newly published volume *Methods in Community-Based Participatory Research for Health* (Israel et al., 2005), former Surgeon General

David Satcher described the design used for the development of goals, objectives, and strategies in Healthy People 2010, illustrating the interaction among determinants of health and other major issues that impact a community's health. The major components of this design include (a) the individual and his or her behavior, (b) the physical and social environment including health care, and (c) the various policies that impact this interaction. Satcher further explains:

> In order to reach the goals of improving quality as well as increasing years of healthy life and eliminating disparities in health among different racial, ethnic, and socio-economic groups, we must target all the determinant of health where disparities have their roots. We must close the gaps that exist in access to quality healthcare, practice of healthy lifestyles, quality of physical and social environments, and policies that impact these areas. (Israel et al., 2005, xiii-xiv)

The kinds of health disparity issues affecting vulnerable populations that were addressed by the community-academic collaborations could be categorized into four distinct, but not mutually exclusive, areas of focus that parallel the components of the design described by Satcher. Furthermore, the community-academic research partnerships were found to exert a positive influence on the goal of reducing and eliminating health disparities by increasing the relevance of health research and increasing the effectiveness of interventions that were developed and implemented with the process.

Although advances have been made in terms of involving the community in research, few examples exist where communities were given the opportunity to determine and pursue their own research agenda. As is reflected in our review of the literature, it is infrequent for the communities to control the research process. Traditionally, the academic researcher identifies funding sources, responds to requests for proposals, and then approaches communities for involvement (Wallerstein et al., 2005). Funding agencies rarely allow non-academic researchers to function as a principal investigator. To move this field even further forward in the face of formidable obstacles, such as resource inequities and existing power imbalances, academic researchers must be willing to let go of control and power while still assisting their community partners to become independent. Furthermore, funding agencies must be willing to modify their policies so that community partners can function as principal investigators and have administrative control of these cooperative project budgets.

In addition, despite the fact that it promises to be a successful strategy in reducing disparities in health status and health care, there has been insufficient achievement in increasing the numbers of health professionals and academic researchers that are from vulnerable populations. To achieve greater strides in positively affecting the health of vulnerable populations, policies need to be put into action that ensure the increased representation of vulnerable populations in positions that direct the use of the nation's limited health research resources.

## REFERENCES

Anderko, L., & Uscian, M. (2002). Academic-community partnerships as a strategy for positive change in the sexual behavior of rural college-aged students. The Nursing Clinics of North America, 37, 341–349.

Angell, K. L., Kreshka, M. A., McCoy, R., Donnelly, P., Turner-Cobb, J. M., Graddy, K. et al. (2003). Psychosocial intervention for rural women with breast cancer: The Sierra-Stanford Partnership. Journal of General Internal Medicine, 18, 499–507.

Caldwell, C. H., Zimmerman, M. A., & Isichei, P. A. (2001). Forging collaborative partnerships to enhance family health: An assessment of strengths and challenges in conducting community-based research. Journal of Public Health Management & Practice, 7, 1–9.

Cotter, J. J., Welleford, E. A., Vesley-Massey, K., & Thurston, M. O. (2003). Collaborative community-based research and innovation. Family & Community Health, 26, 329–337.

Crist, J. D., & Escandon-Dominguez, S. (2003). Identifying and recruiting Mexican American partners and sustaining community partnerships. The Journal of Transcultural Nursing, 14, 266–271.

DeMarco, R., & Johnsen, C. (2003). Taking action in communities: Women living with HIV/AIDS lead the way. Journal of Community Health Nursing, 20, 51–62.

Erwin, K., Blumenthal, D. S., Chapel, T., & Allwood, L. V. (2004). Building an academic-community partnership for increasing representation of minorities in the health professions. Journal of Health Care for the Poor and Underserved, 15, 589–602.

Forti, E. M., & Koerber, M. (2002). An outreach intervention for older rural African Americans. The Journal of Rural Health, 18, 407–415.

Galea, S., Factor, S. H., Bonner, S., Foley, M., Freudenberg, N., Latka, M., et al. (2001). Collaboration among community members, local health service providers, and researchers in an urban research center in Harlem, New York. Public Health Report, 116, 530–539.

Grinstead, O. A., Zack, B., & Faigeles, B. (1999). Collaborative research to prevent HIV among male prison inmates and their female partners. Health Education and Behavior, 26, 225–238.

Hackbarth, D. P., Schnopp-Wyatt, D., Katz, D., Williams, J., Silvestri, B., & Pfleger, M. (2001). Collaborative research and action to control the geographic placement of outdoor advertising of alcohol and tobacco products in Chicago. Public Health Report, 116, 558–567.

Haire-Joshu, D., Brownson, R. C., Schechtman, K., Nanney, M. S., Houston, C., & Auslander, W. (2001). A community research partnership to improve the diet of African Americans. American Journal of Health Behavior, 25, 140–146.

Israel, B.A., Eng, E., Schulz, A. J., & Parker, E. A. (Eds.). (2005). Methods on community-based participatory research for health. San Francisco: Jossey-Bass.

Israel, B. A., Schulz, A. J., Parker, E. A., & Becker, A. B. (1998). Review of community-based research: Assessing partnership approaches to improve public health. Annual Review of Public Health, 19, 173–202.

Lesser, J., Verdugo, R. L., Koniak-Griffin, D., Tello, J., Kappos, B., & Cumberland, W. G. (2005). Respecting and protecting our relationships: A community research HIV prevention program for teen fathers and mothers. *AIDS Education & Prevention, 17*(4), 347–360.

Levine, D. M., Bone, L. R., Hill, M. N., Stallings, R., Gelber, A. C., Barker, A., et al. (2003). The effectiveness of a community/academic health center partnership in decreasing the level of blood pressure in an urban African-American population. *Ethnicity and Disease, 13,* 354–361.

Maciak, B. J., Guzman, R., Santiago, A., Villalobos, G., & Israel, B. A. (1999). Establishing LA VIDA: A community-based partnership to prevent intimate violence against Latina women. *Health Education and Behavior, 26,* 821–840.

Meade, C. D., & Calvo, A. (2001). Developing community-academic partnerships to enhance breast health among rural and Hispanic migrant and seasonal farmworker women. *Oncology Nursing Forum, 28,* 1577–1584.

Minkler, M., & Wallerstein, N. (Eds.). (2003). *Community-based participatory research for health.* San Francisco: Jossey-Bass.

Northridge, M. E., Vallone, D., Merzel, C., Greene, D., Shepard, P., Cohall, A. T., et al. (2000). The adolescent years: An academic-community partnership in Harlem comes of age. *Journal of Public Health Management & Practice, 6,* 53–60.

O'Neil, J., Elias, B., & Wastesicoot, J. (2005). Building a health research relationship between First Nations and the University in Manitoba. *Canadian Journal of Public Health, 96*(Suppl. 1), S9–S12.

Parker, E. A., Israel, B. A., Williams, M., Brakefield-Caldwell, W., Lewis, T. C., Robins, T., et al. (2003). Community action against asthma: Examining the partnership process of a community-based participatory research project. *Journal of General Internal Medicine, 18,* 558–567.

Parra-Medina, D., D'Antonio, A., Smith, S. M., Levin, S., Kirkner, G., & Mayer-Davis, E. (2004). Successful recruitment and retention strategies for a randomized weight management trial for people with diabetes living in rural, medically underserved counties of South Carolina: The POWER study. *The Journal of the American Dietetic Association, 104,* 70–75.

Perera, F. P., Illman, S. M., Kinney, P. L., Whyatt, R. M., Kelvin, E. A., Shepard, P., et al. (2002). The challenge of preventing environmentally related disease in young children: Community-based research in New York City. *Environmental Health Perspectives, 110,* 197–204.

Portillo, C. J., & Waters, C. (2004). Community partnerships: The cornerstone of community health research. *Annual Review of Nursing Research, 22,* 315–329.

Quandt, S. A., Arcury, T. A., & Pell, A. I. (2001). Something for everyone? A community and academic partnership to address farmworker pesticide exposure in North Carolina. *Environmental Health Perspectives, 109*(Suppl 3), 435–441.

Schulz, A. J., Israel, B. A., Parker, E. A., Lockett, M., Hill, Y., & Wills, R. (2001). The East Side Village Health Worker Partnership: Integrating research with action to reduce health disparities. *Public Health Reports, 116,* 548–557.

Taylor, K. L., Turner, R. O., Davis, J. L., III, Johnson, L., Schwartz, M. D., Kerner, J., et al. (2001). Improving knowledge of the prostate cancer screening dilemma among African American men: An academic-community partnership in Washington, DC. *Public Health Reports, 116,* 590–598.

Tello, J. (1998). El hombre noble buscando balance: The noble man searching for balance. In R. Carrillo & J. Tello (Eds.), *Family violence and men of color: Healing the wounded male spirit* (pp. 31–52). New York: Springer Publishing.

VanDevanter, N., Hennessy, M., Howard, J. M., Bleakley, A., Peake, M., Millet, S., et al. (2002). Developing a collaborative community, academic, health department partnership for STD prevention: The Gonorrhea Community Action Project in Harlem. *Journal of Public Health Management & Practice, 8*, 62–68.

Wallerstein, N., Duran, B., Minkler, M., & Foley. (2005). Developing and maintaining partnerships with communities. In B. A. Israel, E. Eng, A. J. Schulz, & Parker, E. A. (Eds.), *Methods in community-based participatory research for health* (pp. 31–51). San Francisco: Jossey-Bass.

# Chapter 12

## Vulnerable Populations in Thailand: Giving Voice to Women Living With HIV/AIDS

Adeline Nyamathi, Chandice Covington,
and Malaika Mutere

### ABSTRACT

*Thailand was the first Asian country hit by the AIDS epidemic, and in the 1990s reported the fastest spread of HIV/AIDS in the world. According to Thailand's Ministry of Public Health, women, primarily between the child-bearing ages of 15 and 49, are increasingly becoming infected with HIV. A number of factors contribute to the increasing AIDS epidemic, including the rise of the commercial sex industry in Thailand; social disparities that have existed between men and women throughout Thailand's history; and the gender-expectations faced by Thai women toward family and society.*

*Thailand enjoys one of the oldest, reputedly successful primary health care delivery systems in the world; one that relies on community health workers to reach the most rural of populations. In the mid-1990s, day care centers were established at district hospitals by the Thai government to provide medical, psychological, and social care to people living with HIV/AIDS (PWA). Buddhist temples also provide a source of alternative care for PWAs. However, the AIDS policy of the Thai government relies on families to care for the country's sick.*

*Although poor women are a vulnerable population in Thailand, they are changing the paradigm of AIDS stigma while providing a significant cost-savings to the Thai government in their caregiving activities. Based on existing nursing studies on Thailand, this chapter gives voice to poor Thai women living with HIV/AIDS, and examines how they make sense of their gendered contract with society and religion while being HIV/AIDS caregivers, patients, or both.*

**Keywords: HIV/AIDS; Thailand; commercial sex industry; vulnerable populations; women**

# INTRODUCTION

Thailand, a population of 62 million, was the first Asian country hit by the AIDS pandemic; this country also reported the fastest spread of HIV/AIDS in the world by the 1990s. Thailand's Ministry of Public Health indicates that women are increasingly becoming infected with HIV, with the proportion of men to women infected with HIV increasing from 97:3 in 1988 to approximately 60:40 in 2005. The HIV/AIDS epidemic in Thailand has emanated from both the high-risk sexual behaviors of men who visit the numerous commercial sex workers (CSWs) in Thailand (Wawer, Podhisita, Kanungsukkasem, Pramualtrana, & McNamara, 1996) and the increased use of illegal injection drugs (Mastro et al. 1994). Although prostitution is frowned upon in Thailand, CSWs generate significant foreign income to society while helping to support the financial obligations of their families. The majority (86%) of Thai women infected with HIV are between the ages of 15 and 49, with an increasing prevalence among pregnant women in some areas (Songwathana, 2001).

In Thailand, HIV in women has been associated with dirt, danger, and death. These associations have led to a profound stigma for infected mothers in seeking care and support. Moreover, as part of the Buddhist view that AIDS is a disease of Karma *(rok khong khon mee k am)*, in that infected persons deserved their fate, HIV-infected Thai women have had to carry the dual demands of survival and maternal caregiving single-handedly. HIV-positive Thai mothers are often overwhelmed by feelings of guilt, grief, emotional pain, and exhaustion; all of which effect their emotional responses to already stressful situations complicated by poverty (Andrews, Williams, & Neil, 1993; Weiler, 1995). Desperate for support from family, friends, and community, poor HIV-positive mothers often experience a profound sense of isolation (Shayne & Kaplan, 1991) and powerlessness over the disease and the associated social stigma, which in turn effects their maternal role-taking process. Coming from a vulnerable population framework where poor outcomes are associated with limited resources and such populations are at high risk for morbidity and premature mortality (Flaskerud & Winslow, 1998), the experiences of poor HIV-infected Thai women need to be better understood by health care providers.

The purpose of this chapter is to highlight some of the key nursing studies conducted from 1990 to 2005 in Thailand, a developing country plagued with a high HIV/AIDS prevalence. A computerized literature retrieval was conducted with Entrez PubMed and CINAHL database searches using keywords HIV/AIDS, Thailand, and nursing. The search resulted in 198 articles published between 1988 and November 2005. PubMed provides access to bibliographic information that includes Medline and OldMedline, covering over 4,800 journals published in the United States and more than 70 other countries primarily from pre-1966 to the present. Citations in Medline are from journals selected for inclusion in the database. CINAHL is a literature resource for nursing and allied health professionals that provides indexing for 2,719 journals from the fields of nursing and allied health. The database contains more than 1 million records dating back to 1982.

From this search, a specific review for those articles where primarily nursing professionals conducted qualitative studies and the essence of the investigation focused on nursing phenomena revealed 10 articles for review. Our focus on qualitative studies was based on the fact that an understanding of the cultural and social context of HIV/AIDS and of women in Thailand is foundational and critical to ongoing studies of caregiving and survival. Those selected articles, as shown in a Table 12.1, were published between 1992 and 2004, and form the set for review.

## Social Status of Poor HIV-Infected Women in Thailand

Numerous studies characterize a main feature of Thailand's social structure as giving second class status to women, particularly those who are poor and vulnerable. In an analysis of the growth of prostitution in Thailand, Muecke (1992) concludes that Thai ideologies of family and religion are being prostituted for material rewards as is evident in the country's economic progress. Muecke (1992) examines the heterosexual transmission of AIDS through female prostitution in contemporary lowland, village-level Buddhist Thai society as a socio-cultural phenomenon. Although illegal, prostitution enables women to fulfill traditional cultural functions of daughters through remittances provided to the families at home and as merit-making activities, all of which paradoxically helps conserve

**TABLE 12.1** Selected Research Studies Reviewed

| References | Sample / Setting | Study Design | Recommendations |
|---|---|---|---|
| Bechtel & Apakapakal, 1999 | • 5, HIV+, mean age 27 + 5 years<br>• Buddhist temple in Southern Thailand | Narrative study over 2 months; four 90-minute sessions per informant; unstructured telling of their story | A systematic effort by nursing organizations encouraging *krengjai* is needed to promote culturally holistic interventions |
| Boonpongmanee et al., 2003 | • 77 HIV- / 79 HIV+ pregnant women; mean age 29 / 26<br>• Bangkok & Nonthaburi | Predictive model testing design included comparison group of HIV- pregnant women to help interpret findings | Findings on the relationships of depression, resourcefulness, & prenatal self-care can help nurses provide more effective services & counseling |
| Jirapaet, 2001 | • 39 low-income HIV+ mothers representing each month of infant age from 1–12 months; 18–40 age range<br>• Bangkok & suburbs | Qualitative, unstructured, in-depth phenomenological 2-hour interviews over 8 months; two per mother; concluded with negative sentence to authenticate data | HIV+ mothers need more access to private consultation, a regular provider, confidentiality, & respectful treatment in health care settings |
| Kauffman & Myers, 1997 | • Seven VHVs & villagers<br>• Northeast Thailand | Ethnographic field study over 2 weeks: participant observation; focus groups; semi-structured interviews; informal interviews | While still a vital part of Thailand's PHC system, the VHV role needs to adapt to the needs of an increasingly urbanized community |
| Kespichayawattana & VanLandingham, 2003 | • 394 HIV+ household parents / 376 HIV- household parents<br>• Chiang Mai, phichit, & Rayong provinces | Comparison of health outcomes between affected & matched nonaffected parents using survey data; & between principal & nonprincipal care-givers (18 interviews of affected parents) | Adverse health outcomes of affected parents/caregivers call for management of pain, sleep, anxiety, & other forms of palliative care; need health care training & financial assistance |

| Author, Year | Sample/Setting | Methods | Findings |
|---|---|---|---|
| Muecke, 1992 | • Unspecified<br>• Chiang Mai Province, Northern Thailand | Case studies, some from 5 years of longitudinal anthropological study; participant observation; review of media & texts | Concludes that ideologies of family & religion are being prostituted for material rewards in Thailand in the form of increasing CSWs |
| Muecke, 2001 | • Non-clinical mothers & children from larger ongoing study<br>• Chiang Mai Province, Northern Thailand | Semi-structured & open-ended interviews; supplementary data obtained from HCPs, NGOS, AIDS organizations, & Health Ministry officials | The progress of AIDS in Chiang Mai reconfirms gender & class biases by Thai society at large |
| Nilmanat & Street, 2004 | • Eight caregivers, 2 HIV+, 27–61 age range<br>• Songkhla Province, Southern Thailand | Longitudinal narrative study over 8 months; interviews-conversations; participant observation; & field notes | Dominant care-giver theme: "search for a cure" aimed to reunify & balance fragmented lives with a more holistic & palliative AIDS care approach |
| Songwathana, 2001 | • 15 caregivers, 9 HIV+ 6 HIV, 21–50 age range<br>• Southern Thailand | Narrative study; in-depth interviews; participant observation; qualitative analysis following Spradley | Research is needed on role of men in sharing care-giving. Interventions are needed to address the needs of HIV+ care-giving women |
| Tsunekawa et al., 2004 | • 271 DCC members at 9 district hospitals<br>• 29.5%<br>• Chiang Mai Province, Northern Thailand | Cross-sectional survey using DCC-employed research nurses to conduct interviewer-administered questionnaire: 47 multiple choice questions & verbal clarifications as needed | PWA benefit from DCC services; services would be enhanced by physical exams & administration of meds; Thailand's expansion of ART should define DCC role & address access barriers for PWA |

institutions of the government, which benefits from the lucrative, tourist-fueled sex industry, the family, and Buddhism.

Muecke (1992) draws from Thailand's history to connect this particular aspect to current social norms and their health implications. From the 15th century, Thai laws codified male authority over women and, until the late 19th century, men could legally sell or give wives or daughters away without their consent as a gift to a superior or as debt payment. Men could also purchase slave women as so-called lesser or minor wives; traditional Thai polygamy was an acceptable custom, which provided men access to more than one woman. These customs and laws collectively set a precedent for the current practice where family members, especially daughters, are sold for economic gain. It is conservatively estimated that no fewer than 1 million of Thailand's population are female prostitutes, over 20,000 of whom are under the age of 15.

## Research Methodologies

Until the mid-1970s, the major ethnographies of Thai society were conducted almost exclusively by foreign male ethnographers (Muecke, 1992); thus the earlier literature tended to overlook social disparities for females. Much of the data in this chapter derives from ethnographic nursing studies, where data were gathered through qualitative systematic inquiry using the researcher as instrument. Progressive in-depth interviews were conducted (e.g., structured demographic data, semi-structured interviews, focused conversations, and mutual dialogue or casual conversations); participant observations and extensive field notes were made; and qualitative analyses were applied to the data that included extensive Thai-English and English-Thai translations to ensure fidelity to original intent and participant meaning. Jirapaet (2001) employed Patton's (1980) phenomenological method of interviewing, which began with an open-ended question and elicited storytelling by informants through unstructured, in-depth interviews. Songwathana (2001) employed a constant comparative method following Spradley (1979) in performing a qualitative analysis of data.

Boonpongmanee, Zauszniewski, and Morris (2003) tested Rosenbaum's theory of learned resourcefulness, a predictive model testing design, in their examination of self-care in HIV-positive pregnant women with evident depression. Among other findings, they suggest that a qualitative study would be helpful to gain more insight into cultural meanings of learned resourcefulness in Thailand. As many argue, modern medicine splits the diseased body from the ill person's life and daily experiences, which is why Nilmanat and Street (2004) advocate that health care professionals pay attention to their clients' stories, referred to as illness narratives. These narratives offer patients the opportunity to reframe their experiences, construct new contexts, and fit their so-called illness (disruption of an ongoing life) into a temporary framework. In Nilmanat and Street's study (2004) their key informants (primary care-givers) are aware that health professionals hold different views of sickness, and therefore would often withhold information on their participation in spiritual or traditional healing rites during medical visits.

## Impact of Culture on HIV/AIDS in Thailand

The cultural concept of *krengjai*, consistent with the concepts of Buddhism, describes and governs family and social order through the maintenance of harmonious relationships. To fully understand the HIV/AIDS experience of women in Thailand, it is important to understand how the concept of *krengjai* works within Thai society (Bechtel & Apakupakul, 1999). Illness, along with a pervasive sense of isolation, creates chaos for a Thai families' sense of harmony, and harshly threatens their social support system or *krengjai*. To make matters worse, the stigma of HIV/AIDS, which is profound in Thailand, akin to leprosy, requires the physically debilitated and infected person to be isolated from family and society. Thus, the impact on caregiving activities is profound.

Vichit-Vadakan's (1994) review of Thai women in social changes notes that opportunities for wage labor in cities created distances that altered the traditional Thai family structure. The Thai family has typically been a modified extended structure based around a matrilineal residence, to which married daughters bring husbands to work and live until the daughter's family grows large and breaks away to form a new family unit. Although women are the center of the Thai family and the major agents of socialization in their children's lives, they are still second class to men in society, providing supporting and subservient roles, which are never direct or overt.

## Studies of the Health Care System in Thailand

Thailand enjoys a government-supported primary health care (PHC) system that is reputed to be one of the world's oldest successful health care delivery systems. PHC began in Chiang Mai in 1966 as a successful pilot project to develop a model of community participation in resolving health issues. This system was implemented through partnerships of community residents, health workers, and health care professionals using a combination of appropriate technology, local resources, and government support to provide culturally appropriate interventions for the communities' health-priorities.

Kauffman and Myers (1997) performed an ethnographic field study in 1994 to look at the role of the Community Health Worker (CHW) or, as Thai's commonly refer to him or her, Village Health Volunteer (VHV), as the backbone of the PHC system in Thailand. Through systematic inquiry over a 2-week period in Thailand's largest, poorest, least developed region, these authors explored the implementation and acceptance of the role of VHV to determine whether current PHC methods effectively lead to universal health care. Areas of assessment included how the VHV role was implemented and how their role was understood and accepted by villagers. This study was designed to provide information for evaluation and revision of the existing PHC model, and to help other planners avoid hurdles to community acceptance and utilization of VHV.

Through qualitative analysis of their ethnographic data, Kauffman and Myers conclude that rapid urbanization and increased technology provided greater access for villagers to secondary and tertiary services. Therefore, use of VHV services and the importance of their role, as outlined by Thailand's PHC model, diminished exponentially as an entrée into the PHC system. VHVs themselves expressed difficulty in obtaining continuing education to remain current on treatment practices. Villagers reported minimal use of VHV services and most were unable to identify who the VHVs were, opting instead for self-treatment and self-referral for health concerns based on information obtained from radio and television. Kauffman and Myers suggest that the VHV role needs to be adapted accordingly with help from, and in collaboration between, U.S. nurses and those in Thailand's urban centers.

In another evaluation of how Thailand's health care system is addressing the needs of the sick, in particular people living with HIV/AIDS (PWA), Tsunekawa et al. (2004) studied day care centers (DCCs) which, as a result of Thai government policy, were established at district hospitals in 1995 to provide medical, psychological, and social care to PWA. This cross-sectional study of 271 DCC members at nine well-established hospitals in the Chiang Mai province, attempted to assess the psychosocial and economic impact of DCC services to PWA, and to determine the extent to which DCCs were making a difference in the lives of PWA.

Tsunekawa et al. (2004) evaluated the socioeconomic and demographic background data of PWA and their reasons for attending DCCs, their use of the medical services, the cost of attending DCCs, and how DCCs changed their lives. Registration at DCCs is voluntary for people who are diagnosed as HIV positive. Monthly meetings at DCCs included activities such as breathing exercises, massage, group sharing of experiences, counseling, and Buddhist teachings. These authors concluded that the services provided by DCCs benefited PWA, particularly in areas of educational and mutual psychological support. However, barriers preventing PWA access to utilize DCCs were apparent, some of which included economic and geographic issues. Tsunekawa and colleagues suggest that these issues call for a more comprehensive examination on the role of DCCs, and that the role of DCCs needs to be clearly defined within the planned expansion of antiretroviral therapy in Thailand. They recommend enhancing DCC's medical services by including physical examinations and administering medications such as IPT-cotrimoxazole and antiretroviral therapy.

## Voices of the Thai Poor: Living With HIV/AIDS as Caregivers, Patients, or Both

The Thai government's AIDS policy relies on families to care for the country's sick (Muecke, 2001), validating the premise made by Kespichayawattana and VanLandingham (2003) that "the economic, social, and familial context in which this caregiving occurs in Thailand and in other developing countries is vastly different from the situation in the developing world" (p. 217). Muecke (2001) similarly acknowledges the role of wealth in Thai women's health: "Although wealth probably is not protecting Thai women from receiving the HIV from their husbands, it can protect them from the stigmatizing label of HIV/AIDS, and it can buy them care to promote the quality and duration of their lives" (p. 36). A number of nursing studies exist that reflect the voice of the Thai poor as they experience living with HIV/AIDS, as patients, caregivers, or both.

In an exploratory ethnographic study, Muecke (1992) examined the experiences of AIDS caregivers, very poor to lower middle class, non-clinical urban informants drawn from Chiang Mai, Thailand's province of highest AIDS mortality. Data were obtained from mothers and children by semi structured interviews, in the informant's home or workplace, followed by a varying number of open-ended interviews. Supplementary data were obtained by open-ended interviews with health care providers, AIDS nongovernmental organizations (NGOs), and Ministry of Health officials. Muecke translated Thai recordings into English and field researchers checked translations for accuracy of interpretation.

The research questions raised were the following: (a) Who are the home and community caregivers for PWAs? (b) What kind of care do they give? and (c) What is the impact of caregiving on the caregiver(s)? Findings revealed that among caregivers, parents, overwhelmingly mothers—followed by wives, then grandmothers, and then sisters—considered it their place and duty to care for adult children or husbands sick with AIDS. They also believed that caring for their ailing family members provided moral and spiritual benefit in the form of building positive karma for themselves. The most intimate and physical care for PWA came from women, who were also most likely to sacrifice their jobs and food-obtaining activities in order to care for the men in the family who are dying of AIDS. In addressing the question of who will care for women when they get AIDS, Muecke (2001) notes:

It is not clear how families will cope financially, emotionally or socially as more AIDS widows and children become sick, but it is likely that the burdens will be even heavier on families who have already witnessed the suffering of the disease and spent their emotional and financial resources in caring for one who died from it. (p. 33)

Women, in particular those who are poor, were changing the paradigm of AIDS stigma while providing significant cost-savings to the Thai government in their caregiving activities. Motivating factors for women as AIDS caregivers included social, cultural, and moral predisposition; family ties (mother to son or daughter, daughter to parent, sister to brother/sister, and wife to husband); and lack of other support for PWA who are poor.

Bechtel and Apakupakul (1999) conducted a qualitative study of the experiences of five individuals experiencing HIV disease in rural southern Thailand. Isolated from family and social networks, each participant told their story over a 2-month period in an average of four 90-minute sessions, and explored their tenuous relationship with *krengjai*, a sense of order which is essential to Thai's sense of harmony for family and society. All participants lived in a Buddhist *wat* or temple, as a source of alternative care. Each conversation began with the researcher asking the participants their feelings about having AIDS.

Findings of the study, which incorporated additional data from the subject's family and friends, revealed the significant loss of identity these persons experienced within their families and society, and the subsequent isolation and partial reconnection with society, either through their original families or new emerging families in the *wat*. Clearly, HIV disease was found to interrupt economic and social patterns, to cause chaos and mistrust, and to limit adaptability and adjustment to family crisis as separation ensued, with loss of *krengjai*. Inability to cope with this disintegration increased utilization of already scarce resources and aggravated the cycle of poverty and despair.

Re-establishing *krengjai* was a consistent focus. All participants felt the need to incorporate into their social networks and fulfill a social purpose; they returned part of their earnings from work in the *wat* (as health permitted) back to family to make things right. Men expressed a strong desire to return to birth family. Women adapted by connecting with new familial groupings, relationships made in the *wats*, and as a result of their shared situations, enabled a new sense of *krengjai*. As a profession, nursing is focused on enhancing a holistic environment within the family and community by encouraging *krengjai*.

In a longitudinal narrative case study, Nilmanat and Street (2004) examined the experiences of family members caring for a relative with AIDS in rural southern Thailand's Songkhla Province. The study explored the construction of health-seeking behaviors: how caregivers made sense of illness episodes and how they chose and evaluated particular treatments and care. By means of illness narratives, eight female caregivers (two of whom were unemployed and HIV-positive from spousal contact), ranging in age from 27 to 61, were offered the opportunity to reframe their experiences, construct new contexts, and fit their so-called illness (disruption of an ongoing life) into a temporary framework. Qualitative data collection via semi structured and structured interviews, focused conversations, mutual dialogue, and participant observation captured their social world of being a caregiver; the support system they created to support their beliefs about health, life and death; how they managed and cared for their patients; and what medicines and remedies they provided for their loved one.

The dominant theme of the caregivers' illness narratives was the search for a cure. As caregivers became aware that available medicines and therapies were palliative and not directed at a cure, they sought other sources of cure and adopted alternative remedies and religious practices. Families held a holistic view (mind-body-spirit) of illness and suffering, and believed that illness might be affected by various causes such as pathogens, supernatural affliction, or karma. They made sense of their experiences by combining medical, supernatural, and traditional therapeutic means. Some sought secondary forms of treatment to support medical therapies, and others focused on addressing religious or supernatural causes that might hinder the efficacy of medical treatments. Early health seeking behaviors were dominated by the view that modern medicine held the best hope for a family member with AIDS, and the caregivers' subsequent search for a cure was aimed to heal, bring unity and balance to the fragmented parts of life, and establish a more holistic approach towards AIDS care.

In another ethnographic study, Songwathana (2001) examined the role of women in traditional Thai families, concentrating on personal, kinship, and social obligations of women. Specifically she assessed under what circumstances women take on the caregiver role, and how they cope with this function; particularly if they themselves are HIV-infected. In-depth interviews, participant observations, and qualitative analyses were conducted on 15 women afflicted or affected by HIV/AIDS in southern Thailand, all but one of whom were Buddhist, and six of whom were employed.

The research findings showed that women with HIV/AIDS had multiple roles, in part because the expectation and experience of their caring role remains, even if they are employed. In answer to the research question of how a woman lives with HIV, manages her family, and provides meaningful care for herself, her family, or both, the following narrative themes were elicited:

(1) with HIV, I become patient but miserable; (2) when the income earner is sick, care is my responsibility; (3) when the income earner recovers, I care for the children; (4) when the child is sick, care is our karma; (5) when the income earner is sick again and terminally ill, continuing care keeps my morale high; (6) when the income earner is dead, care is for survival; (7) when I myself am sick, I khit maak [worry very much] with greater suffering; (8) when I am dead, care will be transferred to my mother. (Songwathana, 2001, p. 267)

In Thai culture, women are required to fulfill the expectations of other people's needs because being a woman means to nurture, even if it is at the expense of her own health. The emphasis is on giving (*hai*) and sacrificing (*siasala*). Buddhist beliefs in karma reinforce this sense of responsibility for women, particularly those who were infected by their husbands or those who were taking care of HIV/AIDS patients. The belief that AIDS is the result of their karma made acceptance of responsibility to give care in this life in order to have happiness in a future life, according to Buddhist principles of transmigration and reincarnation. Women's sexuality, vulnerability, responsibility, and caregiving are adversely affected by traditional, persistent gender imbalances and inequalities.

In another study, Kespichayawattana and VanLandingham (2003) explored the potential health effects on older parents (over age 50) caused by living with and caring for their adult HIV-infected children. In Thailand, as in other developing countries with modest health care budgets and high rates of infection, multiple generations live in the same household including PWAs. The researchers compare the health outcomes between affected and matched non-affected parents, and between principal and non-principal caregivers in Thailand to determine whether and to what extent the physical and mental health of older parents declined from close contact and providing care to their ill children.

Village clusters (*tambon*) were chosen within the three provinces of Chiang Mai (AIDS epidemic characterized by relatively high prevalence and long duration); Phichit (maintained low levels of AIDS prevalence); and Rayong (relatively high prevalence and short duration). VHVs acted as intermediaries and helped identify the 394 AIDS-affected families based on AIDS deaths that had occurred 6 months to 3 years prior to the interview period, as well as 376 control households, matched by age, marital, and socioeconomic status of the parent(s), that had not experienced an AIDS death within the same timeframe.

The range of caregiving tasks performed by AIDS-affected parents included: shopping; food preparation; feeding; dishwashing; bathing; helping with toileting; dressing; laundry; watching over; lifting and moving (e.g., from bed to chair); preparing and giving medicines; cleaning wounds; providing transportation to the clinic or hospital; consulting with health care providers; and helping to apply for welfare benefits. The more physically strenuous and time-consuming tasks were carried out by significantly more parents, mostly mothers, who co-resided with PWAs than by those who did not. This extensive output of care directly resulted in older parents suffering adverse health outcomes. Conversely, the suffering of PWAs would be much worse without these massive inputs of time, energy, and money by their parents.

Lower levels of overall happiness were reported by parents who had an adult child die from AIDS, compared to the control households. During the period of caregiving, parents of children with AIDS reported high levels of anxiety, insomnia, fatigue, muscle strain, and head and stomach aches. To address the needs found in this study, Kespichayawattana and VanLandingham (2003) recommended a variety of programs, such as: anxiety, pain and sleep management programs for parents; accessing social support networks; government and private financial assistance for PWAs and their families; training workshops on cleaning wounds and administering medications for caregivers; and training local health personnel to identify and treat older people who are suffering from caregiving strains.

Pregnant Thai women constitute the fastest-growing segment of people diagnosed with HIV/AIDS (Boonpongmanee et al., 2003). HIV infection with pregnancy increases a woman's risk for depression due to changes in maternal identity, tasks, as well as the physical alterations (Rubin, 1984). Poor health-related behaviors such as smoking, consumption of alcohol and cocaine, and poor weight gain help give rise to symptoms of depression during pregnancy (Walker, Cooney, & Riggs, 1999). In a study of pregnant HIV-positive Thai women, Panuwatsuk (1998) found that women reported no condom use with partners, no exercise during pregnancy, and over-the-counter drug use.

Using Rosenbaum's theory of learned resourcefulness, Boonpongmanee et al. (2003) revealed the direct effects of depression and resourcefulness on prenatal self-care as well as the mediating effects of resourcefulness on depression and self-care. Resourcefulness is learned through experience, instruction, and modeling and, for HIV-positive pregnant women, may serve as a repertoire of coping skills to help manage symptoms of depression and perform self-care. Research findings indicate direct effects of depression and resourcefulness on prenatal self-care. The effect of depression on prenatal self-care was mediated by resourcefulness. HIV status did not predict prenatal self-care.

These findings support the usefulness of learned resourcefulness theory (Rosenbaum, 1990) for studying depression and prenatal self-care among pregnant women who are either HIV-positive or HIV-negative. Boonpongmanee and associates (2003) suggest that these findings can help nurses provide effective services to pregnant Thai women, including teaching resourcefulness to enhance prenatal self-care. The authors also suggest that formative studies involving in-depth interviews can significantly help in gaining more insight into the meanings of learned resourcefulness in Thai culture.

Recently, the influence of HIV on Thai women after childbirth has been addressed in several studies. Jirapaet (2001) explored factors affecting maternal role attainment of HIV-infected Thai women. Maternal role attainment is a process by which the mother achieves competence in the maternal role and comfort with her identity as a mother through integrating the mothering behaviors into her established role set (Mercer, 1985). Most mothers attain this role completely by well before the end of the first postpartum year (Grace, 1993; Mercer, 1985; Mercer & Ferketich, 1995).

In Jirapaet's sample of 39 informants, aged 18–40, heterosexual transmission was identified as the factor for HIV infection. Seventy-four percent were infected by their husbands, and 26% had a history of prostitution. From the informants' storytelling, Jirapaet identified the following six essential themes or descriptive factors that commonly fuel HIV-positive mothers to attain competency in their maternal roles while surviving with the infection:

1. Setting a purpose for life to raise an infant: Over 50% of mothers attempted suicide after first being identified as HIV-positive, but found motivation to live after aiming their life goals toward responsibility for their infants' well-being. When presented with the choice of therapeutic abortion, all chose to continue their pregnancies and have sterilization after the labor—a decision that was strongly influenced by a husband or grandmother.

2. Keeping secrets from others: All the women identified that secrecy was necessary to ensure safety for their infants and themselves. Informants feared rejection or expulsion from home and community, as well as the negative associations and unpleasant consequences that would follow disclosure through family members, such as stigmatizing the infants.

3. Normalization: Normalization was described by informants as the need to feel and live as if nothing has happened. This occurred through partial denial wherein mothers, if they were symptom free, could easily maintain verbal denial. However, behaviorally, their actions showed considerable regard to protecting their infants from infection. Alternatively, the women could achieve normalization by possessing a positive attitude toward life.

4. Quality of support from others: More significant than the number of supportive persons in their support networks is the quality of support the women receive. Most common true companions were an HIV-infected husband, a parent (especially the mother), or a sister.

5. Having hope for an HIV cure: One hundred percent of mothers were Buddhist and believed in the process of karma. Herbal remedies also provided hope for a cure.

6. Health services environment: Even in the presence of benefits, 98% of the HIV-positive mothers avoided using health services, even though they described health care providers as important and reliable sources of information, and potential aids to preserving their physical and mental health and meeting their infants' needs. The avoidance of health services was due to lack of accessible and pleasant health services, and the failure on the health services part to protect the anonymity of the women. Low income mothers with no health coverage

had to use government health care agencies, which the majority felt provided unpleasant service (e.g., "impolite talk," "scolding and acting sarcastic"), lacked a stable care provider, and personal privacy. In addition, hospital regulations required notation of the mother's HIV status on her infant's immunization record, which carried the risk of being disclosed to other family members, thus creating a continual source of worry (Jirapaet, 2001, pp. 28–30).

The implications of this study are that in order to encourage low-income HIV-positive mothers to access health care, providers need to ease the HIV-positive mothers' transition to maternal role attainment through providing more understanding of her struggle and needs; by creating accessibility to a regular provider and private consultation; by being more cordial and constructive in outreach activities; by including the mothers' most trusted people in the caring system; and by demonstrating an ethical concern for the mothers' confidentiality.

## Design and Methodological Limitations

Nilmanat and Street (2004) argue that modern medicine splits the diseased body from the ill person's life and daily experiences, and note that Thai caregivers are aware that health professionals hold different views of sickness than they do, even though the search for a cure is a shared concern of both. Perceptions of illness, hospitalization, isolation, and adaptation between both groups differ in significant ways, largely along cultural lines. These differences in perception play out adversely in therapeutic settings. Existing instruments dealing with coping and adaptation are Western oriented, and are seen by some as inappropriate in Thailand. Boonpongmanee et al. (2003) attempt a predictive model testing design using Rosenbaum's theory of learned resourcefulness, and among other things, conclude that qualitative studies are needed to gain more insight into the cultural meanings of learned resourcefulness in Thailand.

## SUMMARY

Thailand's HIV/AIDS crisis presents some interesting challenges to the nursing profession, in terms of how it views itself; its role in non-Western cultures; and how it would operate within existing health policies. Although the Ministry of Public Health in Thailand established DCCs at district hospitals to provide services to PWAs, the Thai government AIDS policy nevertheless relies on families to care for the country's sick, in part because of a lack of inpatient beds. Cultural factors dictate that women bear the burden of caregiving for those families unable to afford professional nursing and medical care. Poor women living with HIV/AIDS provide a tremendous cost-savings to the Thai government but their numbers and caregiving activities are often overlooked within the professional ranks of health-care providers, even in terms of providing them much-needed basic health care training as advised by Kespichayawattana and VanLandingham (2003). Most of the highlighted studies in this chapter, as presented in Table 12.1, were based on qualitative data and provided important cultural insights which challenge Western sciences to be more inclusive and holistic. Indeed non-Western knowledge systems have much to offer the healing profession. As Muecke (2001) suggests, poor Thai women are changing the paradigm of AIDS stigma, and as Bechtel and Apakupakul (1999) suggest, "A holistic and systematic effort by professional nursing organizations to promote family and community strengths by encouraging *krengjai* should be undertaken" (p. 474). In Bechtel and Apakupakul's view, this mechanism will effectively reduce patterns of morbidity and mortality from AIDS, and will enhance women's and children's health worldwide.

## REFERENCES

Andrews, S., Williams, A. B., & Neil, K. (1993). The mother-child relationship in the HIV-1 positive family. *Nursing Research, 25*(3), 193–198.

Bechtel, G. A., & Apakupakul, N. (1999). AIDS in southern Thailand: Stories of *krengjai* and social connections. *Journal of Advanced Nursing, 29*(2), 471–475.

Boonpongmanee, C., Zauszniewski, J. A., & Morris, D. L. (2003). Resourcefulness and self-care in pregnant women with HIV. *Western Journal of Nursing Research, 25*(1), 75–92.

Flaskerud, J. H., & Winslow, B. J. (1998). Conceptualizing vulnerable populations health-related research. *Nursing Research, 47*(2), 69–78.

Grace, J. T. (1993). Mothers' self-reports of parenthood across the first 6 months postpartum. *Research in Nursing & Health, 16*, 431–439.

Jirapaet, V. (2001). Factors affecting maternal role attainment among low-income, Thai, HIV-positive mothers. *Journal of Transcultural Nursing, 12*(1), 25–33.

Kauffman, K. A., & Myers, D. H. (1997). The changing role of village health volunteers in Northeast Thailand: An ethnographic field study. *International Journal of Nursing Studies, 34*(4), 249–255.

Kespichayawattana, J., & VanLandingham, M. (2003). Effects of coresidence and caregiving on health of Thai parents of adult children with AIDS. *Journal of Nursing Scholarship, 35*(3), 217–224.

Mastro, T. D., Kitayaporn, D., Weniger, B. G., Vanichseni, S., Laosunthorn, V., Uneklabh, T., et al. (1994). Estimating the number of HIV-infected injection drug users in Bangkok: A capture-recapture method. *American Journal of Public Health, 84*, 1094–1099.

Mercer, R. T. (1985). The process of maternal role attainment over the first year. *Nursing Research, 34*, 198–204.

Mercer, R. T., & Ferketich, S. L. (1995). Experienced and inexperienced mothers' maternal competence during infancy. *Research in Nursing & Health, 18*(4), 333–343.

Muecke, M. A. (1992). Mother sold food, daughter sells her body: The cultural continuity of prostitution. *Social Science Medicine, 35*(7), 891–901.

Muecke, M. (2001). Women's work: Volunteer AIDS care giving in Northern Thailand. *Women & Health, 33*(1/2), 21–37.

Nilmanat, K., & Street, A. (2004). Search for a cure: Narratives of Thai family caregivers living with a person with AIDS. *Social Science & Medicine, 59,* 1003–1010.

Panuwatsuk, P. (1998). *A study of self-care in HIV-seropositive pregnant women during pregnancy.* Unpublished master's thesis, Mahidol, Thailand.

Patton, M. Q. (1980). *Qualitative evaluation methods.* London: Sage, Ltd.

Rosenbaum, M. (1990). The role of learned resourcefulness in the self-control of health behavior. In M. Rosenbaum (Ed.), *Learned resourcefulness: On coping skills, self-control, and adaptive behavior* (pp. 3–30). New York: Springer Publishing.

Rubin, R. (1984). *Maternal identity and the maternal experience.* New York: Springer Publishing.

Shayne, V. T., & Kaplan, B. J. (1991). Double victims: Poor women and AIDS. *Women & Health, 17,* 21–37.

Songwathana, P. (2001) Women and AIDS caregiving: Women's work? *Health Care for Women International, 22,* 263–279.

Spradley, J. P. (1979). *The ethnographic interview.* New York: Holt, Rinehart and Winston.

Tsunekawa, K., Moolphate, S., Yanai, H., Yamada, N., Summanapan, S., & Ngamvithayapong, J. (2004). Care for people living with HIV/AIDS: An assessment of day care centers in Northern Thailand. *AIDS Patient Care & STDs, 18*(5), 305–314.

Vichit-Vadakan, J. (1994). Women and the family in Thailand in the midst of social change. *Law & Society Review, 28*(3), 515–524.

Walker, L. O., Cooney, A. T., & Riggs, M. W. (1999). Psychosocial and demographic factors related to health behaviors in the 1st trimester. *Journal of Obstetric, Gynecologic, & Neonatal Nursing, 28,* 606–614.

Wawer, M. J., Podhisita, C., Kanungsukkasem, U., Pramualtrana, A., & McNamara, R. (1996). Origins and working conditions of female sex workers in urban Thailand: Consequences of social context for HIV transmission. *Social Science & Medicine, 42,* 453–462.

Weiler, J. B. (1995). Respite care for HIV-affected families. *Social Work in Health Care, 21,* 55–67.

# Index

# Contents of Previous 10 Volumes

## VOLUME 22: Eliminating Health Disparities Among Racial and Ethnic Minorities in the United States

# Vulnerable Older Adults

## *Health Care Needs and Interventions*

### Patricia M. Burbank, DNSc, RN, Editor

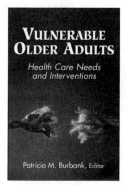

*"It has been said that one measure of a society is the care it provides to its most vulnerable members. By taking on this challenge, Burbank and her colleagues have opened the door to addressing the needs of the most vulnerable among our older population."*
—**Mathy Mezey**, RN, EdD, FAAN

Based on the concept that vulnerability in the older populace encompasses those who are at increased risk for physical and psychosocial health problems, this book takes a closer look at vulnerability and how it affects five specific populations within the elderly: those incarcerated in prisons; the homeless; gay, lesbian, bisexual, and transgender people; those who are HIV positive or living with AIDS; and the frail.

Physical and psychosocial health care issues and needs are addressed as well as interventions and resources that can be implemented to care for these very specific populations and their requirements for successful physical and mental health care. The unique challenges of hospice care in prisons, the lack of services that cater to homeless older people, and the overall attitude towards helping elderly gay, lesbian, bisexual, or transgender people are some of the increasingly important issues covered.

**Unique Features Include:**

• Summary of the latest research and theoretical approaches to give health professionals a concise picture of health care needs of these older adult populations

• Interdisciplinary approach to care, cultural considerations, and neglect and abuse

• Discussion of strategies and resources for caring for older adults with dementia for each vulnerable population

2006 · 304pp · 978-0-8261-0208-9 · hardcover

**11 West 42nd Street, New York, NY 10036-8002** • **Fax: 212-941-7842**
**Order Toll-Free: 877-687-7476** • **Order Online: www.springerpub.com**

9174